HOT TOPICS

D1534877

GERD / Dyspepsia

DATE DUE

NOV 2 2 2005	
SEP 2 1 2006	
JUN 2 8 2010	
SEP 49 2010	
OCT 1 2 2010	
NOV 0 9 2010	

HOT TOPICS

GERD / Dyspepsia

Ronnie Fass, MD, FACP, FACG

Staff Physician
Department of Internal Medicine/Gastroenterology
and Director, GI Motility Laboratory
Southern Arizona Veterans Administration Health Care System
Associate Professor of Medicine
University of Arizona School of Medicine
Director, GI Motility Laboratory
University of Arizona Health Sciences Center
Tucson, Arizona

HANLEY & BELFUS
An Affiliate of Elsevier

HANLEY & BELFUS, INC.
An Affiliate of Elsevier

The Curtis Center
Independence Square West
Philadelphia, Pennsylvania 19106

Note to the reader: Although the information in this book has been carefully reviewed for correctness of dosage and indications, neither the editor, nor the authors, nor the publisher can accept any legal responsibility for any errors or omissions that may be made. No warranty is expressed or implied with respect to the material contained herein. Before prescribing any drug, the reader must review the manufacturer's current product information (package inserts) for accepted indications, absolute dosage recommendations, and other information pertinent to the safe and effective use of the product described.

Library of Congress Control Number: 2003096254

GERD / DYSPEPSIA: HOT TOPICS   ISBN 1-56053-582-2

Printed in the United States of America

Last digit is the print number: 9 8 7 6 5 4 3 2 1

Contents

Contributors

Peter Bytzer, MD, PhD
Associate Professor and Head, Department of Medical Gastroenterology, Glostrup University Hospital, Glostrup, Denmark

Brooks D. Cash, MD
Assistant Professor, Department of Medicine, Uniformed Services University of the Health Sciences, Bethesda; Staff Gastroenterologist, National Naval Medicine Center, Bethesda, Maryland

Mai-Sie Chan, MD
Resident, Department of Internal Medicine, Santa Clara Valley Medical Center, San Jose, California

William D. Chey, MD
Associate Professor, Division of Gastroenterology, University of Michigan, Ann Arbor, Michigan

Roy Dekel, MD
Research Fellow, The Neuro-Enteric Clinical Research Group, Southern Arizona Veterans Administration Health Care System, Tucson, Arizona

Hashem B. El-Serag, MD, MPH
Head, GI Outcomes Research, Gastroenterology and Health Services Research, and Staff Physician, Houston Veterans Administration Medical Center, Houston; Assistant Professor, Department of Medicine, Baylor College of Medicine, Houston, Texas

Ronnie Fass, MD, FACP, FACG
Staff Physician, Department of Internal Medicine/Gastroenterology, and Director, GI Motility Laboratories, Southern Arizona Veterans Administration Health Care System, Tucson; Associate Professor, University of Arizona School of Medicine, Tucson; Director, GI Motility Laboratories, University of Arizona Health Sciences Center, Tucson, Arizona

Ofer Feder, MD
Fellow in Gastroenterology, Division of Gastroenterology and Hepatology, University of North Carolina School of Medicine, Chapel Hill; Clinical Instructor, University of North Carolina Hospitals, Chapel Hill, North Carolina

Robert S. Fisher, MD
Professor, Department of Medicine, and Chief, Gastroenterology Section, Temple University School of Medicine, Philadelphia, Pennsylvania

Frank Friedenberg, MD
Associate Professor, Department of Medicine, Gastroenterology Section, Temple University School of Medicine, Philadelphia, Pennsylvania

Eyal Gal, MD
Physician, Department of Gastroenterology, Rabin Medical Center, Beilinson Campus, Tel Aviv University, Petach Tikva, Israel

Lauren B. Gerson, MD, MSc
Assistant Professor, Department of Medicine, Division of Gastroenterology and Hepatology, Stanford University School of Medicine, Stanford; Attending Physician, Stanford University Hospital, Stanford, California

Howard Hampel, MD, PhD
Fellow in Gastroenterology, Department of Gastroenterology/Medicine, Baylor College of Medicine, Houston, Texas

Ikuo Hirano, MD
Assistant Professor, Department of Gastroenterology, Northwestern University, Feinberg School of Medicine, Chicago, Illinois

Michael P. Jones, MD
Assistant Professor, Department of Gastroenterology, and Director, Gastroenterology Laboratory, Northwestern University, Feinberg School of Medicine, Chicago, Illinois

Sunil Joseph, MD

Brian E. Lacy, MD, PhD
Associate Professor, Department of Medicine, Division of Digestive Diseases, Johns Hopkins Medical Institutions, Baltimore, Maryland

Uri Ladabaum, MD, MS
Assistant Clinical Professor, and Director, Gastrointestinal Motility Program, Division of Gastroenterology, Department of Medicine, University of California School of Medicine, San Francisco, California

Kwang-Jae Lee, MD, PhD

Yaron Niv, MD
Associate Professor, Department of Gastroenterology, Rabin Medical Center, Beilinson Campus, Tel Aviv University, Petach Tikva, Israel

Jaime A. Oviedo, MD
Clinical Instructor, Department of Medicine, Section of Gastroenterology, Boston University School of Medicine, Boston; Staff Physician, Boston Medical Center, Boston, Massachusetts

Henry P. Parkman, MD
Associate Professor, Department of Medicine, Temple University School of Medicine, Philadelphia, Pennsylvania

Richard E. Sampliner, MD
Professor, Department of Medicine/Gastroenterology, University of Arizona School of Medicine, Tucson; Chief of Gastroenterology, Southern Arizona Veterans Administration Health Care System, Tucson, Arizona

Nicholas J. Shaheen, MD, MPH
Director, Center for Esophageal Diseases and Swallowing, and Attending Physician, University of North Carolina Hospitals, Chapel Hill; Assistant Professor of Medicine and Epidemiology, Division of Gastroenterology and Hepatology, University of North Carolina School of Medicine, Chapel Hill, North Carolina

Hrair P. Simonian, MD
Fellow in Gastroenterology, Department of Medicine, Temple University School of Medicine, Philadelphia, Pennsylvania

Amnon Sonnenberg, MD, MSc
Professor, Department of Medicine, Oregon Health & Science University, Portland; Staff Physician, Portland Veterans Administration Medical Center, Portland, Oregon

Jan Tack, MD, PhD
Professor, Department of Internal Medicine, University of Leuven, Leuven, Belgium

George Triadafilopoulos, MD
Professor, Department of Medicine, Division of Gastroenterology and Hepatology, Stanford University School of Medicine, Stanford; Chief, Gastroenterology Section, Palo Alto Veterans Administration Health Care System, Palo Alto, California

Michael F. Vaezi, MD, PhD
Staff, Center for Swallowing and Esophageal Disorders, Department of Gastroenterology and Hepatology, Cleveland Clinic Foundation, Cleveland, Ohio

Nimish Vakil, MD
Aurora Sinai Medical Center, Milwaukee, Wisconsin

Marcelo F. Vela, MD
Fellow, Department of Gastroenterology and Hepatology, Cleveland Clinic Foundation, Cleveland, Ohio

J. Patrick Waring, MD
Clinical Professor, Emory University School of Medicine, Atlanta, Georgia

Harland S. Winter, MD
Associate Professor, Department of Pediatrics, Harvard Medical School, Boston; Director, Pediatric Inflammatory Bowel Disease Program, Division of Pediatric GI and Nutrition, and Pediatrician, Massachusetts General Hospital, Boston, Massachusetts

M. Michael Wolfe, MD
Professor, Department of Medicine, Section of Gastroenterology, and Research Professor, Department of Physiology and Biophysics, Boston University School of Medicine, Boston; Chief, Section of Gastroenterology, Boston Medical Center, Boston, Massachusetts

Benjamin Chun-Yu Wong, MD
Associate Professor, Department of Medicine, University of Hong Kong; Honorary Consultant, Queen Mary Hospital, Hong Kong

Wai-Man Wong, MD
Honorary Clinical Associate Professor, Department of Medicine, University of Hong Kong; Medical and Health Officer, Queen Mary Hospital, Hong Kong

Ronald W. Yeh, MD
Fellow in Gastroenterology, Department of Medicine, Division of Gastroenterology and Hepatology, Stanford University School of Medicine, Stanford; Fellow in Gastroenterology, Stanford University Hospital, Stanford, California

Qian Yuan, MD, PhD
Instructor in Pediatrics, Harvard Medical School, and Clinical Fellow, Harvard Program in Pediatric Gastroenterology and Nutrition, Boston Children's Hospital, Boston, Massachusetts

Preface

Gastroesophageal reflux disease and dyspepsia are currently hot areas of interest. Research in gastroesophageal reflux disease, the new epidemic of this millennium, has significantly evolved in the last decade, leading to greater understanding of the disease's epidemiology, pathophysiology, and complications. Revelations about diagnosis have encouraged the implementation of new techniques. Non-erosive reflux disease has been established as a major area of interest, and atypical/extra-esophageal manifestations of gastroesophageal reflux disease remain an area of intense research. New treatments have been implemented for Barrett's esophagus, and deeper understanding of the evolution of the disorder as well as its progression to cancer has been achieved. New tools have been developed to assess quality of life and cost issues. Patient subgroups, such as those with systemic disorders, children, and the elderly, have been recognized to have unique manifestations of the disease. Novel treatment approaches to GERD recently have been put forth, and new surgical and endoscopic techniques are underway.

The area of dyspepsia has also significantly progressed in the last decade. The spectrum of the problem is now more readily recognized. Several studies have proposed a cost-effective approach to dyspepsia. Different mechanisms that contribute to the disorder have been identified, including gastric acid, motility, accommodation, *Helicobacter pylori,* and visceral hyperalgesia. New therapeutic modalities have been proposed and some have been studied. A plethora of compounds designed to treat dyspepsia are currently in the pipeline.

The rapid evolution in understanding of gastroesophageal reflux disease and dyspepsia in the last decade was the impetus for writing this book. A group of esteemed experts in both fields agreed to summarize the current available literature and present their own views and vision.

I am deeply indebted to my colleagues, who took time from their busy schedules and produced up-to-date chapters. This book is intended to serve primary care physicians, internists, surgeons, subspecialists (ENT docs, pulmonologists, and others), as well as gastroenterologists. We've emphasized easy-to-read chapters, simple and clear algorithms, and take-home messages. My hope is that you will use this book on a regu-lar basis for clinical purposes and that it will serve as a first-line text for gastroesophageal reflux disease and dyspepsia.

Ronnie Fass, MD
EDITOR

Dedication

To my wife Shira
and my children—Ofer, Hagar, & Sharon—
the loves of my life.

Epidemiologic Aspects in the Occurrence and Natural History of Gastroesophageal Reflux Disease

chapter
1

Amnon Sonnenberg, M.D., M.Sc.

By studying the epidemiology of gastroesophageal reflux disease (GERD), gastroenterologists and epidemiologists strive to understand which factors and mechanisms are primarily responsible for the disease. Like most other diseases, the development of GERD depends on the interplay between environmental risk factors and genetically determined physiologic mechanisms. Besides the onset of the disease, its progression through various stages of severity is also influenced by such an interplay between exogenous and endogenous risk factors. The exact nature of many environmental risk factors is still unknown. To learn about these risk factors, epidemiologists study the variation of a disease among distinct populations and subgroups of populations characterized by different age, gender, ethnicity, geography, history, season, occupation, and health status. If striking disease variations become associated with any such characteristics, one can then try to make inferences about the nature of the underlying risk factors and, thus, gain etiologic insights about disease mechanisms. For instance, the marked geographic variation in the occurrence of GERD and its negative correlation with the spread of *Helicobacter pylori* infection suggests that *H. pylori*–induced gastritis protects against GERD. Similarly, one can speculate that the higher prevalence of GERD among men possibly relates to their larger stomachs and the resulting increased acid output when compared to women.

The **clinical epidemiology** of GERD deals with the diverse manifestations of the disease, the progression of GERD through consecutive

1

stages, and disease-related complications affecting the esophagus and adjacent organs. Whereas the clinical epidemiology of GERD is mostly focused on the natural history and factors that modulate its course, the **descriptive epidemiology** of GERD is more concerned with its general prevalence in the population, its demographic, geographic, and temporal variation, and its association with other disease conditions. This chapter touches on both of these aspects of GERD epidemiology.

Disease Definition and Clinical Presentation

The term *gastroesophageal reflux disease,* or *GERD,* is used to describe the symptoms and changes of the esophageal mucosa that result from reflux of gastric contents into the esophagus (Table 1). GERD patients present with a variety of general symptoms, but the individual patient usually presents with only a subset of symptoms. The symptoms may be experienced daily, weekly, or only a few times per month. With respect to GERD, individual symptoms carry a sensitivity and specificity that, in general, do not exceed 65% and 80%, respectively.[1,2] The frequency and severity of symptoms from gastroesophageal reflux correlate only poorly with the extent of mucosal changes seen during endoscopic examination of the esophagus.[3]

Most commonly used grading systems for GERD are based on modifications of the Savary-Miller classification.[3,4] Subjects with reflux symptoms but no macroscopically visible lesions are said to have reflux disease without esophagitis, sometimes referred to as grade 0. Peptic esophagitis is graded according to the extent and severity of macroscopically visible erosions: single patchy, large confluent, or circumferential erosions representing grade I, II, or III, respectively. The term *complicated esophagitis,* or *grade IV,* relates to esophagitis accompanied by Barrett's mucosa, ulcers, or strictures. The synonyms *Barrett's esophagus, epithelium,* and *metaplasia* refer to the replacement of esophageal squamous epithelium by a gastric type of columnar epithelium with

TABLE 1. Spectrum of Gastroesophageal Reflux Disease	
Organ	**Types of Disease Manifestation**
General symptoms	Belching, heartburn, regurgitation, chest pain, dysphagia, pharyngeal soreness, hoarseness, coughing
Esophagus	Erosion, ulcer, stricture, Barrett's metaplasia, adenocarcinoma
Throat	Pharyngitis, laryngitis, sinusitis, aphonia, laryngeal stenosis, cancer
Mouth	Tooth decay, gingivitis
Lung	Asthma, chronic obstructive pulmonary disease, pneumonia

intestinal metaplasia that reaches 3 cm or more above the lower esophageal sphincter. A cutoff length of 2 or 3 cm is used to distinguish between long and short segments of Barrett's esophagus. In general, Barrett's epithelium is more susceptible than the regular squamous epithelium of the esophagus to the development of deep esophageal ulcers or peptic strictures. Barrett's epithelium is considered a premalignant lesion, and its presence is associated with an increased risk for progression into esophageal adenocarcinoma.

The original classification of disease severity established by Savary and Miller was based on the assumption that GERD progressed through different stages of disease severity. Hiatal hernia was perceived as a facilitator for acid reflux into the esophagus. After initial exposure of the esophageal mucosa to gastric contents resulting in symptoms only, patients would develop single esophageal erosions. Prolonged exposure to larger amounts of acid would cause more extensive damage with larger confluent erosions or even ulcers. In some patients, healing of the large erosions or ulcers would eventually result in scarring and formation of a peptic strictures. In this picture, Barrett's esophagus represented the end result of large confluent erosions that failed to heal over by regular squamous epithelium. There are several clear-cut clinical observations, however, that speak against this scheme. In a random population of GERD patients, for instance, the severity of GERD does not correlate with the individual length of case history.[5] Moreover, in clinical practice, one rarely, if ever, observes patients progress through consecutive disease stages. Most patients present to their physician at the onset of their disease already with the most severe stage that they will ever reach. If the concept of GERD progression through consecutive stages truly applies, such progression must occur within a short time period at the very onset of the disease. Nevertheless, the striking similarities in the epidemiology, pathophysiology, and clinical presentation of diverse GERD types provide strong evidence that they all represent different expressions of the same underlying disease process. Figure 1 illustrates the comorbid occurrence of various GERD forms in identical patients.[6]

In addition to damage inflicted on the esophageal mucosa, gastric contents can spill in the pharynx, larynx, mouth, and lung. A variety of extraesophageal manifestations of GERD are listed in Table 1. Most pharyngeal and laryngeal diseases reflect mucosal damage and ensuing inflammation secondary to the refluxate.[7,8] In patients with copious amounts of acidic reflux into their mouth, the dental enamel may become resolved by the changed oral acidic milieu.[9] In a subgroup of patients with asthma, the disease seems to be precipitated solely by gastroesophageal reflux and aspiration of acidic juice.[10,11]

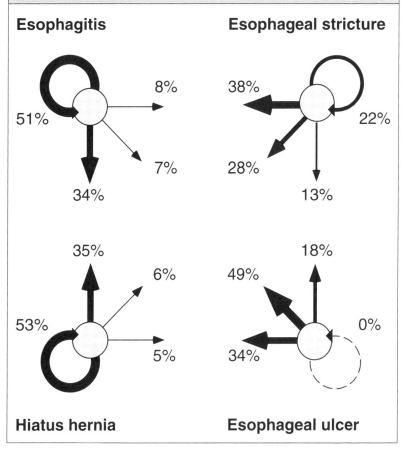

Figure 1. Comorbid associations between four forms of gastroesophageal reflux disease (GERD), each *arrow* representing one association. The percentage describes the fraction of patients with one form of GERD (where the arrow starts) who also suffer from a second form of GERD (to which the arrow points). The *circular arrows* represent patients who have one form of GERD as their sole presentation. (Adapted from El-Serag HB, Sonnenberg A: Associations among different forms of gastroesophageal reflux disease in US veterans. Gut 41:594–599, 1997.)

Prevalence and Incidence Rates

Estimates for the prevalence of various manifestations of GERD are listed in Table 2. The prevalence of GERD varies markedly between different populations.[15,16] During the past three decades the prevalence of GERD has increased more than twofold, and previously reported data

TABLE 2. Prevalence of Gastroesophageal Reflux Disease	
Disease Type	**Prevalence, %**
All GERD[12,13]	40
Weekly symptoms[14]	14
Daily symptoms[14]	4–7
Erosive esophagitis[16,17]	1.2–2.4
Peptic stricture[17,18]	0.10
Barrett's metaplasia[19]	0.40
Esophageal adenocarcinoma	0.0025

may no longer apply to present day populations.[17] With all these caveats in mind, one should consider the data cited as crude estimates only. The SEER cancer registries indicate that 7000 people die annually from esophageal adenocarcinoma, which translates into a mortality rate of 25 deaths per million living population.[18] Considering the overall high prevalence of GERD, fortunately, this most severe outcome of GERD is extremely rare.

The prevalence data for manifestations of reflux disease in the middle range of the disease spectrum are less well characterized. In general, patients with severe and frequent symptoms tend to suffer from more severe forms of GERD. However, such a relationship shows only as a statistical phenomenon in large patient series. Symptoms are poor (insensitive and unspecific) indicators to predict disease severity in the individual patient.[1–3] Therefore, a study trying to assess the true population prevalence of erosive esophagitis and its complications could not rely on symptoms alone and would need to subject a large group of asymptomatic and symptomatic persons to upper gastrointestinal endoscopy. For obvious reasons, such a study would be expensive to conduct and difficult to justify.

A recent study from China estimated a 5% prevalence rate of erosive esophagitis.[19] Of those patients presenting with symptoms suggestive of GERD, 18.5% were found to have erosive esophagitis. A Swedish study reported an incidence of 120 new cases of erosive esophagitis per 100,000 per year.[20] Assuming a case history of 10 to 20 years yields crude estimates of 1.2% to 2.4% for the prevalence rate. Because symptomatic patients are more likely to undergo endoscopy, however, incidence and prevalence rates based largely on routine endoscopy reports overestimate the true prevalence of erosive esophagitis in the general population. For these reasons the lower rate may represent a better estimate the true prevalence. Ulcers or strictures are found in less than 10% of all patients with erosive esophagitis.[20,21] Therefore, a prevalence estimate of 0.1% is shown in Table 2. Lastly, a post-mortem study from

Olmsted County in Minnesota found a prevalence rate of 0.4% for Barrett's esophagus.[15]

Demographic, Temporal, and Geographic Variations

Only mild forms of GERD without mucosal damage are found slightly more often in women than in men. All other, more severe forms of GERD characterized by erosive esophagitis, esophageal ulcer, or stricture are far more common in men than in women. All forms of GERD affect people of European ethnicity more often than African Americans or Native Americans. The prevalence of GERD increases with age. Similar demographic patterns characterize the epidemiology of all GERD manifestations, including esophageal adenocarcinoma.[22] The demographic shift from men to women, whites to blacks, and young to old are usually more pronounced in severe than in mild forms of GERD. The typical patient with peptic stricture or Barrett's esophagus, for instance, is an elderly white male. By contrast, Barrett's esophagus is rarely found in female African Americans. In the United States, these variations by age, gender, and ethnicity are revealed similarly by different types of morbidity parameters, that is, prevalence data, physician visits, hospitalizations, and death rates.[22] The prevalence of GERD is high among residents of developed countries in North America and Europe but relatively low among those of developing countries in Africa and Asia.[16]

Between 1970 and 1987, the rates of hospitalizations in the National Hospital Discharge Survey secondary to erosive esophagitis rose twofold in men and women alike.[22] A less striking increase also occurred in cases of esophageal strictures. The rise in hospitalization for esophagitis was not matched by an equal rise in surgical procedures, as the rate of surgical repair of hiatal hernia declined during the identical time period. The time trends from the National Hospital Discharge Survey are corroborated by similar trends of hospitalizations among US military veterans and US mortality rates taken from the Vital Statistics registries.[17]

In the veteran population, as in many other populations, patients with gastric and duodenal ulcer showed a significant decline in hospitalization rates between 1970 and 1995, the decline being more pronounced in duodenal than in gastric ulcer cases. The hospitalization rates for gastric and duodenal ulcer were similar among whites and other ethnic groups. In striking contrast with the behavior of peptic ulcer, the hospital discharges involving GERD rose four-fold and seven-fold among whites and non-whites, respectively, during the same time period.

Similar to gastric and duodenal ulcer, gastric cancer is also strongly associated with upper gastrointestinal infection by *H. pylori*. Gastric cancer shows an epidemiologic pattern quite similar to that of gastric ulcer and, to a lesser degree, duodenal ulcer. The same way that esophageal adenocarcinoma represents the extreme outcome of reflux disease, gastric cancer may be perceived as the extreme outcome at the very end of a disease spectrum that extends from the first infection through *H. pylori* to gastritis and peptic ulcer disease.[23] The opposing time trends of peptic ulcer and GERD is exemplified by the opposing time trends of their corresponding cancer types. While hospitalization resulting from cancer of the gastric corpus and antrum declined between 1968 and 1995, hospitalization from esophageal adenocarcinoma increased during the same time period (Fig. 2). Both cancer types also show opposing patterns with respect to their ethnic distribution, gastric cancer being less and esophageal adenocarcinoma being more common among whites than among any other ethnic group.

Risk Factors

The risk factors that influence the occurrence and natural history of GERD can be grouped into two large categories, that is, *exogenous* (or

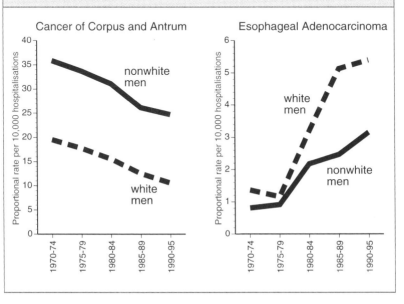

Figure 2. Time trends of hospitalization for gastric cancer of the corpus or antrum (*left*) and esophageal adenocarcinoma/cancer of the cardia (*right*). Data points represent the average of consecutive time periods as shown on the x-axis. (Adapted from El-Serag HB, Sonnenberg A: Opposing time trends of peptic ulcer and reflux disease. Gut 43:327–333, 1998.)

TABLE 3.   Environmental Risk Factors for Gastroesophageal Reflux Disease

Risk Factor	Mechanism of Risk
Smoking	Weakened LES? (small risk)
Alcohol	Mucosal damage? (small risk)
Medications	Weakening of LES, mucosal damage
Meals and specific foods	Gastric distension, weakening of LES, irritation of esophageal mucosa
Helicobacter pylori	Beneficial influence as corpus gastritis reduces acid output
Naso-gastric tubes	Conduit for acid reflux in supine patients
Abdominal trauma	Disruption of diaphragm?

LES = lower esophageal sphincter

environmental) risk factors (Table 3) and *endogenous* risk factors. The endogenous risk factors comprise, first, genetically predetermined variations in upper gastrointestinal physiology that favor the development of GERD and, second, the occurrence of other comorbid disease conditions that disrupt normal esophageal physiology to promote GERD. Currently, most existing research in GERD epidemiology is devoted to the elucidation of new risk factors. This research area holds the promise that one day we will discover new risk factors to gain a better understanding of GERD etiology and its natural history. Rather than discuss each and every risk factor, the subsequent sections focus on those risk factors that seem most important or that have garnered most attention in the recent medical literature.

Acid Output

Hydrochloric acid is the main noxious constituent of the refluxate swept through the incompetent lower esophageal sphincter into the esophagus. The name *gastroesophageal reflux* places gastric contents and especially gastric acid in the center of GERD etiology. The obvious success of innumerable clinical trials using antisecretory medications, such as histamine-2 antagonists or proton pump inhibitors, to heal GERD confirms the overwhelming relevance of acid in precipitating the GERD and its associated mucosal lesions. Many trials have also established a clear correlation between the extent of acid inhibition and the clinical success in relieving GERD symptoms and healing mucosal damage.[24]

The role of acid can also be established by direct measurement. In our own study, for instance, esophageal function was tested in a large group of GERD patients by 24-hour intraesophageal pH-monitoring and esophageal manometry.[25] The group consisted of 228 patients with nonerosive reflux disease, 170 patients with erosive esophagitis, 235 patients with Barrett's esophagus, and 30 patients with high-grade dysplasia or esophageal adenocarcinoma. The results are presented in Figure 3. The number of reflux episodes increased significantly with increasing severity of reflux disease, including high-grade dysplasia and cancer. The percentage of acid contact time also increased with increasing severity of reflux disease. The other parameters of pH-monitoring (not shown in the figure), such as acid contact time in the supine and upright positions, frequency of reflux episodes over 5 minutes, and length of the longest reflux episode, were highly correlated with the total acid contact time and revealed a similar pattern when compared among the four patient groups. Lastly, the average pressure of the lower esophageal sphincter decreased significantly among the four groups. Similar results have been published by many other investigators.[26,27] They all attest to the significance of acid in the development of mucosal damage and the function of the lower esophageal sphincter as a pressure barrier to keep gastric acid out of the esophagus.

Bar graphs tend to obscure the large variation that one encounters in measuring esophageal function. Although the average values may change consistently with disease severity, one observes a large overlap between the results of pH-monitoring among patients with varying disease severity (Fig. 4).[28] Hirschowitz[29] found that basal and stimulated acid or pepsin output did not correlate with the presence or severity of esophagitis. His subsequent studies also showed similar acid and pepsin outputs among patients with peptic stricture or Barrett's esophagus and matched control subjects.[30,31] In essence, it has remained impossible to predict disease severity based on the amount of gastric acid output or the outcomes of pH-monitoring and esophageal manometry.

Bile Reflux

Another potential risk factor that has been explored to explain the differences in the clinical presentation of GERD is intraesophageal bile reflux.[26,32–34] Vaezi et al.[26] found a positive relationship between bile reflux and disease severity; that is, more bile reflux was measured among patients with severe than mild forms of GERD (Fig. 5). In their patient population, the amount of bile reflux also strongly correlated with the amount of acid reflux into the esophagus. Large amounts of gastric volume constituted the primary means to sweep bile into the esophagus. Overall, the results of their analysis closely resembled similar types of data obtained through previous measurements of intraesophageal acid alone. No new dimension was added to the picture of GERD pathophysiology by the possibility of measuring bile reflux. Patients with prolonged acid contact time were also characterized by similarly increased bile exposure. However, the data did not help in delineating a new

Figure 3. Frequency of reflux episodes, acid contact time, and the lower esophageal sphincter pressure among patients with various grades of gastroesophageal reflux disease (GERD). The bars represent the mean and the standard error of each group. The differences among the four groups with respect to all three parameters were significant at $P < 0.0001$ when tested by ANOVA. NERD = nonerosive reflux disease; HGD/CA = high-grade dysplasia or esophageal adenocarcinoma. (Adapted from Avidan B, Sonnenberg A, Schell TG, et al: Hiatal hernia size, Barrett's length, and severity of acid reflux are all risk factors for esophageal adenocarcinoma. Am J Gastroenterol 97:1930–1936, 2002.)

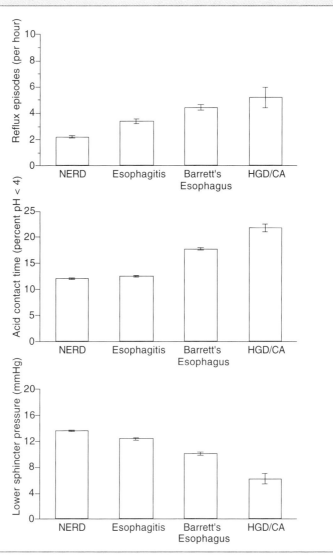

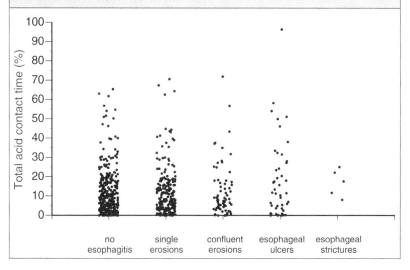

Figure 4. Total acid contact time in patients with various grades of erosive reflux esophagitis. (Adapted from Avidan B, Sonnenberg A, Schell TG, et al: Acid reflux is a poor predictor for the severity of erosive reflux esophagitis. Dig Dis Sci 47:2565–2573, 2002.)

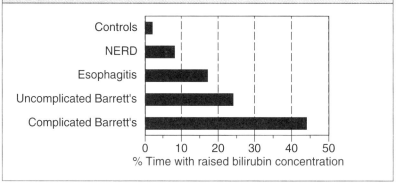

Figure 5. Duodenogastroesophageal reflux in healthy control subjects and four patient groups with increasing severity of reflux disease. NERD = nonerosive reflux disease. (Adapted from Valzi MF, Richter JE: Role of acid and duodenogastroesophageal reflux in gastroesophageal reflux disease. Gastroenterology 111:1192–1199, 1996.)

group of patients, for instance, those with low acid contact time, in whom a markedly increased high bile reflux would have explained an otherwise puzzling severe form of GERD.

After partial gastrectomy, with removal of the pylorus and antrum, duodenal contents flow easily backwards through the small gastric remnant, and under the right conditions, into the esophagus. The partial gastrectomy (or any gastric surgery that leads to bile reflux) can serve as an epidemiologic model to assess the role of duodenogastroesophageal reflux in cases of Barrett's esophagus and Barrett's adenocarcinoma. In our study, two case populations of 650 subjects with short-segment Barrett's esophagus and 366 subjects with long-segment Barrett's esophagus were compared to a control population of 3047 subjects without GERD. The comparison concerned any previous history of gastric surgery[35] among case and control subjects. We did not find gastric surgery for benign peptic ulcer disease to be a risk factor for either type of Barrett's esophagus (Fig. 6). This lack of association casts doubts on the ability of bile without accompanying acid to damage the esophageal mucosa.

The syndrome name "Saint's triad" alludes to the concomitant occurrence of gallstones, hiatal hernia, and diverticulosis.[36] Speculations about the relationship between gallstone and reflux disease have persevered in the medical literature, probably because of the existence of such a catchy eponym as "Saint's triad" and its initial description by such a respected epidemiologist as Burkitt (from Burkitt's lymphoma). Cholelithiasis and cholecystectomy have been claimed to affect the antropyloric barrier.[37,38] The loss of the reservoir function for bile after removal of the gallbladder leads to changes in the dynamics of bile flow. Instead of the intermittent meal-induced bile flow, a continuous flow ensues that may affect antroduodenal motility and promote duodenogastric reflux.[39] In a recent case-control study, therefore, we assessed the relationships between the occurrence of gallstones and the presence of hiatal hernia or GERD.[40] Our own analysis failed to establish any significant relationships between gallstones and hiatal hernia, or gallstones and GERD. Consistent with a previous study by Manifold and coworkers,[41] the absence of association pertained similarly to the diagnosis of asymptomatic gallstones, as well as to a past history of symptomatic gallstones for which cholecystectomy had been performed. Moreover, the presence of gallstones in patients with hiatal hernia did not increase the risk for harboring GERD.

Helicobacter pylori

Because *H. pylori* plays an essential role in the pathogenesis of gastric ulcer, duodenal ulcer, and gastric cancer, the general decline of its infection rate in Western societies provides the most likely explanation

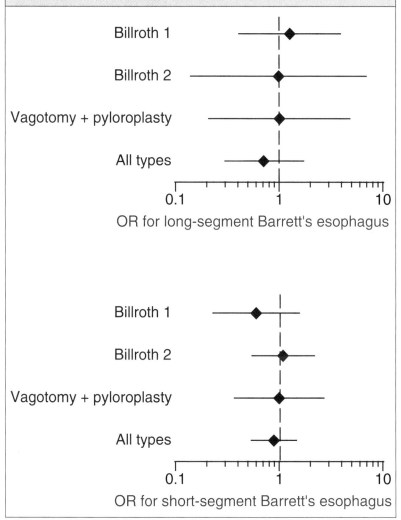

Figure 6. Odds ratio (OR) for the development of long-segment (*upper panel*) or short-segment (*lower panel*) Barrett's esophagus associated with different types of gastric surgery. (Data taken from Avidan B, Sonnenberg A, Schell TG, et al: Gastric surgery is not a risk for Barrett's esophagus or esophageal adenocarcinoma. Gastroenterology 121:1281–1285, 2001.)

for the falling time trends of these three diseases. The acquisition of *H. pylori* infection results in the development of acute gastritis that, if left untreated, gives way to chronic gastroduodenitis.[42] Both types of peptic ulcer and gastric cancer are all strongly correlated with a gastroduodenal infection by *H. pylori*[43,44] Antral gastritis, found mostly in patients with duodenal ulcer, leaves the ability to secrete acid unaffected or even increases gastric acid output by compromising somatostatin secretion of the D-cells and its inhibitory effect on gastrin output. In contradistinction with antral gastritis, gastritis that involves large areas of the gastric body (corpus) results in partial atrophy of the acid-secreting mucosa and hypochlorhydria.[45,46]

In general, patients with an endoscopically diagnosed reflux esophagitis are less likely to harbor active or chronic corpus gastritis than patients without esophagitis.[47–49] Figure 7 shows data from our series of consecutive patients undergoing esophagogastroduodenoscopy for various upper gastrointestinal symptoms.[49] The patient population was composed of 116 case subjects with and 148 control subjects without erosive esophagitis. The severity of acute or chronic gastritis in the gastric body, characterized by polymorphonuclear cells and lymphocytes, respectively, were both inversely related to the prevalence rate of erosive esophagitis. Overall, patients with erosive esophagitis showed a significantly lower prevalence rate of gastritis in the body of their stomach. The occurrence and severity of *H. pylori*–induced gastritis may be more

Figure 7. Prevalence rates of various grades of acute (*left panel*) or chronic gastritis (*right panel*) of the gastric body in 116 case subjects with and in 148 control subjects without erosive esophagitis. The differences in the prevalence rates of acute and chronic gastritis among case and control subjects were both statistically significant. (Data from El-Serag HB, Sonnenberg A, Jamal MM, et al: Corpus gastritis is protective against reflux esophagitis. Gut 45:181–185, 1999.)

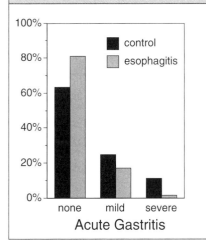

Acute Gastritis

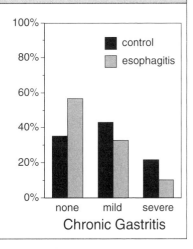

Chronic Gastritis

important than the actual colonization of the upper gastrointestinal mucosa by the bacterium itself.

Whereas the inverse relationship between gastritis and esophagitis is relatively easy to establish, the relationship between gastric colonization by *H. pylori* itself and its protective influence against GERD appears to be far more tenuous.[49,50] Some authors have claimed that not all *Helicobacter* infections but only those by *Helicobacter* strains with the cytotoxin-associated gene A (*cagA*) pathogenicity island protect against reflux disease.[51,52] In some patients, the hypochlorhydria secondary to corpus gastritis becomes reversible, once the infection with *H. pylori* has been treated with antibiotics.[45,46] Labenz and colleagues[53] followed patients with duodenal ulcer after antibiotic cure of *H. pylori* infection for 3 years. The incidence of reflux esophagitis was 25.8% after eradication of *H. pylori,* compared with 12.9% in patients with persistent infection. Not all authors have been able to confirm such a dramatic effect of *Helicobacter* eradication on GERD, however.[54,55] Besides being responsible for the decline of peptic ulcer and gastric cancer, therefore, the time trends *H. pylori* infection also offer a possible explanation for the rise of GERD and esophageal adenocarcinoma. The opposing time trends of peptic ulcer and gastric cancer on one side versus GERD and esophageal adenocarcinoma on the other side suggest that *Helicobacter pylori* infection may be protect against GERD.

An additional piece of evidence to support the role of *H. pylori* in GERD is provided by the remarkable differences among ethnic groups. While people of color in the United States incurred substantially reduced hospitalization and mortality rates related to GERD or esophageal adenocarcinoma, they suffered more from gastric cancer than whites.[21] In general, people of color in the United States tend to harbor higher rates of infection with *H. pylori* acquired at a younger age than whites.[56] Again, this pattern translates into prolonged time periods of chronic gastritis and a greater chance of developing mucosal atrophy of the gastric body associated with reduced acid output. Gastric atrophy and reduced acid output mean a greater risk for gastric cancer and a smaller risk for GERD and esophageal adenocarcinoma, respectively. The geographic distribution of GERD could also relate to the geographic distribution of *H. pylori*. In developed countries the decline in *H. pylori* infection is likely to have resulted in an increased susceptibility to developing to GERD.

Hiatal Hernia

Endoscopic, radiographic and manometric studies have reported that 50 to 94% of patients with reflux disease have hiatal hernia, whereas a far lower percentage of subjects without reflux disease have hiatal hernia.[57–59] In several of our epidemiologic studies, the presence of hiatal hernia turned out to be the predictor variable with the strongest influence on mucosal disease severity, exceeding those of acid reflux, lower esophageal sphincter pressure, or any of the demographic characteristics.[25,28,60] Hiatal hernia is also known to be more common in patients with Barrett's esophagus than in healthy control subjects.[61,62] The significance of hiatal hernia in cases of Barrett's esophagus was emphasized in a study by Cameron,[63] showing that 96% of his patients harbored a hiatal hernia. In addition, the hiatus sac tended to be longer and wider in subjects with than in those without Barrett's esophagus. The results of our studies corroborated these previous reports. Even in comparison with patients suffering from nonerosive reflux disease, the existence of a hiatal hernia stood out as a highly significant risk factor for both the presence and the overall length of Barrett's esophagus. In Barrett's esophagus as in erosive esophagitis, hiatal hernia proved to be more influential than either the reduced tone of the lower esophageal sphincter or the percentage of total acid contact time.

Hiatal hernia has always been thought to influence the development of GERD by facilitating gastroesophageal reflux. The occurrence of hiatal hernia has been associated with an impairment of lower esophageal sphincter tone and clearance of esophageal acid.[64,65] Hiatal hernia has been assumed to act only as an indirect mediator of other more crucial mechanisms, such as increased access of acid to the esophageal mucosa, as well as delayed esophageal clearance of the acid. The findings from the epidemiologic studies cited, however, cast doubt on the long-accepted mechanisms by which hiatal hernia causes esophagitis, since neither the pressure of the lower esophageal sphincter nor the esophageal mucosal acid exposure compared in magnitude with the overwhelming importance of hiatal hernia in influencing disease severity. It is difficult to reconcile a secondary permissive role of hiatal hernia with its more powerful influence in comparison with the other risk factors. By contradistinction, the overall stronger influence associated with hiatal hernia leads one to speculate that the hiatal hernia itself might affect the occurrence of erosive esophagitis beyond that of simply facilitating acid reflux.

Currently, there is no clear-cut answer to this seeming discrepancy. In the presence of hiatal hernia, for instance, the shortened longitudinal muscle fibers could compromise mucosal blood supply by compression of the arterioles and small vessels. Hiatal hernia could also act in transmitting intragastric pressure directly into the esophagus and expose the mucosa of the distal esophagus to strong abrasive forces during episodes of retching or vomiting. Such additional mechanisms would not negate the general relevance of acid in the occurrence of erosive reflux esophagitis, but they could help to reconcile the obvious discrepancy between the relevance of hiatal hernia and the parameters of acid reflux in predicting disease severity.

Associated Diseases

Other diagnoses can be linked to GERD through three different mechanisms. As listed in Table 1, a variety of diseases of the throat, mouth, and lung stem from the same underlying disease process that affects primarily the esophagus. Frequent occurrence of nighttime reflux can irritate the pharyngeal and laryngeal structures and result in laryngitis, hoarseness, or aphonia. Aspiration of gastric contents has been associated with asthma, chronic obstructive lung disease, pneumonia, and bronchiectasies.[7,8,10,11]

A second group of diagnoses is linked to GERD by the type of medications used for their treatment, some of which affect esophageal function and its mucosal integrity. Most of these drugs impair esophageal motility, delay esophageal clearance of refluxed acid, and reduce lower esophageal sphincter tone. This applies to calcium antagonists, anticholinergics, α- and β-blockers, and progesterone. Alendronate (and other biphosphonates), doxycycline, potassium chloride, and nonsteroidal anti-inflammatory drugs act directly on the esophageal mucosa by disrupting tissue resistance and leading to erosions or pill-induced ulcers. Several studies have suggested that more severe forms of peptic esophagitis, associated with large confluent erosions, strictures, and Barrett's esophagus, are more common in patients on chronic consumption of nonsteroidal anti-inflammatory drugs.[66–70] In the veterans population, many of the diseases commonly treated with nonsteroidal anti-inflammatory drugs, such as osteoarthritis, back pain, or tension headache, were associated with a small but significant odds ratio of about 1.4 for reflux esophagitis.[68]

In a third group of diagnoses, the disease-specific process itself interferes with the normal esophageal physiology and facilitates increased exposure of the esophageal mucosa to acid. This group of medical conditions are listed in Table 4. For instance, esophageal clearance is markedly impaired in CRST syndrome and systemic sclerosis, because muscle atrophy results in dysfunction of the lower sphincter and aperistalsis of the tubular esophagus.[71–75] Among the population of US military veterans, we found systemic sclerosis to be associated with a sixfold increased risk for erosive esophagitis.[16] In cases of Sjögren's syndrome, reduced or absent salivary secretion interferes with normal esophageal clearance and also results in an increased risk for erosive esophagitis.[68] Zollinger-Ellison syndrome provides the only striking ex-

TABLE 4. Medical Conditions Associated with Gastoesophageal Reflux Disease

Associated Condition	Mechanism of Risk
Obesity	Increased intra-abdominal pressure
Diabetes mellitus	Delayed gastric emptying
Zollinger-Ellison syndrome	Increased acid output
Pregnancy	Increased intra-abdominal pressure, weakened LES
Myotomy in achalasia	Destroyed LES
CRST syndrome	Impaired peristalsis
Sicca syndrome	Impaired esophageal clearance
Psychiatric disease	Impaired esophageal motility
Mental retardation of childhood	Impaired esophageal motility
LES = lower esophageal sphincter	

ample for a positive association between the amount of acid output and mucosal damage to the esophageal mucosa.[76] Severe neuropsychiatric diseases of childhood, such as Down syndrome and cerebral palsy, are associated with particularly severe forms of GERD, frequently accompanied by long segments of Barrett's metaplasia and tight peptic strictures.[77,78] A host of psychiatric disease in adults also predispose to an increased occurrence of GERD.[79,80]

Key Points: GERD

- ⤷ Gastric acid and its reflux into the esophagus are the main risk factors for GERD.
- ⤷ Acid inhibition has had therapeutic success in the clinical management of GERD.
- ⤷ *Helicobacter pylori* reduces the risk of GERD by causing corpus gastritis and reducing gastric acid output.
- ⤷ The geographic and temporal trends of *H. pylori* infection among human populations may be ultimately responsible for much of the apparent GERD epidemiology.
- ⤷ The ethnic variation of GERD-related disease may also stem from underlying variations in *H. pylori* infection.
- ⤷ The gender-specific variation of GERD may involve the association of a larger surface area with a higher acid output in men, but probably involves other factors as well.
- ⤷ Most epidemiologic studies have shown hiatal hernia to exert an influence far and beyond its role in facilitating acid reflux and delaying esophageal clearance.

Suggested Reading

1. Klauser AG, Schindlbeck NE, Müller-Lissner SA: Symptoms in gastro-oesophageal reflux disease. Lancet 335:205–208, 1990.
2. Avidan B, Sonnenberg A, Schnell TG, et al: There are no reliable symptoms for erosive esophagitis or Barrett's esophagus: Endoscopic diagnosis still essential. Aliment Pharm Ther 16:735–742, 2002.
3. Lundell LR, Dent J, Bennet JR, et al: Endoscopic assessment of oesophagitis: Clinical and functional correlates and further validation of the Los Angeles classification. Gut 45:172–180, 1999.
4. Savary M, Miller G: The esophagus: Handbook and atlas of endoscopy. Solothurn, Switzerland, Gassmann, 1978.
5. Sonnenberg A, El-Serag HB: Clinical epidemiology and natural history of gastroesophageal reflux disease. Yale J Biol Med 72:81–92, 1999.
6. El-Serag HB, Sonnenberg A: Associations among different forms of gastroesophageal reflux disease. Gut 41:594–599, 1997.
7. El-Serag HB, Sonnenberg A: Extraesophageal complications of gastroesophageal reflux disease in US veterans. Gastroenterology 113:755–760, 1997.
8. El-Serag HB, Hepworth EJ, Lee P, et al: Gastroesophageal reflux disease is a risk factor for laryngeal cancer. Am J Gastroenterol 96:2013–2018, 2001.
9. Schroeder PL, Filler SJ, Ramirez B, et al: Dental erosion and reflux disease. Ann Intern Med 122:809–815, 1995.
10. Avidan B, Sonnenberg A, Schnell TG, et al: Temporal associations between coughing or wheezing and acid reflux in asthmatics. Gut 49:767–772, 2001.
11. Sontag JS, Schnell TG, Miller TQ, et al: Prevalence of esophagitis in asthmatics. Gut 33:872–876, 1992.
12. Gallup organization: A Gallup survey on heartburn across America. Princeton, NJ, The Gallup Organization, 1988.
13. Locke GR III, Talley NJ, Fett SL, et al: Prevalence and clinical spectrum of gastroesophageal reflux: A population-based study in Olmsted County, Minnesota. Gastroenterology 112:1448–1456, 1997.
14. Nebel OT, Fornes MF, Castell DO: Symptomatic gastroesophageal reflux: Incidence and precipitating factors. Am J Dig Dis 21:953–956, 1976.
15. El-Serag HB: The epidemic of esophageal adenocarcinoma. Gastroenterol Clin North Am 31:421–440, 2002.
16. Chang CS, Poon SK, Lien HC, et al: The incidence of reflux esophagitis among the Chinese. Am J Gastroenterol 92:668–671, 1997.
17. Lööf L, Götell P, Elfberg B: The incidence of reflux oesophagitis: A study of endoscopy reports from a defined catchment area in Sweden. Scand J Gastroenterol 28:113–118, 1993.
18. Ollyo JB, Monnier P, Fontolliet C, et al: The natural history, prevalence and incidence of reflux oesophagitis. Gullet 3:3–10, 1993.
19. Cameron AJ, Zinsmeister AR, Ballard DJ, et al: Prevalence of columnar-lined (Barrett's) esophagus: Comparison of population-based clinical and autopsy findings. Gastroenterology 99:918–922, 1990.
20. Sonnenberg A: Epidemiologie und Spontanverlauf der Refluxkrankheit. In Blum AL, Siewert JR (eds): Refluxtherapie. Berlin, Springer-Verlag, 1981, pp 85–106.
21. El-Serag HB, Sonnenberg A: Opposing time trends of peptic ulcer and reflux disease. Gut 43:327–333, 1998.
22. Sonnenberg A: Esophageal diseases. In Everhart JE (ed): Digestive diseases in the United States: Epidemiology and impact. US Department of Health and Human Ser-

vices, NIH publication no 94–1447. Washington, DC, US Government Printing Office, 1994, pp 299–356.

23. Molloy RM, Sonnenberg A: The relationship between gastric cancer and previous peptic ulcer disease. Gut 40:247–252, 1997.

24. Chiba N, De Gara CJ, Wilkinson JM, et al: Speed of healing and symptom relief in grade II to IV gastroesophageal reflux disease: A meta-analysis. Gastroenterology 112:1798–1810, 1997.

25. Avidan B, Sonnenberg A, Schnell TG, et al: Hiatal hernia size, Barrett's length, and severity of acid reflux are all risk factors for esophageal adenocarcinoma. Am J Gastroenterol 97:1930–1936, 2002.

26. Vaezi MF, Richter JE: Role of acid and duodenogastroesophageal reflux in gastroesophageal reflux disease. Gastroenterology 111:1192–1199, 1996.

27. Kahrilas PJ, Dodds WJ, Hogan WJ, et al: Esophageal peristaltic dysfunction in peptic esophagitis. Gastroenterology 91:897–904, 1986.

28. Avidan B, Sonnenberg A, Schnell TG, et al: Acid reflux is a poor predictor for the severity of erosive reflux esophagitis. Dig Dis Sci: 47:2565–2573, 2002.

29. Hirschowitz BI: A critical analysis, with appropriate controls, of gastric acid and pepsin secretion in clinical esophagitis. Gastroenterology 101:1149–1158, 1991.

30. Hirschowitz BI: Gastric secretion of acid and pepsin in patients with esophageal stricture and appropriate controls. Dig Dis Sci 41:2115–2122, 1996.

31. Hirschowitz BI: Gastric acid and pepsin secretion in patients with Barrett's esophagus and appropriate controls. Dig Dis Sci 41:1384–1391, 1996.

32. Champion G, Richter JE, Vaezi MF, et al: Duodenogastroesophageal reflux: Relationship to pH and importance in Barrett's esophagus. Gastroenterology 107:747–754, 1994.

33. Menges M, Müller M, Zeitz M: Increased acid and bile reflux in Barrett's esophagus compared to reflux esophagitis, and effect of proton pump inhibitor therapy. Am J Gastroenterol 96:331–337, 2001.

34. Kauer WKH, Burdiles P, Ireland AP, et al: Does duodenal juice reflux into the esophagus of patients with complicated GERD? Evaluation of a fiberoptic sensor for bilirubin. Am J Surg 169:98–104, 1995.

35. Avidan B, Sonnenberg A, Schnell TG, et al: Gastric surgery is not a risk for Barrett's esophagus or esophageal adenocarcinoma. Gastroenterology 121:1281–1285, 2001.

36. Burkitt DP, Walker ARP: Saint's triad: confirmation and explanation. S Afr Med J 50:2136–2138, 1976.

37. Svensson JO, Gelin J, Svanvik J: Gallstones, cholecystectomy, and duodenogastric reflux of bile acid. Scand J Gastroenterol 21:181–187, 1986.

38. Cabrol J, Navarro X, Simo-Deu J, et al: Evaluation of duodenogastric reflux in gallstone disease before and after simple cholecystectomy. Am J Surg 160:283–286, 1990.

39. Pedrikis G, Wilson P, Hinder R, et al: Altered antroduodenal motility after cholecystectomy. Am J Surg 168:609–615, 1994.

40. Avidan B, Sonnenberg A, Schnell TG, et al: No association between gallstones and gastroesophageal reflux disease. Am J Gastroenterol 96:2858–2862, 2001.

41. Manifold DK, Chi B, Anggiansah A, et al: Effect of cholecystectomy on gastroesophageal and duodenogastric reflux. Am J Gastroenterol 95:2746–2750, 2000.

42. Sipponen P: Long-term consequences of gastroduodenal inflammation. Eur J Gastroenterol Hepatol 4(Suppl 2):S25–S29, 1992.

43. Parsonnet J, Friedman GD, Vandersteen DP, et al: *Helicobacter pylori* infection and the risk of gastric carcinoma. N Engl J Med 325:1127–1131, 1991.

44. Nomura A, Stemmermann GN, Chyou PH, et al: *Helicobacter pylori* infection and the risk for duodenal and gastric ulceration. Ann Intern Med 120:977–981, 1994.

45. El-Omar EM, Oien K, El-Nujumi A, et al: *Helicobacter pylori* infection and chronic gastric acid hyposecretion. Gastroenterology 113:15–24, 1997.
46. Gutierrez O, Melo M, Segura AM, et al: Cure of *Helicobacter pylori* infection improves gastric acid secretion in patients with corpus gastritis. Scand J Gastroenterol 32:664–668, 1997.
47. Ohara S, Sekine H, Iijima K, et al: Gastric mucosal atrophy and prevalence of *Helicobacter pylori* in reflux esophagitis of the elderly [in Japanese]. Nippon Shokakibyo Gakkai Zasshi Japan J Gastroenterol 93:235–239, 1996.
48. Wu JCY, Sung JJY, Ng EKW, et al: Prevalence and distribution of *Helicobacter pylori* in gastroesophageal reflux disease: A study from the east. Am J Gastroenterol 94:1790–1794, 1999.
49. El-Serag HB, Sonnenberg A, Jamal MM, et al: Corpus gastritis is protective against reflux esophagitis. Gut 45:181–185, 1999.
50. Newton M, Bryan R, Burnham WR, et al: Evaluation of *Helicobacter pylori* in reflux oesophagitis and Barrett's esophagus. Gut 40:9–13, 1997.
51. Vicari JJ, Peek RM, Falk GW, et al: The seroprevalence of *cagA*-positive *Helicobacter pylori* strains in the spectrum of gastroesophageal reflux disease. Gastroenterology 115:50–57, 1998.
52. Warburton-Timms VJ, Charlett A, Valori RM, et al: The significance of *cagA*+ *Helicobacter pylori* in reflux oesophagitis. Gut 49:341–346, 2002.
53. Labenz J, Blum AL, Bayerdörffer E, et al: Curing *Helicobacter pylori* infection in patients with duodenal ulcer may provoke reflux esophagitis. Gastroenterology 112:1442–1447, 1997.
54. Fallone CA, Barkun AN, Friedman G, et al: Is *Helicobacter pylori* eradication associated with gastroesophageal reflux disease? Am J Gastroenterol 95:914–920, 2000.
55. Moayyedi P, Bardhan C, Young L, et al: *Helicobacter pylori* eradication does not exacerbate reflux symptoms in gastroesophageal reflux disease. Gastroenterology 121:1120–1126, 2001.
56. Malaty HM, Evans DG, Evans DJ, et al: *Helicobacter pylori* in Hispanics: Comparison with blacks and whites of similar age and socioeconomic class. Gastroenterology 103:813–816, 1992.
57. Sloan S, Kahrilas PJ: Impairment of esophageal emptying with hiatal hernia. Gastroenterology 100:596–605, 1991.
58. Kahrilas PJ, Lin S, Chen J, et al: The effect of hiatus hernia on gastro-esophageal junction pressure. Gut 44:476–482, 1999.
59. Peterson H, Johannessen T, Sandvik AK: Relationship between endoscopic hiatus hernia and gastroesophageal reflux symptoms. Scand J Gastroenterol 26:921–926, 1991.
60. Avidan B, Sonnenberg A, Schnell TG, et al: Hiatal hernia and acid reflux frequency predict presence and length of Barrett's esophagus. Dig Dis Sci 47:256–264, 2002.
61. Borrie J, Goldwater L: Columnar-cell lined esophagus: Assessment of etiology and treatment. J Thorac Cardiovasc Surg 71:825–834, 1976.
62. Robbins AH, Vincent ME, Saini M: Revised radiologic concepts of Barrett's esophagus. Gastrointest Radiol 3:377–381, 1978.
63. Cameron AJ: Barrett's esophagus: prevalence and size of hiatal hernia. Am J Gastroenterol 94:2054–2059, 1999.
64. Kahrilas PJ, Dodds WJ, Kern HM, et al: Esophageal peristaltic dysfunction in peptic esophagitis. Gastroenterology 91:897–904, 1986.
65. Mittal RK, Balaban DH: The esophagogastric junction. N Engl J Med 336:924–932, 1997.
66. Wilkins WE, Ridley MG, Pozniak AL: Benign stricture of the oesophagus: Role on non-steroidal anti-inflammatory drugs. Gut 25:478–480, 1984.

67. Lanas A, Hirschowitz BI: Significant role of aspirin use in patients with esophagitis. J Clin Gastroenterol 13:622–627, 1991.
68. El-Serag HB, Sonnenberg A: Non-steroidal anti-inflammatory drugs represent risk factors of erosions and peptic strictures of the esophagus. Am J Gastroenterol 92:57–60, 1997.
69. Avidan B, Sonnenberg A, Schnell TG, et al. Risk factors of esophagitis in arthritic patients. Eur J Gastroenterol Hepatol 13:1095–1099, 2001.
70. Avidan B, Sonnenberg A, Schnell TG, et al: Risk factors for erosive reflux esophagitis: A case-control study. Am J Gastroenterol 96:41–46, 2001.
71. Recht MP, Levin MS, Katzka DA, et al: Barrett's esophagus in scleroderma: Increased prevalence and radiographic findings. Gastrointest Radiol 13:1–5, 1988.
72. Treacy WL, Bagenstoss A, Slocumb CH, et al: Scleroderma of the esophagus. Ann Intern Med 59:351–356, 1963.
73. Saladin TA, French AB, Zarasafonetis CJD, et al: Esophageal motor abnormalities in scleroderma and related diseases. Am J Dig Dis 11:522–535, 1966.
74. Weston S, Thumshirn M, Wiste J, et al: Clinical and upper gastrointestinal motility features in systemic sclerosis and related disorders. Am J Gastroenterol 93:1085–1089, 1998.
75. Ergun GA: Esophageal abnormalities in systemic disease. In Castell DO (ed): The Esophagus. Boston, Little, Brown, 1992, pp 367–381.
76. Miller LS, Vinayek R, Frucht H, et al: Reflux esophagitis in patients with Zollinger-Ellison syndrome. Gastroenterology 98:341–346, 1990.
77. Clouse RE, Lustman PJ: Psychiatric illness and contraction abnormalities of the esophagus. N Engl J Med 309:1337–1342, 1983.
78. Snyder JD, Goldman H: Barrett's esophagus in children and young adults: Frequent association with mental retardation. Dig Dis Sci 35:1185–1189, 1990.
79. Avidan B, Sonnenberg A, Giblovich H, et al: Reflux symptoms are associated with psychiatric disease. Aliment Pharm Ther 15:1907–1912, 2001.
80. Böhmer CJM, Klinkenberg-Knol EC, Niezen-de Boer MC, et al: Gastroesophageal reflux disease in intellectually disabled individuals: How often, how serious, how manageable? Am J Gastroenterol 95:1868–1872, 2000.

The Pathophysiology of Gastroesophageal Reflux Disease

Marcelo F. Vela, M.D.
Michael F. Vaezi, M.D., Ph.D.

Gastroesophageal reflux disease (GERD) is a common clinical problem affecting all segments of the population. Nearly 20% of Americans experience heartburn or acid regurgitation weekly, with an annual prevalence of up to 59%.[1] Traditionally, treatment of reflux has focused on the most offending agent, gastric acid. However, other factors may also play important roles in the development of GERD and esophageal mucosal damage (Fig. 1). Harmful ingredients to the esophageal mucosa include gastric agents (acid and pepsin) and duodenal agents (conjugated and unconjugated bile acids and trypsin). The injury caused by these agents occurs after they traverse the esophagogastric junction and bathe the esophageal mucosa. This is usually prevented by the lower esophageal sphincter (LES), which, in concert with the crural diaphragm, constitutes the key barrier to reflux of gastroduodenal contents. The esophagogastric junction may be breached as a result of transient lower esophageal relaxations, hypotensive LES, or other mechanisms associated with the presence of a hiatal hernia. Once the esophageal mucosa is exposed to the damaging effect of gastroduodenal agents, luminal protection is provided by esophageal clearance (through peristalsis and acid neutralization) as well as by mechanisms of epithelial defense and repair, which are important in preventing mucosal injury. Failure of these protective mechanisms may lead to complications of GERD, including esophagitis, stricture, or Barrett's esophagus. Finally, in some individuals, a genetic component may be a contributor in predisposing to GERD.

Normally, there is a balance between these aggressive and defensive mechanisms. GERD results when this balance is lost, favoring aggressive factors. This chapter examines the interplay between the mechanisms contributing to the pathogenesis of GERD.

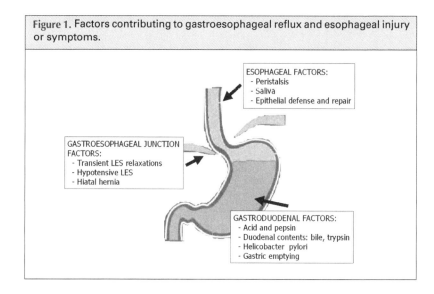

Figure 1. Factors contributing to gastroesophageal reflux and esophageal injury or symptoms.

ESOPHAGEAL FACTORS:
- Peristalsis
- Saliva
- Epithelial defense and repair

GASTROESOPHAGEAL JUNCTION FACTORS:
- Transient LES relaxations
- Hypotensive LES
- Hiatal hernia

GASTRODUODENAL FACTORS:
- Acid and pepsin
- Duodenal contents: bile, trypsin
- Helicobacter pylori
- Gastric emptying

Gastroduodenal Factors

The most injurious gastric components are acid, produced by the parietal cells, and pepsin, produced by the gastric chief cells. As commonly encountered during endoscopy, gastric contents may be mixed with duodenal material containing bile acids and trypsin. Therefore, when there is reflux of gastric contents into the esophagus, it may be a combination of gastric and duodenal agents contributing to the pathogenesis of GERD. Other factors that contribute to the pathogenesis of GERD in the stomach are *Helicobacter pylori*, which can have an impact on gastric acid secretion and the degree of gastric emptying (Fig. 2).

Gastric Agents

Acid and Pepsin. Substantial experimental and clinical evidence strongly supports the importance of acid and pepsin in GERD.[2] Animal experiments have shown that acid alone may cause injury to the esophageal mucosa only at very low pH values (pH 1–2). On the other hand, the combination of acid and even small concentrations of pepsin results in macroscopic as well as microscopic esophageal injury (See Fig. 2).[3] Acid results in cellular damage because a high concentration of hydrogen ions impairs cell volume regulation, leading to edema and ultimately necrosis.[4] In an acidic milieu (pH < 4), pepsin can damage the esophagus because of its proteolytic properties, whereas it is inactive at a pH > 4.[5] Early investigations[6] measuring distal esophageal acid expo-

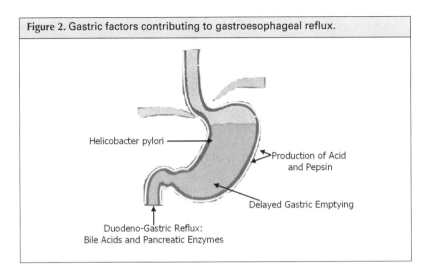

Figure 2. Gastric factors contributing to gastroesophageal reflux.

sure have shown good correlation between symptomatic heartburn and esophageal exposure to reflux material with pH < 4. Additionally, a series of studies[7-11] have shown that patients with various grades of esophagitis, including Barrett's esophagus, have increased frequency and duration of esophageal exposure to refluxate with pH < 4.

Interestingly, while increased exposure to acid in the esophagus has been clearly demonstrated in subjects with GERD, production of acid in the stomach is not increased in these patients. This was demonstrated by Hirschowitz et al,[12] who found that basal and pentagastrin-stimulated secretion of gastric acid and pepsin was similar between GERD patients and healthy control subjects. Therefore, the abnormal esophageal acid exposure in cases of GERD identified on ambulatory pH monitoring is most likely due to failure of the gastroesophageal barrier and poor esophageal clearance (discussed later). That said, there is a small number of patients, such as those with Zollinger-Ellison syndrome, in whom hypersecretion of acid leads to increased gastroesophageal reflux.[13]

The frequency and duration of esophageal acid exposure are not always predictive of the degree of esophageal mucosal injury. This suggests the importance of other factors, including duodenogastroesophageal reflux and mechanisms of luminal clearance and epithelial defense and repair.

Duodenal Agents

Bile acids and pancreatic enzymes may migrate from the duodenum, across the pylorus, and into the stomach, where they intermix with gastric secretions. The role of duodenal contents, specifically bile acids and the pancreatic enzyme trypsin, in the development of esophageal mucosal injury is controversial and the subject of many in vitro animal studies.[14-18] These studies suggest that the esophageal mucosal damage is dependent on the conjugation state of the bile acids. Conjugated forms are injurious at an acidic pH, whereas unconjugated forms are harmful at alkaline pH ranges. The way in which bile produces mucosal injury is not well understood; proposed mechanisms include cell damage through solubilization of the mucosal lipid membranes and intramucosal damage after entry of bile salts into the cell. Trypsin, like pepsin, harms through proteolysis and is most injurious at a pH of 5–8.[19]

The clinical evidence for the possible damaging effects of duodenogastroesophageal reflux on the esophageal mucosa remains controversial. However, recent studies by Vaezi and Richter[20] using the ambulatory bilirubin monitoring device (Bilitec) suggests that duodenogastroesophageal reflux parallels acid reflux in the clinical spectrum of GERD, being highest in patients with Barrett's esophagus (Fig. 3). Furthermore, these investigators found that simultaneous esophageal exposure to both acid and duodenogastroesophageal reflux was the most prevalent reflux pattern, occurring in 95% of patients with Barrett's esophagus and 79% of GERD patients. In fact, they found a strong correlation (R = 0.73) between acid and duodenogastroesophageal reflux in control subjects, reflux patients, and those with Barrett's esophagus. Thus, these studies support the earlier findings in animals that suggested

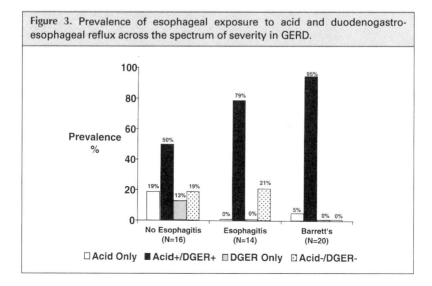

Figure 3. Prevalence of esophageal exposure to acid and duodenogastroesophageal reflux across the spectrum of severity in GERD.

a possible synergy between gastric acid and bile acids in the development of esophagitis and Barrett's esophagus.

The role of duodenogastroesophageal reflux in producing esophageal mucosal injury, in the absence of acid reflux, was not clarified until recently. Studies by Marshall et al[21] using prolonged pH and bilirubin monitoring in 38 patients with GERD found that duodenogastroesophageal reflux in the absence of acid reflux was a rare event (7%) in patients without prior gastric surgery. Additionally, Sears et al[22] studied 13 partial gastrectomy patients with reflux symptoms and found increased duodenogastroesophageal reflux by Bilitec monitoring in 77% of patients. Endoscopic esophagitis, however, was present only in those who had concomitant acid reflux. Subsequently, Vaezi et al[23] confirmed these observations and found that only 24% of upper gastrointestinal symptoms reported by partial gastrectomy patients were due to duodenogastroesophageal reflux in the absence of acid reflux. These studies show that duodenogastroesophageal reflux without excessive acid reflux can cause reflux symptoms but does not usually produce esophagitis.

Therefore, studies suggest that acid and pepsin are by far the main culprits behind mucosal injury. Duodenal contents contribute to mucosal damage in the presence of acid and pepsin but in their absence may not be injurious. However, reflux of nonacidic gastroduodenal contents may be responsible for continued symptoms in some patients treated with acid-suppressing medications. Using combined pH and bilirubin monitoring, Koek et al[24] showed that in 15 symptomatic patients treated with proton pump inhibitors, bile reflux elicited GERD symptoms. In a study using the recently developed technique of combined intraluminal impedance and pH, which allows measurement of both acid and nonacid reflux, Vela et al[25] reported that in a group of subjects with frequent heartburn studied in the postprandial period, omeprazole significantly decreased the number of acid reflux episodes; however, nonacid reflux continued to occur and was responsible for some symptoms.

The importance of bile and nonacid reflux in symptomatic patients, particularly those with adequate acid suppression, awaits further study. Studies using multichannel intraluminal impedance, which is capable of differentiating between liquid and gas, as well as acid and nonacid reflux, are likely to expand our knowledge in this area.

Gastric Emptying

Delayed gastric emptying may result in increased gastroesophageal reflux by triggering transient LES relaxations, which constitute one of the main mechanisms underlying reflux, as explained subsequently. Although studies evaluating the relationship between gastric emptying and reflux have yielded conflicting results,[26] a recent study suggests that the rate of proximal stomach emptying may have a more significant effect on reflux. Stacher et al[27] measured gastric emptying of a semisolid meal and performed 24-hour pH monitoring in 71 patients with symptoms of both delayed gastric emptying and reflux; they found that slow proximal but not distal gastric emptying correlated with increased 24-hour and postprandial esophageal acid exposure.

Helicobacter pylori

It has been suggested that H. pylori, known to be a risk factor for peptic ulcer disease and gastric cancer, may protect against GERD because the corpus gastritis caused by this bacterium results in decreased gastric acid production. Conversely, eradication of H. pylori has been shown to increase basal gastric acidity and basal gastric acid output.[28] A large epidemiologic study found that between 1975 and 1995, hospitalizations for GERD and esophageal adenocarcinoma in the United States rose significantly, whereas hospitalizations for peptic ulcer disease and gastric cancer fell; the authors hypothesized that the opposing trends for these diseases were due to the declining rate of H. pylori infection in the Western population.[29] In another report, Labenz et al[30] described a group of 450 patients with duodenal ulcer who received treatment for H. pylori infection; 3 years after therapy, the incidence of reflux esophagitis was twice as high in the group with successful eradication (26%) compared to those with persistent infection (13%), suggesting again that H. pylori may protect against reflux. Subsequent studies found a similar prevalence of H. pylori infection for GERD patients and control subjects; however, the presence of the cagA[+] strain of H. pylori was protective against more severe forms of GERD, such as Barrett's esophagus.[31,32]

Other investigations have yielded conflicting results regarding the relationship of H. pylori and GERD. Vakil et al[33] assessed 242 patients with duodenal ulcer who received treatment for H. pylori infection in four randomized controlled trials and found no increase in the incidence of GERD in patients with successful H. pylori erradication. More recently, an analysis of eight double-blind prospective trials of H. pylori therapy in 1165 patients with duodenal ulcer found that eradication of this bacterium does not lead to the development of esophagitis or worsening of symptoms in patients with preexisting GERD.[34]

Although the clinical importance of H. pylori in the setting of GERD is still a matter of debate, in some individuals corpus gastritis due to H. pylori, particularly the cagA[+] strain, may protect against reflux by decreasing gastric acid production. However, currently there are no recommendations regarding the need to diagnose or treat *H. pylori* infection in patients with GERD.

Gastroesophageal Junction Factors

Reflux of gastric contents into the esophagus is prevented by two mechanisms at the gastroesophageal junction: (1) the LES, a high-pressure zone in the distal esophagus, and (2) the crural diaphragm, which serves to augment the high pressure at the gastroesophageal junction. Failure of one or both of these complimentary mechanisms may lead to abnormal esophageal exposure to injurious gastroduodenal contents, resulting in esophageal mucosal damage or symptoms of GERD. In cases of mild to moderate nonerosive reflux disease, the basal LES pressure and the crural diaphragm anatomy are frequently normal,[35] and many recent studies have established that transient lower esophageal sphincter relaxations are the major mechanism of reflux in normal subjects and patients with reflux disease.[36,37]

Transient Lower Esophageal Sphincter Relaxations

McNally et al[38] first reported non-swallow-induced LES relaxation as a mechanism of belching in 1964. It was not until 1980, however, that transient lower esophageal sphincter relaxations were related to GERD.[39] Transient lower esophageal relaxations are spontaneous, swallow-independent relaxations of the LES associated with relaxation of the crural diaphragm; they are induced by gastric distention, through a vagally mediated pathway (Fig. 4) that integrates stimulating and inhibiting factors and, when a threshold of excitation is reached, signals the LES and crural diaphragm to relax. In addition to gastric distention, pharyngeal intubation or stimulation may increase the rate of transient lower esophageal sphincter relaxations (see Fig. 4).[40]

Transient lower esophageal sphincter relaxations constitute the most common mechanism of reflux in both healthy subjects and GERD patients.[36,37] Transient lower esophageal sphincter relaxations account for well over 90% of reflux episodes in healthy individuals,[36] and their contribution to reflux decreases as one moves across the spectrum of disease severity from normal to nonerosive GERD to reflux with endoscopic esophagitis. Thus, in patients with severe disease, in whom hiatal hernias are very common, other mechanisms (such as low basal LES pressure) become increasingly important. A study evaluating the mechanisms responsible for reflux episodes over a 24-hour period in patients with and without hiatal hernia showed that in patients with moderate-sized to large hiatal hernia, the relative contribution of transient lower

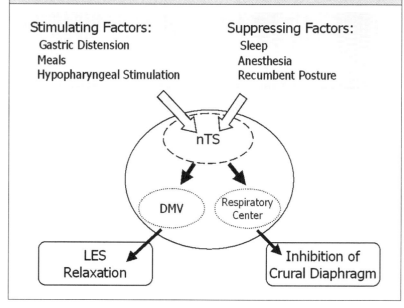

Figure 4. Mediation and control of transient lower esophagus relaxations. nTS = nucleus tractus solitarius, DMV = dorsal motor vagus nucleus, LES = lower esophageal sphincter. (Modified from Holloway RH: Systemic pharmacomodulation of transient lower esophageal sphincter relaxations. Am J Med 111: 1785–1855, 2001.)

esophageal sphincter relaxations to reflux is smaller, with significant amounts of reflux caused by hypotensive LES, swallow-related LES relaxations, deep inspiration, and straining.[41]

Pharmacologic inhibition of transient lower esophageal sphincter relaxations may provide a novel alternative to acid suppression in the treatment of GERD. Using combined pH and bilirubin monitoring to evaluate 15 symptomatic patients with normal findings of pH monitoring but pathologic bile reflux while being treated with proton pump inhibitors, Koek et al[24] documented a decrease in bile reflux and symptoms after treatment with the GABA-B agonist baclofen, which decreases gastroesophageal reflux by inhibiting transient lower esophageal sphincter relaxations.[24] Two studies have used combined intraluminal impedance and pH to assess acid and nonacid reflux and their associated symptoms after pharmacologic manipulation. Vela et al[25] reported that in a group of subjects with frequent heartburn studied in the postprandial period, omeprazole significantly decreased the number of acid reflux episodes; however, nonacid reflux continued to occur and was responsible for some symptoms. In a subsequent study of postprandial reflux in patients with heartburn, these investigators showed that baclofen was able to decrease both acid and nonacid reflux as well as their associated symptoms in the postprandial period.[42] Whether these medications are effective in cases of severe GERD with accompanying hiatal hernia remains to be determined.

Hypotensive Lower Esophageal Sphincters

Although transient lower esophageal sphincter relaxation is the major mechanism of reflux, a low LES pressure is an important mechanism of reflux in patients with severe GERD. A hypotensive LES (i.e., with a basal pressure < 10 mm Hg) may allow gastric contents to reflux freely into the esophagus, resulting in esophagitis or GERD symptoms. The mechanism by which low LES pressure results in reflux is not completely understood. One possibility is that a combination of a low pressure in LES and hiatal hernia is required for the development of erosive esophagitis. The larger the hernia is, the wider the esophageal hiatus is, and the more likely it is that the crural diaphragm component of the sphincter is incompetent.

Most patients with GERD have a normal LES pressure, but a small number, particularly those with severe GERD and erosive esophagitis, usually have a low LES pressure. The degree of endoscopic injury appears to correlate with LES pressure. For example, patients with scleroderma who often have severe esophagitis also have very low LES pressures. Myogenic and neurogenic failure, whether primary or secondary to acid injury, have been proposed as explanations for the low LES pressure, but the mechanism responsible for this has not been well established.[43] Additionally, a low LES pressure can result from external factors, such as gastric distension, foods (chocolate, alcohol), smoking, or medication.

Hiatal Hernia

In general, *hiatal hernia* refers to herniation of portions of the abdominal cavity through the esophageal hiatus of the diaphragm. There are four types of hiatal hernia, the most common of which is a sliding hernia (type I), with a prevalence of 10% to 80%.[44] Types II, III, and IV are variants of paraesophageal hernias that are less common, and together they account for a small percentage of all hiatal hernias.[45]

There has been significant controversy with respect to the relationship between hiatal hernia, heartburn, and esophagitis. Hiatal hernia is considered significant mainly because of its association with GERD. Most patients with moderate to severe gastroesophageal reflux disease have a type I hiatal hernia.[46] Furthermore, as shown in a study of 66 GERD patients and 16 control subjects who underwent endoscopy, manometry, and pH monitoring, hiatal hernia size correlates with the severity of esophagitis.[47]

The herniation of a portion of the stomach into the thoracic cavity can promote reflux in several different ways. Gastric acid present in the hernia sac may easily reflux into the esophagus during swallow-associated relaxations, as the antireflux effect of the crural diaphragm is lost with displacement of the esophagogastric junction. Additionally, patients with hiatal hernia have a lower threshold for triggering of transient lower esophageal sphincter relaxations elicited by gastric distension.[48] Finally, as explained earlier, patients with hernia have a higher proportion of reflux resulting from hypotensive LES, swallow-related LES relaxation, deep inspiration, and straining.[41] How hiatal hernias develop remains unexplained; animal[49] and human[50] studies suggest that hernias may be caused by shortening of the esophagus due to acid injury.

Esophageal Factors

Antireflux barriers are the first line of defense against the reflux of injurious gastroduodenal contents. They are designed to limit the frequency and volume of refluxates. Once these barriers are breached, a second line of defense, esophageal clearance, protects the esophagus by emptying gastric contents through peristalsis and neutralizing residual intraluminal acid by means of bicarbonate present in saliva and other secretions. Each of these factors that promote clearance to prevent mucosal damage is examined in this section (Fig. 5).

Esophageal Clearance

Clearance of acid from the esophagus is a two–step process that involves emptying of esophageal refluxate by gravity and peristalsis (primary and/or secondary) followed by neutralization of acid in the esophageal lumen by bicarbonate present in saliva or secreted by esophageal submucosal glands.[51]

Abnormal Peristalsis

Defective primary peristalsis (also known as *ineffective esophageal motility*), characterized by either absent or low-amplitude (< 30 mm Hg) contractions in the distal esophagus, can result in impaired esophageal volume clearance.[52] Furthermore, ineffective esophageal motility is the main motility abnormality in GERD patients,[53] and peristaltic dysfunction becomes more common as the severity of esophagitis increases, being present in 50% of patients with severe esophagitis.[54]

Although primary peristalsis (swallow-induced) is by far the most common motor event seen after reflux (up to 90% of the time), sec-

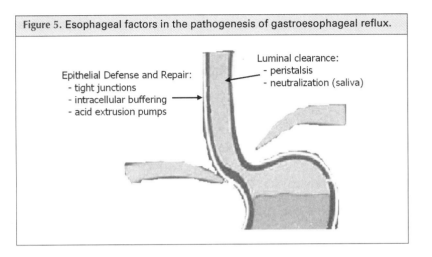

Figure 5. Esophageal factors in the pathogenesis of gastroesophageal reflux.

Epithelial Defense and Repair:
- tight junctions
- intracellular buffering
- acid extrusion pumps

Luminal clearance:
- peristalsis
- neutralization (saliva)

ondary peristalsis elicited by distention of the esophagus may play a role in esophageal clearing during sleep, when spontaneous swallowing is significantly decreased.[55] Abnormal secondary peristalsis, though less studied than primary peristalsis, has been reported in GERD patients. Studies comparing GERD patients to healthy control subjects have shown that secondary peristalsis was less frequently triggered in patients with GERD;[56] additionally, the duration and amplitude of secondary peristaltic contractions are decreased in GERD patients.[57]

Whether the defective peristalsis seen in GERD patients is a consequence of chronic reflux-related injury or is present as a primary smooth muscle abnormality that contributes to the development of GERD is not well understood. Animal models of esophagitis have shown that acute acid injury produces a reduction in LES pressure that is reversible upon resolution of the inflammation.[58,59] However, healing of esophagitis has not resulted in reversion of defects in primary peristalsis in patients with chronic reflux treated with proton pump inhibitors[60] or antireflux surgery.[61] Likewise, defects in secondary peristalsis did not disappear after successful antireflux surgery.[56] These findings suggest that the defective peristalsis seen in chronic GERD patients constitutes either a primary motility abnormality or an irreversible injury due to chronic exposure to acid.

Acid Neutralization

The second step in esophageal clearance, after emptying of the esophagus through gravity and peristalsis, consists of de-acidifying the intraluminal milieu by bicarbonate present mainly in saliva and, to a lesser degree, secreted by the esophageal submucosal glands. Additionally, saliva contains a number of growth factors, including epidermal growth factor, which have the potential to enhance mucosal repair, provide cytoprotection against irritants, and decrease the permeability of the esophageal mucosa to hydrogen ions.[62]

Conditions under which production of saliva is impaired may lead to defective acid neutralization in the esophagus. For example, prolonged esophageal acid exposure has been shown in patients with chronic xerostomia.[63] Additionally, studies have shown that smoking can contribute to GERD by an anticholinergic effect that decreases production of saliva and results in significant increases in acid clearance time in comparison to nonsmokers.[64] Conversely, smoking cessation is associated with significant improvements in salivary bicarbonate secretion.[65] However, studies have not convincingly shown that there is a decrease in salivary production of patients with GERD. For example, basal and citric acid–stimulated salivary secretion were shown to be similar between healthy control subjects and patients with esophagitis.[66] Hence, although external factors such as smoking or alcohol[67] may result in hyposalivation, GERD patients may not have impairment in saliva production. However, the decrease in spontaneous swallowing seen during sleep can result in delayed acid clearance and prolonged episodes of reflux during the night.[68] Thus, as impaired esophageal emptying prolongs acid clearance, reduced salivary rate due to exogenous (smoking, medications) or endogenous (disease states or sleep periods) factors may play a permissive role in the pathophysiology of GERD.

Epithelial Defense and Repair

Increased exposure to acid, due to a combination of frequent reflux episodes and poor esophageal clearance, can lead to mucosal damage. The esophageal epithelium constitutes a structural barrier to diffusion of acid and pepsin because of tight junctions and an intercellular glycoprotein matrix that, together, result in high epithelial electrical resistance, which limits the entry of acid into the tissue. GERD develops when refluxed acidic gastroduodenal contents damage the esophageal intercellular junctions, which then allow easier access for hydrogen ions to come into contact with afferent nerves in the esophageal epithelium, which may result in the sensation of heartburn in patients with GERD. Once hydrogen ions enter the cell, phosphates, protein, and carbonic anhydrase–derived bicarbonate act as buffers; when this intracellular buffering capacity is exhausted, esophageal epithelial cells can resort to extrusion of acid by two transmembrane pumps: a Na/H exchanger and a sodium-dependent Cl/HCO_3 exchanger.[5] When the epithelium is finally overwhelmed by an acid load, intracellular pH falls, leading to cell injury, defects in volume regulation, further impairment of the epithelial defense mechanisms with a resulting increase in permeability to acid, and, ultimately, cell death and necrosis.[69] Repeated acid exposure may cause continued cell death with subsequent mucosal erosion and the endoscopic appearance of erosive GERD.

Subsequent to mucosal injury and once high esophageal acid exposure is under control, epithelial repair may be carried out through cell replication and subsequent migration into the injured area.[4] Depending on the degree of preservation of the stratum germinativum, the proliferation of cells directed toward epithelial repair, characterized histologically by basal cell hyperplasia, can lead to reappearance or normal epithelium or result in further pathologic conditions, such as stricture or Barrett's esophagus.[69]

Genetic Factors

Although the role that genetic factors play in the etiology of GERD is not yet well understood, it has been suggested that there may be a genetic basis for GERD and some of its complications.[70] Pooling the results of several case reports of familial aggregation of GERD and Barrett's esophagus, Romero and Lock[71] described that out of 88 relatives of index cases, 28% had Barrett's esophagus and 42% had esophagitis or heartburn.

Case Control Studies. Three case-control studies evaluated the prevalence of symptoms of reflux among relatives of GERD patients. Romero et al[72] found that the prevalence of reflux symptoms among relatives of patients with endoscopic esophagitis was not increased in comparison to control subjects. In contrast, Trudgill et al[73] examined the prevalence of reflux symptoms in first-degree relatives of index cases with varying severity of GERD (defined by presence of symptoms, abnormal acid exposure on pH study, peptic stricture, and Barrett's esophagus) and used patients with no dyspeptic symptoms as control subjects. They found that the frequency of reflux symptoms was significantly higher in relatives of patients with an abnormal pH study or with Barrett's esophagus. More recently, Chak et al[74] found that individuals with Barrett's esophagus and esophageal adenocarcinoma are more likely to have a positive family history of Barrett's esophagus and esophageal adenocarcinoma compared to control subjects without Barrett's esophagus or adenocarcinoma. This issue continues to be of interest, and future studies are needed to further clarify the role of genetics in GERD.

Twin Studies. In the only published large study of twins examining the presence of reflux symptoms, Cameron et al[75] conducted telephone interviews with 8401 pairs of twins and found higher concordance rates for monozygotic twins (31%) than for same-sex dizygotic twins (14%);

although the reliability of the telephone interview has been called into question, this study supports a role for genetics in the etiology of reflux.

Linkage Studies. In 2000, a study designed to search for a genetic locus for severe pediatric GERD in five families suggested that a gene for severe pediatric GERD maps to chromosome 13q14.[76] However, a subsequent study of a different group of five families with an autosomal dominant pattern of pediatric reflux excluded the importance of this locus.[77] The differences between these results has been attributed to inclusion of older children (over 1 year of age) and the more rigorous phenotyping used in the second study. Overall, the data available to date suggest genetic heterogeneity in familial pediatric gastroesophageal disease. Further linkage studies in pediatric and adult GERD populations will likely contribute to our understanding of this disease and its different presentations, including Barrett's esophagus and esophageal adenocarcinoma.

Key Points: Pathophysiology of Gastroesophageal Reflux Disease

- ∞ The pathophysiology of reflux disease is multifactorial.
- ∞ Pathologic reflux occurs when injurious gastroduodenal contents (acid, pepsin, bile acids) breach the esophagogastric junction because of transient LES relaxations, hypotensive LES, or anatomic disruption (hiatal hernia).
- ∞ After reflux occurs, impaired luminal clearance (peristalsis and acid neutralization) can lead to prolonged exposure to harmful gastroduodenal contents, which ultimately overwhelm the epithelial defenses, resulting in inflammation and symptoms.
- ∞ Healing may lead to re-epithelization with normal tissue or may also result in development of metaplastic tissue (Barrett's esophagus).
- ∞ The contribution of genetics to the disease awaits further study.

Suggested Reading

1. Locke GR, Talley NJ, Fett SL, et al: Prevalence and clinical spectrum of gastroesophageal reflux: A population-based study in Olmstead County, Minnesota. Gastroenterology 112:1448–1456, 1997.
2. Vaezi MF, Singh S, Richter JE: Role of acid and duodenogastric reflux in esophageal mucosal injury: A review of animal and human studies. Gastroenterology 108:1897–1907, 1995.

3. Goldberg HI, Dodds WJ, Gee S, et al: Role of acid and pepsin in acute experimental esophagitis. Gastroenterology 56:223–230, 1969.
3a. Lillemoe KD, Johnson LF, Harmon JW. Role of the components of gastroduodenal contents in experimental acid esophagitis. Surgery 92:276–284, 1982.
4. Orlando RC: Pathogenesis of gastroesophageal disease. Gastroenterol Clin North Am 31:S35–44, 2002.
5. Orlando RC: Pathophysiology of gastroesophageal reflux disease: Offensive factors and tissue resistance. In Orlando RC (eds): Gastroesophageal Reflux Disease. New York, Marcel Dekker, 2000, pp 165–192.
6. Tuttle SG, Ruffin F, Bettarello A: The physiology of heartburn. Ann Intern Med 55:292, 1961.
7. Gillen P, Keeling P, Byrne PJ, et al: Barrett's esophagus: pH profile. Br J Surg 74:774–776, 1987.
8. Hennessy TPJ. Barrett's esophagus. Br J Surg 72:336–340, 1985.
9. Stein HJ, Siewert JR: Barrett's esophagus: Pathogenesis, epidemiology, functional abnormalities, malignant degeneration, and surgical management. Dysphagia 8:276–288, 1993.
10. Stein HJ, Barlow AP, DeMeester TR, et al: Complications of gastroesophageal reflux disease. Ann Surg 216:35–43, 1992.
11. Zamost BJ, Hirschberg J, Ippoliti AF: Esophagitis in scleroderma: Prevalence and risk factors. Gastroenterology 92:421–428, 1987.
12. Hirschowitz BI: A critical analysis, with appropriate controls, of gastric acid and pepsin secretion in clinical esophagitis. Gastroenterology 101:1149–1158, 1991.
13. Miller LS, Vinayek R, Frucht H, et al: Reflux esophagitis in patients with Zollinger Ellison syndrome. Gastroenterolgy 98:341–346, 1990.
14. Cross FS, Wangesteen OH: Role of bile and pancreatic juice in the production of esophageal erosions and anemia. Proc Soc Exp Biol Med 77:862–866, 1961.
15. Gillison EW, DeCastro VAM, Nyhus LM, et al: The significance of bile in reflux esophagitis. Surg Gynecol Obstet 134:419–424, 1972.
16. Harmon JW, Johnson LF, Maydonovitch CL: Effects of acid and bile salts on the rabbit esophageal mucosa. Dig Dis Sci 26:65–72, 1981.
17. Kivilaakso E, Fromm D, Silen W: Effect of bile salts and related compounds on isolated esophageal mucosa. Surgery 87:280–285, 1980.
18. Moffat RC, Berkas EM: Bile esophagitis. Arch Surg 91:963–966, 1965.
19. Vaezi MF: Duodenogastric reflux. In Castell DO, Richter JE (eds): The Esophagus, 3rd ed. Philadelphia, Lippincot Williams & Wilkins, 1999, pp 421–436.
20. Vaezi MF, Richter JE: Role of acid and duodenogastroesophageal reflux in gastroesophageal reflux disease. Gastroenterology 111:1192–1199, 1996.
21. Marshall RFK, Anggiansah A, Owen WJ, Owen WJ: The relationship between acid and bile reflux and symptoms in gastroesophageal reflux disease. Gut 40:182–187, 1997.
22. Sears RJ, Champion G, Richter JE: Characteristics of partial gastrectomy (PG) patients with esophageal symptoms of doudenogastric reflux. Am J Gastroenterol 90:211–215, 1995.
23. Vaezi MF, Sears R, Richter JE: Double-bilnd placebo-controlled cross-over trial of cisapride in postgastrectomy patients with duodenogastric reflux. Dig Dis Sci 41:754–763, 1996.
24. Koek G, Sifrim D, Degreef T, et al: The GABA B agonist baclofen reduces duodenogastro-esophageal reflux (DGER) and symptoms in patients with reflux disease refractory to proton pump inhibitor therapy. Gastroenterology 120:A-34, 2001.
25. Vela MF, Camacho-Lobato L, Srinivasan R, et al: Intraesophageal impedance and pH

measurement of acid and nonacid reflux: Effect of omeprazole. Gastroenterology 120:1599–1606, 2001.

26. Richter JE: Do we know the cause of reflux disease? Eur J Gastroenterol Hepatol 11:S3–S9, 1999.

27. Stacher G, Lenglinger J, Bergman H, et al: Gastric emptying: A contributory factor in gastro-oesophageal reflux activity? Gut 47:661–666, 2000.

28. Feldman M, Cryer B, Lee E: Effects of *Helicobacter pylori* gastritis on gastric secretion in healthy human beings. Am J Physiol 274:G1011–1017, 1998.

29. El-Serag HB, Sonnenberg A: Opposing trends of peptic ulcer and reflux disease. Gut 43:327–333, 1998.

30. Labenz J, Blum AL, Bayerdorffer E, et al: Curing *Helicobacter pylori* infection in patients with duodenal ulcer may provoke reflux esophagitis. Gastroenterology 112:1442–1447, 1997.

31. Vicari J, Peek R, Falk G, et al: The seroprevalence of cagA-positive *Helicobacter pylori* strains in the spectrum of gastroesophageal disease. Gastroenterology 115:50–57, 1998.

32. Vaezi M, Falk G, Peek R: CagA-positive strains of *Helicobacter pylori* may protect against Barrett's esophagus. Am J Gastroenterol 2206:2206–2211, 2000.

33. Vakil N, Hahn B, McSorley D: Recurrent symptoms and gastro-oesophageal reflux disease in patients with duodenal ulcer treated for *Helicobacter pylori* infection. Aliment Pharmacol Ther 14:45–51, 2000.

34. Laine L, Sugg J: Effect of *Helicobacter pylori* eradication on development of erosive esophagitis and gastroesophageal reflux disease symptoms: A post hoc analysis of eight double blind prospective studies. Am J Gastroenterol 97:2992–2997, 2002.

35. Mittal RK, Chowdry NK, Liu J: Is the sphincter function of crural diaphragm impaired in patients with reflux esophagitis? Gastroenterology 108:A169, 1995.

36. Dodds WJ, Dent J, Hogan WJ, et al: Mechanisms of gatroesophageal reflux in patients with reflux esophagitis. N Engl J Med 307:1547–1552, 1982.

37. Mittal RK, Holloway RH, Penagini R, et al: Transient lower esophageal relaxation. Gastroenterology 109:601–610, 1995.

38. McNally EF, Kelly JE, Ingelfinger FJ: Mechanism of belching: Effects of gastric distention with air. Gastroenterology 46:254, 1964.

39. Dent J: Mechanism of gastroesophageal reflux in recumbent asymptomatic human subjects. J Clin Invest 65:256–267, 1980.

40. Mittal RK, Chiareli C, Liu J, Shaker R: Characteristics of LES relaxation induced stimulation of the pharynx with minute amounts of water. Gastroenterology 111:378–384, 1996.

41. Van Herwaarden MA, Samsom M, Smouth AJPM: Excess gastroesophageal reflux in patients with hiatus hernia is caused by mechanisms other than transient LES relaxations. Gastroenterology 119:1439–1446, 2000.

42. Vela MF, Tutuian R, Katz PO, Castell DO: Baclofen reduces acid and nonacid postprandial gastroesophageal reflux measured by combined multichannel intraluminal impedance and pH. Aliment Pharmacol Ther 17:243–251, 2003.

43. Mittal R: Pathophysiology of gastroesophageal reflux disease: Motility factors. In Castell DO, Richter JE (eds): The Esophagus, 3rd ed. Philadelphia, Lippincott Williams & Wilkins, 1999, pp 397–408.

44. Skinner DB: Hernias. In Berk JE (ed): Gastroenterology, 4th ed. Philadelphia, WB Saunders, 1985, p 705.

45. Peridikis G, Hinder RA: Paraesophageal hiatal hernia. In Nyhus LM, Condon RE (eds): Hernia. Philadelphia, JB Lippincott, 1995, p 544.

46. Mittal R, Balaban R: The esophagogastric Junction. N Engl J Med 336:924–932, 1997.

47. Jones MP, Sloan SS, Rabine JC, et al: Hiatal hernia size is the dominant determinant of esophagitis presence and severity in gastroesophageal reflux disease. Am J Gastroenterol 96:1711–1717, 2001.
48. Kharilas PJ, Shi G, Manka M, Hoehl R: Increased frequency of transient lower esophageal relaxation induced by gastric distension in reflux patients with hiatal hernia. Gastroenterology 118:688–695, 2000.
49. White R, Zhang Y, Morris G, Paterson WG: Esophagitis-related esophageal shortening in opossum is associated with longitudinal muscle hyperresponsiveness. Am J Physiol Gastrointest Liver Physiol 280:G463–G469, 2001.
50. White R, Zhang Y, Morris G, Paterson WG: Esophagitis-related esophageal shortening in opossum is associated with longitudinal muscle hyperresponsiveness. Am J Physiol Gastrointest Liver Physiol 280:G463–G469, 2001.
51. Helms JF, Dodds WJ, Pelc LR, et al: Effect of esophageal emptying and saliva on clearance of acid from the esophagus. N Engl J Med 310:284–288, 1984.
52. Kahrilas PJ, Dodds WJ, Hogan WJ: Effect of peristaltic dysfunction on esophageal volume clearance. Gastroenterology 94:73–80, 1988.
53. Fouad YM, Katz PO, Hatlebakk JG, Castell DO: Ineffective esophageal motility: The most common motility abnormality in patients with GERD-associated respiratory symptoms. Am J Gastroenterol 94:1464–1467, 1999.
54. Kahrilas PJ, Dodds WJ, Hogan WJ, et al: Esophageal peristaltic dysfunction in peptic esophagitis. Gastroenterology 91:897–904, 1986.
55. Holloway RH: Esophageal body motor response to reflux events: Secondary peristalsis. Am J Med 108:20S–26S, 2000.
56. Rydberg L, Ruth M, Lundell L: Characteristics of secondary esophageal peristalsis in operated and non-operated patients with chronic gastro-oesophageal reflux disease. Eur J Gastroenterol Hepatol 12:739–743, 2000.
57. Pai CG: Secondary esophageal peristalsis in gastro-oesophageal reflux disease. J Gastroenterol Hepatol 15:30–34, 2000.
58. Eastwood GL, Castell DO, Higgs RH: Experimental esophagitis in cats impairs lower esophageal sphincter pressure. Gastroenterology 69:146–153, 1975.
59. Higgs RH, Castell DO, Eastwood GL: Studies on the mechanism of esophagitis-induced lower esophageal sphincter hypotension in cats. Gastroenterology 71:51–57, 1976.
60. Timmer R, Breumelhof R, Nadorp JH, Smout AJ: Oesophageal motility and gastro-oesophageal reflux before and after healing of reflux esophagitis: A study using 24 hour ambulatory pH and pressure monitoring. Gut 35:1519–1522, 1994.
61. Rydberg L, Ruth M, Lundell L: Does esophageal motor function improve with time after successful antireflux surgery? Results of a prospective, randomized clinical study. Gut 41:82–86, 1997.
62. Sarosiek J, Feng T, McCallum R: The interrelationship between salivary epidermal growth factor and the functional integrity of the esophageal mucosa. Am J Med Sci 302:359–362, 1991.
63. Korsten MA, Rosman AS, Fishbein S, et al: Chronic xerostomia increases esophageal acid exposure and is associated with esophageal injury. Am J Med 90:701–706, 1991.
64. Kharilas PJ, Gupta RR: The effect of cigarette smoking and salivation on esophageal acid clearance. J Lab Clin Med 114:431–438, 1989.
65. Trudgill NJ, Smith LF, Kershaw J, Riley SA: Impact of smoking cessation on salivary function in healthy volunteers. Scand J Gastroenterol 33:568–571, 1998.
66. Sonnenberg A, Steinkamp U, Weise A, et al: Salivary secretion in reflux esophagitis. Gastroenterology 83:889–885, 1982.
67. Dutta SK, Dukehart M, Narang A: Functional and structural changes in parotid glands of alcoholic cirrhotic patients. Gastroenterology 96:510–518, 1989.

68. Orr WC, Johnson LF, Robinson MG: Effect of sleep on swallowing, esophageal peristalsis, and acid clearance. Gastroenterology 86:814–819, 1984.
69. Orlando RC: Pathophysiology of gastroesophageal reflux disease: Esophageal epithelial resistance. In Castell DO, Richter JE (ed): The Esophagus. Philadelphia, Lippincott, Williams & Wilkins, 1999, pp 409–419.
70. Orenstein SR, Shalaby TM, Barmada MM, et al: Genetics of gastroesophageal disease: A review. J Pediatr Gastroenterol Nutr 34:506–510, 2002.
71. Romero Y, Locke GR III: Is there a GERD gene? Am J Gastroenterol 94:1127–1129, 1999.
72. Romero Y, Cameron AJ, Locke GR, et al: Familial aggregation of gastroesophageal reflux in patients with Barrett's esophagus and esophageal adenocarcinoma. Gastroenterology 113:1449–1456, 1997.
73. Trudgill N, Kapur K, Riley S: Familial clustering of reflux symptoms. Am J Gastroenterol 94:1172–1178, 1999.
74. Chak A, Lee T, Kinnard MF, et al: Familial aggregation of Barrett's esophagus, oesophageal adenocarcinoma, and oesophagogastric junctional adenocarcinoma in caucasian adults. Gut 51:323–328, 2002.
75. Cameron A, Lagergren J, Henriksson C, et al: Gastroesophageal reflux disease in monozygotic and dizygotic twins. Gastroenterology 122:55–59, 2002.
76. Hu FZ, Preston RA, Post JC, et al: Mapping of a gene for severe pediatric gastroesophageal reflux to chromosome 13q14. JAMA 284:325–334, 2000.
77. Orenstein SR, Shalaby TM, Finch R, et al: Autosomal dominant infantile gastroesophageal reflux disease: Exclusion of a 13q14 locus in five well characterized families. Am J Gastroenterol 97:2725–2732, 2002.
78. Holloway RH: Systemic pharmacomodulation of transient lower esophageal sphincter relaxations. Am J Med 111:178S–185S, 2001.

Gastroesophageal Reflux Disease: Diagnosis

chapter 3

Sunil Joseph, M.D., and
Ikuo Hirano, M.D.

Diagnosing gastroesophageal reflux disease (GERD) is a common practice in primary care physicians' offices, given the high prevalence of the condition in the general population. In many individuals with reflux symptoms, quality of life is not significantly impaired to the point where medical care is sought. Other patients with GERD report symptoms that substantially affect their daily routine of eating, exercise, or sleep. Still others may present with "extraesophageal" or atypical reflux symptoms. The purpose of this chapter is to review available diagnostic testing for patients with suspected GERD. Appropriate utilization of the various tests is highly dependent on the clinical presentation. As will be shown, in most cases of GERD, diagnostic testing beyond a clinical history and empiric trial of medications is unnecessary. Finally, novel and emerging techniques for the detection of GERD are discussed.

Clinical Presentation

Modern technology has given us many different modalities to investigate cases of suspected GERD. In most cases, however, a simple, well-taken history is still the best and most cost-effective diagnostic tool. The most typical symptoms associated with GERD are heartburn and acid regurgitation. Heartburn is defined as a retrosternal burning sensation that radiates toward the throat. Acid regurgitation is the effortless return of sour or bitter gastric contents into the mouth in the absence of nausea. When these symptoms are elicited as dominant symptoms, they have been found to have a high specificity but poor sensitivity.[1]

Misinterpretation of the word *heartburn* by patients commonly leads to a delay in the diagnosis of GERD. A structured questionnaire using descriptive language to diagnose GERD was found to increase the efficiency and sensitivity of symptom evaluation.[2] This questionnaire has not been validated for use in the primary care setting, however.

Other symptoms commonly associated with GERD are water brash, odynophagia, dysphagia, and globus sensation. These symptoms have not been shown to have the same degree of specificity as heartburn and regurgitation. **Water brash** is the sudden appearance of slightly sour or salty water in the mouth. This is thought to be secondary to hypersecretion from the salivary glands in the mouth in response to intraesophageal acid exposure. **Odynophagia** is usually a sign of ulcerative esophagitis but is not specific for GERD and is a dominant symptom in pill-induced or infectious esophagitis. **Dysphagia** can be from a formation of a peptic stricture or neoplastic complication of long-standing GERD but can also be a symptom of GERD in the absence of overt mechanical stricture. **Globus sensation** is the constant sensation of a lump in the throat that can be related to GERD. It is important to note that globus generally occurs in the absence of dysphagia. Atypical manifestations of GERD include asthma, cough, hoarseness of throat, and noncardiac chest pain. Although these entities are dealt with more thoroughly in separate chapters, it is important to note that the appropriate diagnostic evaluation of suspected GERD varies based on the presentation (Fig. 1).

A primary care physician's role in suspected GERD is not only to establish the diagnosis but also to exclude possible complications. Complications of GERD include erosive esophagitis, esophageal strictures, Barrett's esophagus, and esophageal adenocarcinoma. Classic warning symptoms that trigger further investigation include weight loss, dysphagia, odynophagia, melena, and hematemesis. Chronicity and frequency of symptoms increase the chance of developing adenocarcinoma of the esophagus, and thus diagnostic testing with endoscopy for Barrett's esophagus may be considered in patients with long-standing disease. Issues surrounding the appropriate use of diagnostic testing for Barrett's esophagus is covered in another chapter. If the diagnosis is evident in the absence of warning symptoms, empiric treatment is appropriate (see Fig. 1). Failed response to acid suppression with proton pump inhibitor (PPI) therapy generally warrants additional testing.

Diagnostic Testing

Several modalities are available to evaluate a patient suspected of having GERD. These include barium esophagraphy, upper endoscopy, the Bernstein test, ambulatory 24-hour pH monitoring, and the acid suppression test. Each test has its own advantages and disadvantages which are discussed below and summarized in Table 1.

Radiologic Studies

Radiologic studies that include the barium esophagram and upper gastrointestinal series are widely available and minimally invasive. Barium

Figure 1. Diagnostic pathways for evaluation of suspected gastroesophageal reflux disease. The appropriate use of diagnostic testing depends on the indication and specific clinical presentation. In addition, within a given indication, the utility of the various recommended tests is variable. EGD = esophagogastric duodenoscopy; GI = gastrointestinal study; PPI = proton pump inhibitor.

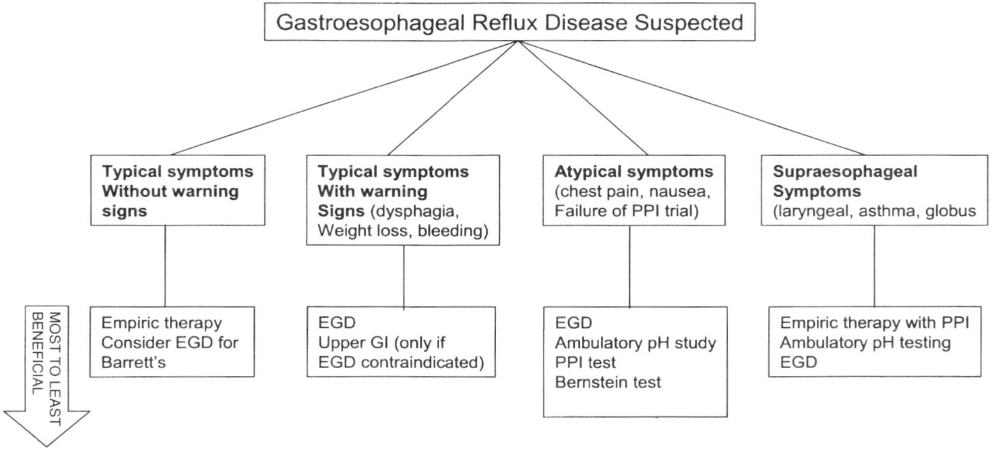

TABLE 1. Available Diagnostic Tests for Gastroesophageal Reflux Disease			
Test	**Advantages**	**Disadvantages**	**Recommended Use**
Endoscopy	Most accurate test for detection of GERD complications Obtains tissue biopsies Treats peptic strictures	Limited sensitivity Invasive procedure Cost	GERD with alarm symptoms Failure of PPI therapy Detection of Barrett's esophagus
Barium swallow	Noninvasive Widely available	Poor sensitivity Poor specificity	Suspect complications of GERD in patients who cannot undergo endoscopy
24-Hour pH monitoring			
• Conventional	Assesses acid exposure Correlation of symptoms and reflux events	Transnasal intubation not well accepted by patients Limitation in activity during study may decrease accuracy	Atypical symptoms Failure of PPI therapy
• Bravo probe	Assesses acid exposure Correlation of symptoms and reflux events Wireless device avoids need for nasal catheter	Requires endoscopy	Atypical symptoms Failure of PPI therapy
PPI Test	Widely available Noninvasive	Subjective outcome Specificity not well defined for patients with atypical and extraesophageal symptoms	Atypical symptoms Extraesophageal symptoms
Bernstein test	Easy to perform May reproduce atypical or infrequent symptoms	Poor sensitivity Limited specificity	Atypical symptoms Infrequent symptoms

GERD = gastroesophageal reflux disease; PPI = proton pump inhibitor.

esophagrams offer the ability to detect gastroesophageal reflux as well as its complications. Radiographic reflux is the movement of barium from the stomach into the esophagus. A major limitation of the barium study is in the differentiation of physiologic and pathologic reflux. Barium studies have detected reflux in up to 20% of normal control subjects and unprovoked, spontaneous reflux in only 26% of patients shown by pH probe to have pathologic degrees of acid reflux.[3] The sensitivity of this study has been increased with the use of provocative maneuvers such as the Valsava maneuver, cough, and abdominal compression but at the expense of specificity.[4] The water siphon test is another provocative maneuver that entails having the subject drink 60 mL of water while in the supine position and then rolling into the right lateral position. This maneuver increased the sensitivity of the barium study to 70% with a specificity of 74% and a positive predictive value of 80%.[3] Overall, even with these provocative maneuvers, barium studies are not recommended for the diagnosis of uncomplicated GERD given their poor sensitivity and specificity.

In terms of complications related to GERD, barium esophagrams have been used to detect reflux esophagitis and strictures. The more common structural abnormalities seen radiographically in patients with reflux esophagitis include mucosal nodularity, thickening of the esophageal folds, erosions and ulcerations, and segmental narrowing due to inflammation, stricture, or neoplasm.[5] However, only two thirds of patients with endoscopically proven reflux esophagitis have radiographic signs of esophagitis. The sensitivity of radiographic detection of esophagitis increases with more severe endoscopic grades of esophagitis. In one study, the sensitivity of barium studies in the diagnosis of mild esophagitis was 26%, whereas with severe esophagitis it was 100%.[6] The detection of esophagitis can be optimized with a combination of multiple radiologic techniques, including mucosal relief, full-column, and double-contrast. Barium studies additionally have a high sensitivity for the detection of peptic strictures, mucosal rings, and adenocarcinoma[7] and can detect a reticular pattern that corresponds with Barrett's esophagus.[8] In spite of the diagnostic capability of radiographic examinations for complications of GERD, endoscopy offers the added advantages of tissue biopsy and therapeutic dilation. Thus, barium studies should be reserved only for GERD patients with suspected complications who are unable to undergo endoscopy.

Bernstein Test

The Bernstein test is often used to detect whether a patient's symptoms are secondary to reflux. The test involves infusing the distal esophagus with either 0.1 N HCl or saline in single blinded manner with assessment of the patient's response. A positive test result is defined as when the patient's symptom or substernal burning pain is reproduced by acid infusion and relieved by normal saline. Patients with GERD may have alterations in tissue resistance and thus have greater chemosensitivity compared with healthy control subjects. Despite this rationale and the ease with which the test can be performed, the Bernstein test has limited sensitivity and specificity as a diagnostic test for suspected GERD. On the other hand, atypical chest pain or somatic complaints attributable to acid reflux may be reproduced during the test. In patients presenting with atypical chest pain, the Bernstein test is reasonably specific for GERD but again lacks sensitivity.[9] Hence, the primary utility of the Bernstein test is in increasing the clinical suspicion that a patient's atypical chest pain is a manifestation of GERD.

Esophageal Manometry

Esophageal manometry has no role in the initial diagnostic evaluation of GERD. Although manometric findings of low basal pressure of the lower esophageal sphincter and transient lower esophageal sphincter relaxations are key features in the pathophysiology of GERD, their detection seldom alters the clinical management of an individual patient. Manometry is, however, used routinely for determining the proper placement of the 24-hour ambulatory pH probe. It is also used to rule out primary and secondary motility disorders prior to antireflux surgery, although the utility of this approach is controversial.[10]

Upper Endoscopy: Conventional and Transnasal

Endoscopy is often considered the first-line test for the diagnosis of GERD with the presence of erosions or ulcerations in the distal esophagus having a high specificity for GERD. Importantly, studies have shown that endoscopic abnormalities are found in less than half of patients with GERD.[11] Thus, the majority of patients with GERD have no endoscopic abnormalities, giving rise to the term *nonerosive reflux disease,* or *NERD,* to describe such patients. Moreover, normal endoscopic findings may on the one hand lead to more extensive, expensive diagnostic testing or, on the other hand, to the incorrect assumption that GERD has been ruled out. To further complicate matters, some patients with initial negative endoscopic findings will develop mucosal lesions during follow-up examinations.[12] Mucosal changes, such as edema, friability, and an irregular squamocolumnar junction that might increase the diagnostic sensitivity of endoscopy are poorly reproducible observations between endoscopists and thus should not be interpreted as esophagitis.[13] Most endoscopic criteria for the diagnosis of GERD rely instead on the detection of erosions or ulcerations (Fig. 2).

The use of esophageal biopsy and histologic analysis was once thought to be an important tool in the diagnosis of reflux disease.[14] Basal cell hyperplasia, increased papillary length of the squamous epithelium, and infiltration by polymorphonuclear leukocytes or eosinophils are some of the findings in distal esophageal biopsies of GERD patients. Recent studies have found these histologic changes in only 30–35% of GERD patients and also in up to 21% of normal control subjects.[15] Given the limited sensitivity of both the gross endoscopic and microscopic changes of GERD, endoscopy should not be used routinely for the sole purpose of diagnosing GERD.

Upper endoscopy has an important role in the evaluation of potential

Figure 2. Endoscopic findings in patients with gastroesophageal reflux disease can vary from normal (*left*), to distal esophageal erosions (*center*), to frank ulceration with stricture formation (*right*). More than half of patients presenting with reflux disease have neither erosions nor ulcerations, forming a group referred to as nonerosive reflux disease patients.

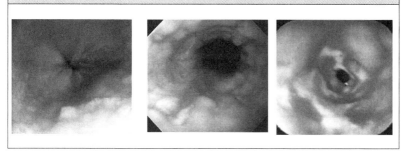

complications associated with GERD. Patients with alarm symptoms that include dysphagia, melena, hematemesis, or weight loss should undergo an endoscopic examination (see Fig. 1). Of available diagnostic testing, endoscopy has the highest sensitivity and specificity for the detection of esophagitis, peptic strictures, Barrett's esophagus, and adenocarcinoma. Findings of advanced grades of esophagitis or evidence of peptic stricture formation would warrant more aggressive therapy with PPIs. Furthermore, endoscopy offers the ability to obtain tissue biopsies for Barrett's esophagus, dysplasia, or carcinoma. Therapeutic interventions including dilation of peptic strictures or palliation of esophageal cancers can also be accomplished. Endoscopy is also reasonable in patients failing to respond to PPI therapy to look for evidence of reflux esophagitis as well as alternate diagnoses that may mimic GERD, such as eosinophilic, pill-induced, or infectious esophagitis. Endoscopy should also be considered in patients with chronic reflux symptoms without warning signs as a screening test for Barrett's epithelium. This controversial topic is covered in a separate chapter.

Transnasal upper endoscopy has emerged as a potential method to evaluate the esophageal mucosa both rapidly and in an ambulatory care setting. The technique involves the use of ultrathin endoscopes that are passed transnasally without the use of conscious sedation. The use of sedation during conventional upper endoscopy adds to the time, personnel, costs, and risks of the procedure. At present, however, both training and patient preferences for being "unaware" of invasive procedures limit the utilization of transnasal endoscopy. Should the increasing incidence of esophageal adenocarcinoma lead to recommendations for increased screening for Barrett's esophagus, the use of such office-based procedures could become more widely accepted. It should be noted that in many countries outside of the United States, conventional upper endoscopy is performed without the use of sedation.

Ambulatory 24-Hour pH Monitoring

Ambulatory 24-hour pH monitoring allows for the quantification of esophageal acid exposure along with the temporal correlation of symptoms. It is not recommended in the initial diagnostic evaluation of typical GERD symptoms but should be reserved for patients with atypical symptoms and for nonresponders to empiric therapy (see Fig. 1). The test involves the transnasal placement of a small, flexible pH recording catheter into the distal esophagus. Esophageal manometry is routinely used to properly position the pH sensor 5 cm proximal to the lower esophageal sphincter. The patient is given a portable data recorder that allows for computerized data analysis at the completion of the test. The patient is also instructed to keep a detailed record of symptoms, meals, and sleep in the diary (Fig. 3). Various schemes have been constructed to analyze pH monitoring, but an intraesophageal pH below 4.0 for more than 4% of the total time is the most commonly used definition of abnormal esophageal acid exposure. This value was obtained by placing the upper limit of normal 2 SD above the mean of the asymptomatic control.[16] Increasing the value above 4% sacrifices sensitivity for specificity.

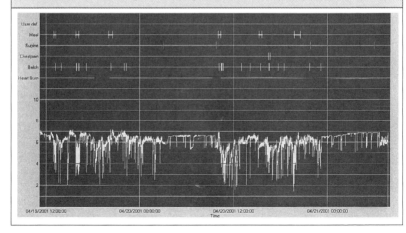

Figure 3. Ambulatory pH testing. The top half of the tracing denotes patient-entered data, including meals, supine body positioning, chest pain, belching, and heartburn. The bottom half of the tracing shows the pH recording over a 48-hour period. pH levels that fall below 4 are considered reflux events. This particular study demonstrates an "upright" refluxer whose reflux events are predominately occurring in the upright rather than supine position.

Although 24-hour pH probe monitoring is considered the "gold standard" for the diagnosis of GERD, many inherent problems with this test limit its applicability and utilization. The sensitivity of the pH probe is thought to range from 77% to 100%, with the highest sensitivities reported in patients with higher grades of esophagitis. However, such patients rarely require pH monitoring, since they are readily identified with endoscopy. Thus, the greatest need for this study lies in patients with nonerosive reflux disease. Studies suggest a limited sensitivity of only 61% to 70% in this population, however.[17] Self-imposed restrictions in the patient's daily activities and dietary habits due to nasal and pharyngeal discomfort from the recording catheter may decrease the occurrence of acid reflux events.[18] In addition, inadvertent cephalad or caudad migration of the pH sensor may yield erroneous results. Other factors involved in symptom generation, including local mucosal sensitivity, mucosal resistance, degree of acidification, and noxious substances in refluxate other than acid may also explain the less than optimal sensitivity of pH testing.

Although the 24-hour pH probe is not considered a useful initial test for the diagnosis of classic GERD, it is an important test in patients with atypical manifestations of GERD, such as asthma, noncardiac chest pain, sore throat, and hoarseness, and in patients who are unresponsive to empiric PPI therapy (see Fig. 1). In the evaluation of such symptoms, it is important to bear in mind that the definition of GERD depends on typical reflux symptoms or mucosal inflammation and not abnormal acid exposure. Detection of abnormal degrees of acid exposure in a patient with atypical symptoms does not prove causality of the association. The high background prevalence of GERD and the inherent limitations of pH testing are important shortcomings in the utilization of pH testing in the diagnosis of atypical symptoms. Compounding the problem further is the paucity of controlled studies that examine the efficacy of pH testing in these selected populations. In patients with suspected reflux laryngitis, it has been shown that a second probe in the proximal esophagus documents reflux episodes that may have been missed by a single distal esophageal probe,[19] although there has been no consensus on the pH criteria that should be used for defining pathologic degrees of proximal acid reflux. Another proposed use of dual probes is in assessing a patient's inadequate response to PPI therapy. A gastric probe is placed 10 cm below the lower esophageal sphincter along with the conventional distal esophageal probe. This allows measurement of the gastric pH to assess the efficacy of acid suppression as well as reflux events and corresponding symptoms.

An advantage of the 24-hour pH test over other diagnostic modalities is the ability to correlate symptoms with acid exposure events. Multiple schemes have been devised to use statistical manipulation to correlate symptoms with acid reflux. The first devised scheme was the symptom index.[20] This involves dividing the number of symptoms associated with pH < 4 by the total number of symptoms, yielding a percentage of symptom episodes that correlate with GERD. The symptom index has important limitations. It does not take into account the total number of reflux episodes. Thus, a patient with only one symptomatic reflux episode will have a symptom index of 100%. In patients with frequent reflux episodes, random, temporal associations between reflux and symptoms may produce a high symptom index in the absence of any true association. The second devised scheme was the symptom sensitivity index.[21] This involves dividing the total number of reflux episodes associated with symptoms by the total number of reflux episodes. This system is also limited and fails to take into account the total number of symptom episodes. Perhaps the best proposed scheme for symptom-reflux correlation is the symptom probability analysis.[22] This involves constructing a contingency table with four fields: (1) positive symptom, positive reflux; (2) negative symptom, positive reflux; (3) positive symptom, negative reflux; and (4) negative symptom, negative reflux. The Fisher's exact test is then applied to calculate the probability that the observed association between reflux and symptoms occurred by chance. To date, none of these schemes have been prospectively validated against an independent parameter of diagnostic accuracy, such as antireflux therapy with symptomatic response.[23] However, it is likely that the use of such symptom indices would improve upon the diagnostic accuracy of pH testing.

Proton Pump Inhibitor Trial

Empiric treatment with PPIs has been suggested to be the "ideal test" for GERD. It is widely available to primary care physicians and is noninvasive, simple, and diagnostic as well as therapeutic. Given the fact that there is no true gold standard for the diagnosis of GERD, coupled with the inconvenience and expense of diagnostic testing, treatment trials are both rational and cost-effective. Although physicians have long used empiric treatment trials as an important aid in establishing a diagnosis of GERD, a number of recent studies have formally examined the use of PPIs in this regard, with promising results.[24–27] A randomized, double-blind, placebo-controlled trial looked at 98 patients with symptoms suggestive of GERD with negative endoscopic findings and compared ambulatory 24-hour pH monitoring versus omeprazole 40 mg PO qd for 2 weeks. In this study, the omeprazole test had a positive and negative predictive value of 68% and 63%, respectively, for the diagnosis of GERD using 24-hour pH testing as the gold standard.[25] A second study comparing omeprazole 40 mg PO q AM and 20 mg PO qhs for 7 days versus 24-hour pH monitoring revealed a specificity of 80% and a sensitivity of 57%.[27] Given the fact that erosive esophagitis is considered definitive evidence of GERD, a third study was conducted comparing 24-hour ambulatory pH monitoring with the omeprazole test in GERD patients with documented esophagitis.[28] The omeprazole test was found to be more sensitive than the total acid exposure score on pH monitoring in diagnosing GERD (83% vs. 60%). Lansoprazole was examined in a prospective, randomized, double-blind study in which patients with GERD symptoms and negative endoscopic findings underwent 24-hour pH monitoring and were given lansoprazole 60 mg orally for 5 days versus placebo using a crossover design.[26] This study revealed a sensitivity of 85% and a test specificity of 73% for lansoprazole.

There are some limitations to the current literature surrounding the PPI trial. First, in interpreting these studies, it is important to note that the sensitivity of the omeprazole test is dependent on how one defines a positive test result. Although the studies defined a positive test result by symptom improvement, the instrument used to measure symptom improvement differed in each study. Secondly, when measuring a subjective outcome such as symptom improvement, a high placebo response rate potentially limits the specificity of the test. Third, various regimens of PPI therapy have been used in the current studies, so there is no current standard as to the optimal dose, frequency, and duration of treatment required for a "positive" PPI test result. Despite this, the simplicity, low cost, and wide availability make the PPI test a valuable means of diagnosing GERD (see Fig. 1). The PPI test has also demonstrated utility in the evaluation of patients presenting with noncardiac chest pain.[24]

New Techniques

Some newer, investigational techniques are currently being developed to aid in the diagnosis of GERD. With the expanding use of PPIs for GERD has come the recognition that a small subset of patients fail to respond to this therapy. Some such patients may suffer from reflux of nonacid material in the form of bland gastric contents or duodenal contents that include pancreatic enzymes and bile. This type of reflux cannot be detected by conventional pH monitoring, which is limited to acid detection. Two methodologies, Bilitec and intraluminal multichannel impedance, are being investigated for the diagnosis of nonacid reflux. The **Bilitec device** employs a fiberoptic probe placed into the esophagus with a portable recording device that is similar to that used for conventional ambulatory pH testing. The Bilitec utilizes the optical properties of bilirubin, the most important pigment in bile, to spectrophotometrically detect its presence in the esophagus, which is suggestive of duodenogastroesophageal reflux.[29] Using such a technique, duodenogastroesophageal reflux has been shown to occur in concert with acid reflux in esophagitis and Barrett's esophagus patients.[30] The second technique, **intraluminal multichannel impedance**, is based on the change of electrical resistance in the esophageal lumen produced by passage of material (food, air, or refluxate) through the axial region of interest. The technique involves the passage of a flexible catheter with a series of axially spaced recording channels into the esophagus. The method has the theoretical advantage of being able to detect acid, alkaline, or neutral reflux events.

The **BRAVO technique** is a novel, catheterless radiotransmitter pH capsule system. This miniature probe is passed transorally via a delivery system into the distal esophagus, where it is clipped to the esophageal mucosa. The delivery system is then removed, leaving the small capsule within the esophagus transmitting a radiosignal to a pager-like receiver worn by the subject. The use of a catheterless system circumvents the problems encountered with limitation in the physical activities and diet that occur using a conventional transnasal pH probe. By being fixed to the esophageal wall, the BRAVO system also avoids potential problems with axial displacement that can occur with the conventional pH catheter. It is likely that the BRAVO pH capsule will also have greater acceptance among patients who have been intolerant of conventional transnasal pH studies.

Key Points: Diagnosis of Gastroesophageal Reflux Disease

- ⇨ The diagnosis of GERD can be challenging given the wide variety of clinical presentations of this common disorder.
- ⇨ Many modalities exist that can establish the diagnosis, but they are rarely required in patients with a classic history of heartburn and regurgitation.
- ⇨ Patients with warning symptoms or signs of potential complications of GERD should undergo endoscopy. Barium studies are rarely indicated.
- ⇨ Ambulatory 24-hour pH monitoring should be limited to patients with atypical symptoms and patients failing to respond to empiric therapy.
- ⇨ A treatment trial with a PPI is effective as both as a diagnostic test and therapeutic intervention.
- ⇨ Newer diagnostic tools are becoming available that will likely further refine our ability to diagnose this common and sometimes vexing disease.

Suggested Reading

1. Klauser AG, Schindlbeck NE, Muller-Lissner SA: Symptoms in gastro-oesophageal reflux disease. Lancet 335:205–2058, 1990.

2. Carlsson R, Dent J, Bolling-Sternevald E, et al: The usefulness of a structured questionnaire in the assessment of symptomatic gastroesophageal reflux disease. Scand J Gastroenterol 33:1023–1029, 1998.

3. Thompson JK, Koehler RE, Richter, JE: Detection of gastroesophageal reflux: Value of barium studies compared with 24-hr pH monitoring [comment]. AJR Am J Roentgenol 162:621–626, 1994.

4. Sellar RJ, De Caestecker JS, Heading RC: Barium radiology: A sensitive test for gastro-oesophageal reflux. Clin Radiol 38:303–307, 1987.

5. Ott DJ: Gastroesophageal reflux disease. Radiol Clin North Am 32:1147–1166, 1994.

6. Ott DJ, et al: Analysis of a multiphasic radiographic examination for detecting reflux esophagitis. Gastrointest Radiol 11:1–6, 1986.

7. Chen YM, Ott DJ, Gelfand DW, Munitz HA: Multiphasic examination of the esophagogastric region for strictures, rings, and hiatal hernia: Evaluation of the individual techniques. Gastrointest Radiol 10:311–316, 1985.

8. Levine MS, Kressel HY, Caroline DF, et al: Barrett esophagus: Reticular pattern of the mucosa. Radiol 147:663–667, 1983.

9. Katz PO, Dalton CB, Richter JE, et al: Esophageal testing of patients with noncardiac chest pain or dysphagia: Results of three years' experience with 1161 patients. Ann Intern Med 106: 593–597, 1987.

10. Kahrilas PJ, Clouse RE, Hogan WJ: American Gastroenterological Association technical review on the clinical use of esophageal manometry. Gastroenterology 107:1865–1884, 1994.

11. Johnsson F, et al: Symptoms and endoscopic findings in the diagnosis of gastroesophageal reflux disease. Scand J Gastroenterol 22:714–718, 1987.

12. Pace F, Santalucia F, Bianchi Porro G: Natural history of gastro-oesophageal reflux disease without oesophagitis. Gut 32:845–848, 1991.

13. Bytzer P, Havelund T, Hansen JM: Interobserver variation in the endoscopic diagnosis of reflux esophagitis. Scand J Gastroenterol 28:119–125, 1993.

14. Ismail-Beigi F, Horton PF, Pope CE 2nd: Histological consequences of gastroesophageal reflux in man. Gastroenterol 58:163–174, 1970.

15. Nandurkar S, et al: Esophageal histology does not provide additional useful information over clinical assessment in identifying reflux patients presenting for esophagogastroduodenoscopy. Dig Dis Sci 45:217–224, 2000.

16. Johnson LF, Demeester TR: Twenty-four-hour pH monitoring of the distal esophagus: A quantitative measure of gastroesophageal reflux. Am J Gastroenterol 62:325–332, 1974.

17. Richter JE: Typical and atypical presentations of gastroesophageal reflux disease: The role of esophageal testing in diagnosis and management. Gastroenterology Clin North Am 25:75–102, 1996.

18. Fass R, et al: Effect of ambulatory 24-hour esophageal pH monitoring on reflux-provoking activities. Dig Dis Sci 44:2263–2269, 1999.

19. Jacob P, Kahrilas PJ, Herzon G: Proximal esophageal pH-metry in patients with 'reflux laryngitis'. Gastroenterology 100:305–310, 1991.

20. Wiener GJ, Richter JE, Copper JB, et al: The symptom index: a clinically important parameter of ambulatory 24-hour esophageal pH monitoring. Am J Gastroenterol 83:358–361, 1988.

21. Breumelhof R, Smout AJ: The symptom sensitivity index: A valuable additional pa-

rameter in 24-hour esophageal pH recording [comment]. Am J Gastroenterol 86: 160–164, 1991.

22. Weusten BL, Roelofs JM, Akkerman ZM, et al: The symptom-association probability: An improved method for symptom analysis of 24-hour esophageal pH data [comment]. Gastroenterology 107:1741–1745, 1994.

23. Kahrilas PJ, Quigley EM: Clinical esophageal pH recording: A technical review for practice guideline development. Gastroenterology 110:1982–1996, 1996.

24. Fass R, Fennerty MB, Ofman JJ, et al: The clinical and economic value of a short course of omeprazole in patients with noncardiac chest pain. Gastroenterology 115:42–49, 1998.

25. Schenk BE, Kuipers EJ, Klinkenbery-Knol EC, et al: Omeprazole as a diagnostic tool in gastroesophageal reflux disease. Am J Gastroenterol 92:1997–2000, 1997.

26. Juul-Hansen P, Rydning A, Jackobsen CD, Hansen T: High-dose proton-pump nhibitors as a diagnostic test of gastro-oesophageal reflux disease in endoscopic-negative patients. Scand J Gastroenterol 36:806–810, 2001.

27. Fass R, Ofman JJ, Gralnek IM, et al: Clinical and economic assessment of the omeprazole test in patients with symptoms suggestive of gastroesophageal reflux disease. Arch Intern Med 159:2161–2168, 1999.

28. Fass R, Ofman JJ, Sampliner RE, et al: The omeprazole test is as sensitive as 24-h oesophageal pH monitoring in diagnosing gastro-oesophageal reflux disease in symptomatic patients with erosive oesophagitis. Aliment Pharmacol Ther 14:389–396, 2000.

29. Tack J, Sifrim D: New techniques for the detection of gastro-oesophageal reflux. Dig Liver Dis 32:S245–248, 2000.

30. Champion G, Richler JE, Valzi MF, et al: Duodenogastroesophageal reflux: Relationship to pH and importance in Barrett's esophagus. Gastroenterology 107:747–754, 1994.

Esophageal Stricture, Ulcer, and Bleeding Complications of Gastroesophageal Reflux Disease

chapter

4

Ofer Feder, M.D. and
Nicholas J. Shaheen, M.D., M.P.H.

Many patients with gastroesophageal reflux disease (GERD) develop complications due to the chronic, relapsing nature of the condition. These complications are thought to be the result of increased acid exposure or vulnerable esophageal epithelium. The practicing gastroenterologist commonly encounters multiple esophageal complications, including stricture formation, ulceration, hemorrhage, and possibly Schatzki's ring. Severe complications of GERD may be observed on the initial evaluation of GERD symptoms.[1] We describe in this chapter the epidemiology, pathogenesis, clinical presentation, diagnosis, and management of these complications. Initially, a brief discussion of esophageal ulceration, esophageal hemorrhage, and Schatzki's ring is presented followed by a discussion at a greater length of esophageal strictures.

Ulceration

Most disruption of esophageal epithelium occurs in the setting of erosive esophagitis. Deep ulcers in the squamous epithelium are rarely encountered in cases of reflux disease (5%). Such esophageal ulcerations tend to be more common in men. When deep ulcers are found in the esophagus, the differential diagnosis is broad and includes those entities listed in Table 1. Careful history taking allows for the exclusion of many causes. Nonpeptic causes of esophageal ulceration are more prevalent in immunocompromised hosts. Assessment of human immunodefi-

TABLE 1.	Differential Diagnosis of Esophageal Ulcers	
Infectious	Viral	
		Cytomegalovirus
		Herpes simplex
		Human immunodeficiency virus
	Bacterial	
		Tuberculosis
		Atypical mycobacteria
	Fungal	
Reflux-induced	Barrett's ulcer	
	Non-Barrett's ulcer	
Mechanical	Mallory-Weiss tear	
	Cameron's ulcer	
Iatrogenic	Nasogastric tube-induced	
	Post-sclerotherapy	
	Post-variceal band ligation	
	Pill-induced	
	Radiation-induced	
	Graft-versus-host disease	
Neoplastic	Benign	
		Leiomyoma
		Lipoma
	Malignant	
		Adenocarcinoma
		Squamous cell carcinoma
		Lymphoma
		Sarcoma
		Nonesophageal primary
Idiopathic	Bullous pemphigoid	
	Epidermolysis bullosa dystrophica	
	Crohn's disease	
	Sarcoid	
	Behçet's disease	

ciency virus status is often useful following the identification of such lesions. The finding of an esophageal lesion as the first indication of human immunodeficiency virus infection was more common prior to the advent of more effective antiretroviral therapies.[2]

A common presenting symptom of esophageal ulceration is odynophagia. Additionally, dysphagia, anorexia, and chest pain are also encountered. Histopathologic review of biopsy specimens obtained at the time of endoscopic examination is essential, because the endoscopic appearance of esophageal ulcer may be similar for different pathogenic mechanisms. Further, depending on the clinical history and lesion appearance, cultures for viral organisms, fungi, atypical mycobacteria, or other pathogens may be appropriate.[3,4] In patients with reflux-associated ulceration and Barrett's esophagus, attention to the presence of ulceration in the region of columnar epithelium is warranted. These *Barrett's ulcers* are often refractory to medical therapy and may be an independent risk factor for development of dysplasia or adenocarcinoma of the esophagus.[5,6] Perforation of a Barrett's ulcer is a rare but well-documented indication for esophageal resection.[5,7,8]

Pill-induced ulcerations are associated with many different medications, including tetracycline, potassium supplements, alendronate, and nonsteroidal anti-inflammatory drugs (NSAIDs).[9] Most pill-induced ulcerations respond to cessation of the offending agent combined with acid suppression. Response failure should prompt an investigation as to other possible causes of ulceration.

Hemorrhage

The finding of erosive esophagitis has been reported in up to 22% of patients undergoing endoscopy for reflux symptoms.[10,11] However, the incidence of hemodynamically significant hemorrhage due to reflux-induced mucosal damage is quite low, reported as less than 2%. Most reported series of patients presenting with acute upper gastrointestinal bleeding demonstrate that less than 10% of patients are suffering from bleeding associated with erosive esophagitis.[12,13] Bleeding resulting from other causes originating within the esophagus (e.g., esophageal varices, Mallory-Weiss tear) accounts for greater than 30% of hemorrhage noted in these series. Certain patient groups are at greater risk for esophageal hemorrhage arising from erosive esophagitis. These include the elderly, institutionalized mentally retarded adults, those with chronic renal insufficiency, and those with concomitant anticoagulant or NSAID use.[14,15] Ulceration associated with a hiatal hernia, known as Cameron's ulcer, is an often unrecognized cause of upper gastrointestinal hemorrhage and chronic anemia.[16] This lesion is thought to be secondary to local ischemic effects in the gastric wall at the level of the diaphragm. Although its development is not due to GERD, the frequent association of hiatal hernia with GERD symptoms warrants consideration of Cameron's ulcer in GERD patients presenting with upper gastrointestinal bleeding. This lesion is easily overlooked at endoscopic examination and may be responsible for the noted increased incidence of iron deficiency anemia in patients with large hiatal hernias.[17,18]

Schatzki's Ring

Schatzki's ring occurs at the junction between squamous esophageal and columnar gastric mucosa. The upper surface of Schatzki's ring is lined by squamous mucosa, and the lower surface is covered by columnar epithelium.[19] The ring is usually quite thin, measuring less than 5 mm in most radiographic views (Fig. 1). Variable invagination of the ring into the esophageal lumen may result in the clinical presentation of dysphagia or esophageal obstruction (Fig. 2).

The origin of Schatzki's ring formation is unclear. Rings may be present congenitally and become symptomatic only in later life. There is some evidence that GERD may be more prevalent in patients with Schatzki's ring.[20] Given that many patients with symptomatic rings lack GERD symptoms, and most GERD patients show no ring formation, any association between the two remains speculative. Also, difficulty differentiating Schatzki's ring from short peptic strictures on endoscopic examination may account for a spurious association between Schatzki's ring and GERD. Treatment of Schatzki's ring is primarily via esophageal bougie dilatation, as is described later in this chapter. Return of dys-

Figure 1. Fluoroscopic image of a Schatzki's ring with food impaction immediately proximal to ring. The patient presented with a 2-day history of dysphagia.

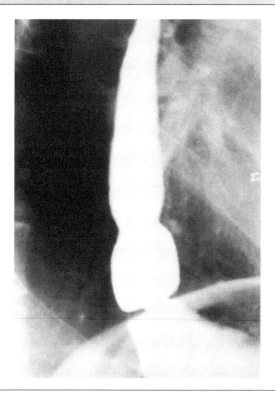

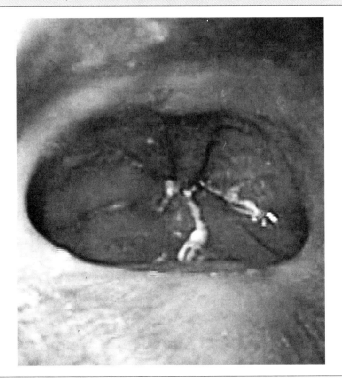

Figure 2. Endoscopic view of a Schatzki's ring.

phagia symptoms associated with ring recurrence is noted in up to 65% of patients, often necessitating repeated treatment.[21,22] Some clinicians advocate four-quadrant biopsies of the ring to facilitate disruption from shearing forces at the time of dilator delivery. Others suggest needle-knife incision of recurrent Schatzki's ring.[23]

Esophageal Peptic Stricture

Epidemiology

Nearly 10% of patients requiring medical evaluation for GERD develop strictures.[24] There are no reliable prognostic factors for stricture development. The severity of GERD only weakly correlates with the propensity to form strictures. The incidence of peptic strictures does increase with age, perhaps reflecting the cumulative effect of prolonged reflux burden.[25] A recent case-control study of patients from the Veterans Administration observed that severe forms of GERD such as esophageal erosions, ulcers, and peptic stricture affected the elderly more often than the young. White race and male sex were also risk factors for stricture formation.[1] It is likely that the association with increased age is because of the increased duration of reflux esophagitis rather than aging itself.

There is an association of stricture formation with conditions treated with aspirin and NSAIDs.[26] In these cases, esophageal injury may be related to direct contact of the medication to the mucosa, as NSAIDs do not seem to worsen GERD.[27] Patients who present with esophageal stricture should be specifically questioned for aspirin or NSAID use.

Pathogenesis

Peptic strictures are typically short, < 1 cm in length, and generally involve the squamocolumnar junction.[28] Their formation appears to be multifactorial, not unlike the pathogenesis of GERD itself. Several observations shed light on the cause of stricture formation in the setting of reflux.[29] GERD patients with strictures appear to be less sensitive to intraesophageal acid exposure than GERD patients without strictures.[30] Additionally, although low resting lower esophageal sphincter (LES) pressures are not consistently seen in patients with uncomplicated GERD, patients with peptic strictures generally do have lower LES pressures relative to those of patients with uncomplicated GERD or control subjects.[31] In fact, a resting LES pressure of less than 8 mm Hg is highly predictive of stricture formation in GERD patients. Further, the presence of hiatal hernia is more common in GERD patients with strictures than in those without.[32] Next, patients with strictures appear to have decreased amplitude and frequency of esophageal peristalsis contributing to decreased acid clearance.[24] Also, those patients who develop strictures have higher levels of acid exposure on 24-hour esophageal pH monitoring than do those with uncomplicated GERD. Other host factors are postulated to contribute but have not been proven, including differences in fibrogenesis and gastric acid hypersecretion. These data suggest that patients with stricture formation suffer more severe reflux. These patients are both less sensitive to the acid and less able to clear refluxate than non-stricture formers with GERD.

Stricture formation occurs in several stages. Early reflux episodes induce mucosal edema and muscular spasm. Clinically, this may be the cause of the so-called ringed or feline esophagus associated with GERD (Fig. 3).[33] The histologic picture at this stage may include basal cell hyperplasia and eosinophilic infiltration of the mucosa. This histologic and clinical appearance is usually reversible with aggressive acid suppression.[34] Continued pathologic acid exposure may lead to ulceration with reactive fibrosis. Extension of this fibrotic reaction into the muscularis

Figure. 3. "Ringed" esophagus, a potential cause of chronic dysphagia, may be caused by GERD.

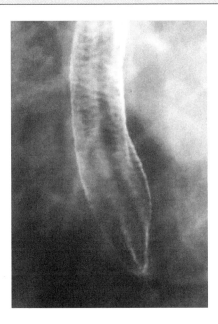

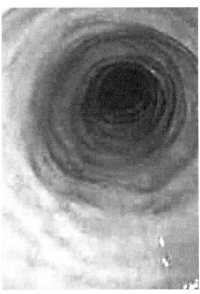

propria impacts the muscular and neuronal elements involved in peristalsis. Thus, impaired esophageal acid clearance and prolonged refluxate dwell times occur. The repetitive nature of the acid exposure and subsequent fibrotic response lead to continued collagen deposition, which over time results in the loss of esophageal luminal caliber and stricture formation.

Presentation

The majority of patients have a history of GERD symptoms that predates their presentation with peptic stricture. However, approximately one third of patients with strictures have no prior history of reflux-type symptoms.[34] This lack of GERD symptoms is attributed to decreased esophageal sensitivity to acid exposure.

The majority of patients presenting with peptic strictures have dysphagia with solid foods. High priority ranking of the symptom of dysphagia is predictive of the presence of an esophageal stricture.[35] Additionally, odynophagia and food impaction are not uncommon presentations.[36]

A patient's subjective localization of the level of an esophageal stricture is highly accurate.[37] Seventy-five percent of patients can localize the level of obstruction to within 4 cm, with 25% localizing the level of obstruction exactly. In a significant subset of patients (15–25%), however, the sensation of dysphagia does not correspond to the level of the obstruction. Patients appear to be most accurate in localizing proximal rather than distal lesions.

Diagnosis

Nearly 70% of strictures result from chronic gastroesophageal reflux. The differential diagnosis for esophageal stricture is broad (Table 2). Most nonpeptic causes of esophageal stricture can be excluded by history. Neoplastic strictures, both squamous cell carcinoma and adenocarcinoma arising near the gastroesophageal junction, may be difficult to differentiate from benign peptic stricture, making it necessary to obtain multiple biopsies of such lesions if they are suspected at the time of endoscopic examination. For any given severity level of acid exposure, patients with strictures are no more likely than those without to have intestinal metaplasia or Barrett's esophagus.[38]

The evaluation of dysphagia commonly includes two diagnostic studies. The first is esophageal contrast radiography (Fig. 4). This imaging modality is sensitive for the detection of mild or early strictures.[39] Stricture morphology can be appreciated, and even distal portions of the stricture may be assessed that could not be visualized by endoscopy. Digestion of solid contrast agents, such as tablets, may further enhance ex-

TABLE 2.	Differential Diagnosis of Esophageal Strictures
Ingestion of caustic substances	Alkali
	Acid
Iatrogenic	Radiation therapy
	Photodynamic therapy
	Post-sclerotherapy
	Post-variceal band ligation
	Pill-induced
	Postoperative
	Chronic nasogastric tube–induced
Idiopathic	Bullous pemphigoid
	Tylosis
	Pemphigus
	Epidermolysis bullosa dystrophica
	Scleroderma
	Crohn's disease
	Sarcoid
	Esophageal webs
	Eosinophilic esophagitis
Acid peptic	Barrett's-associated
	Non-Barrett's-associated
Neoplasia	Adenocarcinoma
	Squamous cell carcinoma
	Nonepithelial tumors
Infectious	Syphilis
	Candida
	Herpes simplex
	Cytomegalovirus
	Tuberculosis

amination sensitivity associated with dysphagia and may be better than endoscopy for identifying subtle acid-induced strictures.[40,41] A second, often complementary evaluation is upper endoscopy. This study has the advantage of being both a diagnostic and a therapeutic modality. Tissue can be obtained at the time of evaluation to exclude malignancy. In tight strictures, passage of even a neonatal endoscope may be impossible without preceding dilatation or fluoroscopic guidance (Fig. 5).

Barium esophagram is an appropriate modality for the initial evaluation of dysphagia. However, many clinicians proceed directly to upper endoscopy.[42] Which modality to choose is often dictated by clinical history. Endoscopy may be especially appropriate in the older patient with weight loss, in whom the pretest probability of significant disease is high. Additionally, such a presentation may require both diagnostic sampling and therapeutic intervention to appropriately address the cause of dysphagia.[43] If upper endoscopy is the initial diagnostic strategy selected, the clinician may occasionally encounter a stricture that

Figure 4. Barium-enhanced radiograph of an esophageal stricture.

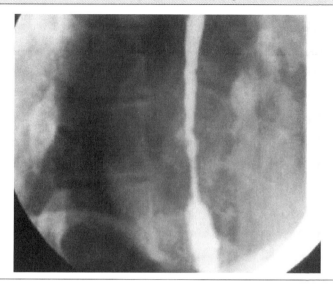

Figure 5. Endoscopic view of a tight esophageal stricture.

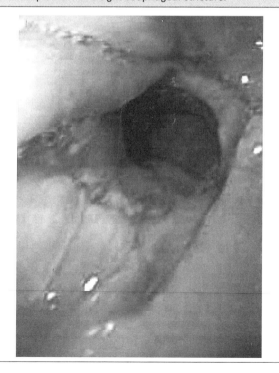

will not allow passage of the endoscope or evaluation of distal morphologic features. Without knowledge of the stricture morphology, it may be wise to defer dilatation until a barium esophagram or fluoroscopic evaluation can be obtained.

Management

Medical

Data are available to support the positive impact of pharmacologic interventions in patients with esophageal peptic strictures. There are several conceptual advantages to aggressive medical treatment of esophageal strictures. Decreasing active inflammation of the esophagus may increase luminal caliber by decreasing associated mucosal edema. Acid suppression may slow or halt the chronic mucosal damage, producing long-term improvement of luminal caliber. Recent evidence suggests that healing coexistent mucosal inflammation may be as important in relieving dysphagia as maintaining an adequate luminal diameter.[44]

The frequency of dilatations needed to achieve adequate luminal caliber is a commonly cited measure in the medical literature by which the efficacy of pharmacologic interventions on peptic strictures is assessed. Using the frequency of dilatation as a measure of the efficacy of interventions presents severe problems. It may hide practitioner-specific differences in performing dilatation, such as the threshold of dysphagia necessary to prompt dilatation. Also, it may fail to identify patient subsets who might be responsive to therapy. For example, any benefit of acid suppression upon early strictures may be obscured by its lack of efficacy in older fibrotic strictures. The perception of dysphagia, and its associated psychological distress, varies from patient to patient. Finally, the placebo effect of medication itself may delay the patient's request for dilatation, regardless of any physiologic effect of the medication. With these caveats in mind, other measures, such as dysphagia scores and endoscopic evaluation of mucosal damage, are utilized to supplement this outcome measure.

The beneficial effect of rigorous acid suppression in patients with peptic stricture is supported by available studies. Earlier data with H_2-receptor antagonists used in patients with strictures failed to demonstrate a decreased need for dilatation.[45,46] More recent data gathered by several investigators have demonstrated that proton pump inhibitors (PPIs) have significant clinical benefits. PPIs decrease the need for recurrent dilatation, promote healing of coexistent esophagitis, and reduce dysphagic symptoms more effectively than H_2-receptor antagonists or placebo.[47–52] Further, PPIs are more cost-effective than H_2-receptor antagonists for management of peptic strictures, despite their increased up-front costs.[53] By coupling dilatations with aggressive acid inhibition, most patients are found to require only a single dilatation, markedly reducing morbidity and the cost of patient management. Therefore, PPIs should be considered first-line pharmacologic therapy for patients with peptic stricture.

Dilatation

The mainstay of medical management of established peptic stricture remains the centuries-old practice of esophageal dilatation. Dilatation was described as early as the 16th century, when wax candles were used. In fact, the term *bougienage* originates from the Algerian town of Bouginhay, a center of the wax candle trade in the Middle Ages.[54] Whalebones with their tips covered with sponge were first described as dilating implements by Sir Thomas Willis in 1674. Blunt-tipped mercury dilators were introduced in 1915 by the British surgeon Arthur Hurst. This design was later modified by Maloney to include a tapered end to allow passage through tight strictures. Eder and Peustow developed an over-the-wire dilation method utilizing oval metal dilators, termed "olives", in 1951. This obsolete system allowed fluoroscopic monitoring. Three types of esophageal dilatation systems are currently commonly used in the United States. Each system and its use is discussed here.

Mercury-Filled Bougienage. This remains a popular and commonly used method for esophageal dilatation despite the advent of more sophisticated systems, because of its simplicity, with no fluoroscopy or guidewires commonly utilized. Costs are therefore relatively low because these adjunct measures are avoided. Furthermore, this established technique has been available for a long time, allowing clinicians to become experienced and confident in its implementation.

Two mercury-filled bougies are commonly available. The first is the Hurst dilator, with a relatively blunt tip, and the second is the Maloney dilator, with a tapered end. The techniques involved for these systems are very similar. Both are dependent on prior assessment of stricture characteristics, specifically caliber and length, accomplished by either barium radiography or endoscopy. The patient is positioned in the recumbent or left lateral decubitus position with the neck slightly hyperextended. The initial dilator is chosen to approximate the same size as the tightest diameter of the stricture. Topical pharyngeal anesthesia and lubrication are utilized. Importantly, systemic sedation is not essential but may be helpful in anxious patients or in those in whom endoscopy is undertaken immediately prior to the dilatation. The dilator is held like a pencil or dart and passed into the hypopharynx over the dorsal surface of the first and second fingers of the nondominant hand (Fig. 6). The patient is instructed to swallow, thereby relaxing the upper esophageal sphincter, allowing the dilator to be passed smoothly into the esopha-

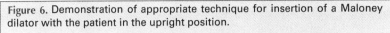

Figure 6. Demonstration of appropriate technique for insertion of a Maloney dilator with the patient in the upright position.

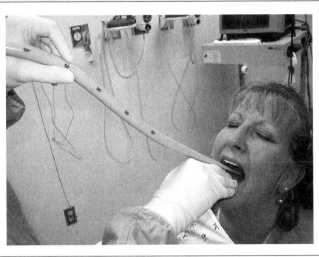

gus with gentle pressure. The dilator is passed forward, such that its maximal diameter travels several centimeters past the most distal extent of the stricture exerting a shearing force. Attention to the depth of bougie passage is especially important with the Maloney dilators, which may encounter resistance with their tapered tip before the maximal diameter of the dilator overcomes the stricture. If the dilator is not completely advanced through the stricture, ineffective bougienage occurs.

This routine is repeated with gradually increasing sizes of dilators, although the optimal number of dilatations performed at a single sitting is not clear. The number of dilators passed is dependent on stricture characteristics, patient tolerance, and the resistance encountered with dilatation. A useful empirical guideline is the "rule of three": no more than three dilatations to resistance should be performed at a single session. However, any time excessive force is required to pass a dilator, it is inadvisable to continue with larger dilators. The goal of dilatation is to accomplish a luminal diameter of 14 mm or more (42 Fr).[55] This diameter generally provides dramatic relief of dysphagia. This goal is usually attainable in fewer than three therapeutic sessions. Symptom resolution can be objectively confirmed by successful passage of a 12 mm diameter barium tablet.[56]

Selection of mercury-filled dilators is predicated on delineation of the stricture characteristics. Patients with short, simple strictures are good candidates for mercury-filled dilators. Similarly, patients with Schatzki's rings or congenital webs are also noted to respond well to a single passage of a large 17 mm (>50 Fr) dilator, frequently becoming asymptomatic.[57] Tight, tortuous strictures are less amenable to this therapy. Not uncommonly, the bougie may impact the shoulder of a complicated or angulated stricture, coiling in the esophagus, and never passing through the stricture zone. The use of mercury-filled dilators should be avoided in patients with strictures associated with adjacent esophageal pseudo-diverticula (Fig. 7); in these patients, wire-guided techniques are more reliably implemented.

A success rate for dysphagia relief greater than 85% is reported in all comers (strictures, rings, and webs) after dilatation. Redilatation rates vary significantly among patients. Forty percent of patients require only one dilatation for symptom relief.[58,59] Some patients require weekly sessions for extended times or scheduled maintenance dilatations to ensure

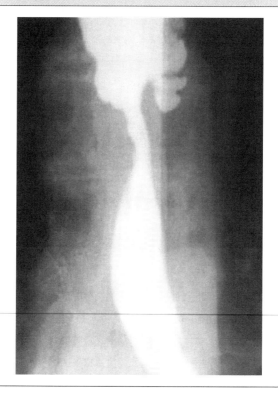

Figure 7. Stricture complicated by pseudodiverticula. Dilatation of this stricture by unguided (fluoroscopic or wire-guided) technique may place the patient at increased risk of perforation.

adequate luminal caliber and to avoid recurrent dysphagia or repeated food bolus impactions. Fluoroscopic guidance has been suggested to improve outcomes; however, the addition to each treatment session of increased cost and radiation exposure makes the technique less attractive.[60–62] Dilatation without fluoroscopy appears safe for most patients.[63] Predictors of the need for recurrent dilatations include fibrous stricture, a maximal dilator size of less than 44 Fr, and more than two initial sessions to relieve dysphagia.[58]

Self-dilatation with mercury-filled dilators has been shown to be effective. This arrangement of self-treatment may be useful and convenient for patients who require frequent regular dilatations of benign peptic strictures to remain symptom free.[64,65] It is critical that patients who undertake such a treatment plan be motivated and receive proper instruction and follow-up to ensure that complications are not encountered.[66] Further, the age and condition of the used dilators should be monitored to avoid cracking or mercury spillage.

Polyvinyl Over-the-Wire Dilators. Commonly encountered are the Savary dilating system (Wilson-Cook, Winston-Salem, NC) and the American Endoscopy dilating system (Bard, Billerica, MA). They differ only slightly in the shape of the dilator and the guidewire design. The Savary system has a radiopaque band at the dilator's widest diameter, whereas the American Endoscopy system has a radiopaque marker along the entire length of the dilator to facilitate fluoroscopic visualization. The techniques involved in dilating with either system are similar.

Before dilatation is undertaken, routine endoscopy is performed. A standard upper endoscope, or in the case of a tight or angulated stricture, a pediatric or neonatal upper endoscope, might be utilized. The diameter of the narrowest portion of the stricture is approximated, using the known diameter of the endoscope as a guide. Next, The spring-tipped end of the guidewire is placed through the endoscope and the wire is advanced under direct visualization (endoscopic or fluoroscopic) into position within the antrum along the greater curve of the antrum. The endoscope is then exchanged, or "traded out," with the guidewire being advanced through the endoscope 5 cm for every 5 cm of endoscope withdrawn. During withdrawal, the position of the wire should be monitored under direct visualization. Suctioning of air during withdrawal, especially within the stomach, helps maintain wire placement. If this wire placement maneuver is completed correctly, the endoscope can be completely withdrawn, leaving approximately 60 to 70 cm of wire in the patient. Attention should be given to the wire markings at the level of the teeth, so that after each dilatation, minimal wire migration can be ensured.

Following wire placement, the dilators are then passed. The patient's mouthpiece should be preselected to allow passage of the largest dilator to be used. Fixation of the wire at the patient's mouth is needed to prevent movement of the noted markings during dilator preparation. The patient's neck should be slightly hyperextended to facilitate dilator passage through the cervical area. The stiff end of the silicone-lubricated wire is inserted into the hollow tip of the dilator, after which the dilator itself is lubricated with a water-based agent. With the dilator held like a pencil in the dominant hand, it is passed over the wire. The assistant should apply gentle traction on the wire, which is held in space by the endoscopy assistant to prevent its migration with the advancement of the dilator. The dilator should be inserted until the maximal diameter of the dilator passes through the stricture zone, exerting its full shearing force. Fluoroscopy is useful to ascertain dilator placement in tight or angulated strictures. The dilator is then withdrawn, while the wire is forwarded through it.

When the dilator is removed, the position of the wire should be reconfirmed. The markings on it should be within 5 cm of the initial starting point. If significant migration has occurred, especially outward, removal of the wire and reinsertion of the endoscope may be necessary to properly replace the wire. Reinsertion of the endoscope directly over the wire should not be done, as this may damage the inner channel of the endoscope. If reinsertion of the endoscope over a guidewire is needed, a plastic biliary catheter should be passed through the scope to protect it, and the wire can then be inserted through the catheter in a retrograde fashion.

The rule of three is a useful guideline as to how many wire-guided dilators may be passed. On the final passage, both the wire and the dilator are removed simultaneously. If resistance to dilator passage is encountered, the wire position should be reassessed to exclude migration and possible dilator impaction on the wire's spring end. Because the dilator tip will not slide over the spring at the end of the wire, impaction of the dilator tip on the spring at the end of the Savary wire is an especially common error in over-the-wire dilatation procedures. When this occurs, the endoscopist may mistake the increased resistance to dilator passage as originating from the stricture itself, as opposed to the wire tip. If the dilator is further advanced over the wire, it may become "stuck" on the spring end of the wire. In such a situation, it is advisable to remove both the dilator and the wire and to replace the wire endoscopically.

Through-the-Scope (TTS) Balloons. These provide effective esophageal stricture dilatation. Various polyethylene balloons ranging in diameter from 4 to 18 mm and in length from 5 to 8.5 cm are available. Data support this technique's efficacy in relief of dysphagia and low complication rates.[67,68] However, some gastroenterologists may use TTS balloons less commonly because of increased costs of single-use balloon catheters or lack of familiarity with this technique relative to older bougienage techniques.

Similar to over-the-wire dilatation, TTS dilatation is initiated following a standard endoscopic evaluation. An inner channel at least 3.2 mm wide is required for balloon passage. The stricture diameter and characteristics are assessed, to select the appropriately sized TTS balloon. The balloon should checked for patency prior to insertion through the endoscope by inflating with water. Dilute (half-strength) contrast material may also be used if fluoroscopy is anticipated. Most balloons have a lifespan of five to 10 uses if handled appropriately.

Balloon selection is paramount. A long, uncomplicated stricture may respond well to dilatation with a single long balloon. On the other hand, shorter balloons may be useful to sequentially dilate a long, angulated stricture so as to minimize perforation risk. The balloon tip is silicone coated to facilitate passage through the endoscope. The rim of the plastic catheter shaft at the base of the balloon should be visible prior to inflation to prevent damage to the endoscope or popping of the balloon. It should be deployed uninflated across the portion of the stricture to be dilated. The balloon may then be slowly inflated. Migration of the balloon is frequently encountered as the balloon fills, causing the balloon to either back out of the stricture zone or advance through it. Frequent balloon repositioning thus may be necessary. Balloons are inflated to their maximal (or graduated) diameters and held in place for 1 to 2 minutes. This may be repeated two to three times. If fluoroscopic evaluation shows obliteration of the stricture waist, dilatation is complete. Complete balloon deflation is required for withdrawal through the endoscope.

The TTS balloons exert a radial force, as opposed to bougies, which provide both radial and shearing force. It was therefore hoped that more aggressive dilatation of strictures might be possible, since damage to tissues might be decreased.[69] Attempts to dilate tight strictures to adequate diameters in a single session have not been as in successful as serial sessions.[67] Thus, as with over-the wire and mercury-filled dilatation techniques, repeated sessions to achieve a desired result are advised.[70] These sessions might combine dilating modalities—for example, utilizing fluoroscopically directed TTS for an initially tight stricture and converting at later sessions to over-the-wire or mercury-filled dilations as the luminal diameter is increased.

Failure to dilate a peptic stricture by antegrade technique is a rare event. There are reports of retrograde dilatation via gastrostomy being successfully performed.[71,72] Results of endoscopic local corticosteroid injections in patients with refractory strictures were not as favorable as those reported in series in which patients are treated with dilatation followed by acid inhibition.[73]

Complications of Dilatation

Potential complications of dilation of peptic stricture include those imposed by the radial and shearing force administered. The main risks of esophageal dilatation include perforation, bleeding, and bacteremia. The bleeding risk is only marginally increased in the presence of a peptic stricture relative to patients undergoing routine endoscopy. Additionally, TTS and over-the-wire dilatations entail concomitant endoscopic risks such as bleeding, perforation, aspiration, and sedation-related complications. However, this risk appears to be similar to that seen in other patients undergoing diagnostic upper endoscopy.

Esophageal perforation is the most morbid complication of esophageal dilatation. Most published series report a low rate of perforation, usually less than 0.5%.[74-78] The risk may be higher for complex strictures. In patients who do suffer perforation, the breach may occur in the cervical esophagus, rather than the stricture zone. This is especially true in older series utilizing Eder-Puestow olives in which the perforation rate may be as high as 14%. Among the current commonly used methods of dilatation, perforation rates appear to be similar.[79] The routine use of fluoroscopy has been suggested to reduce the risk of perforation, although no randomized studies have tested this hypothesis. The use of endoscopy alone in directing dilatation has demonstrated acceptably low complication rates.[78] Risk factors for perforation have been assessed in multiple series and found to include long strictures, tight strictures, large hiatal hernias, and angulated stricture zones.[70,80]

Post-procedural esophageal perforations are best demonstrated by contrast radiography. Multiple views in different patient positions may be required to demonstrate small leaks. Plain radiography demonstrating subcutaneous emphysema or mediastinal air may be suggestive of perforation. Surgical consultation is essential; however, many perforations can be managed medically with good outcomes.

Bleeding following perforation infrequently requires transfusion. It occurs in about 5 in 1000 procedures. It may occur from the dilated stricture zone itself or from proximal mucosa damaged by the shearing force delivered by the push dilator. Repeat endoscopy to assess for focal tear may be necessary, with injection of epinephrine or saline done to tamponade the bleeding. Rarely is operative intervention for bleeding required.

Transient bacteremia following dilatation is not uncommon but is rarely of clinical significance.[81] There have been reported cases of serious infectious complications, however, including endocarditis, meningitis, and brain abscess.[77,82-84] Although there is little evidence to support their use, antibiotics are often given to patients with prosthetic heart valves, a history of endocarditis, or other high-risk profiles, to decrease the risk for infectious complications. The American Society for Gastrointestinal Endoscopy recommends that antibiotic prophylaxis be provided to those high-risk patients undergoing a high risk procedure such as esophageal dilatation.[85] Those conditions that warrant such concern include prosthetic valve placement, history of endocarditis, systemic pulmonary shunt, and synthetic vascular graft less than 1-year old. For all other patient candidates, insufficient data exist to make recommendations. Endoscopists may choose to provide antibiotics on a case-by case basis when esophageal dilatation is planned. This should be tempered by potential adverse drug reactions associated with antibiotic administration.

Comparisons between Dilating Systems

Prospective, randomized comparative studies of the currently utilized dilating systems do not demonstrate a definitive performance benefit of one over the other. Owing to their shared low complication rate, thousands of patients might be necessary to show significant performance differences. A trial comparing Savary dilators to TTS balloons in the treatment of benign esophageal strictures failed to show a difference in efficacy or complication rates, although the need for recurrent dilatation was lower using TTS balloons.[67] A second trial showed that Savary dilators produced less need for subsequent dilatations and larger esophageal diameters 1 year after the initial dilation, when compared with TTS balloons.[68] Given such conflicting results, no recommendation of one system over the other can be made. Importantly, the lower complication rates, improved patient comfort, and equal efficacy seen with Savary dilators as compared with Eder-Puestow olives[86] has prompted the abandonment of this latter system by most clinicians.

Stricture Recurrence after Dilatation

Early studies of dilatation as the primary therapy for peptic stricture prior to the advent of H_2-receptor antagonists or PPIs demonstrated that 40% of patients achieve a sustained response after initial dilatation to the goal diameter.[86–89] Recurrence of stricture was noted in the remaining 60%, necessitating repeat dilatation. In one series before the availability of PPIs, two recurrences of peptic stricture requiring dilatation was predictive of a third stricture recurrence in 94% of patients.[58] However, even with optimal medical management with PPIs, 30% of patients require repeat dilatation within 1 year (Fig. 8).[47] The number of stricture recurrences in the first year appears to predict the likelihood of repeat dilatation during subsequent follow-up.[90] Other predictors of the need for frequent dilatations include weight loss and lack of the sensation of heartburn. Other factors such as age, sex, duration of follow-up, endo-

Figure 8. Repeated dilatations of a stricture may be needed because of recurrent dysphagia, despite the use of PPIs. The shown stricture was dilated three times over the course of a year. (*continued*)

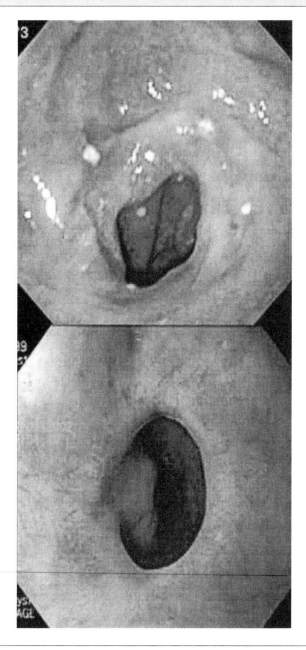

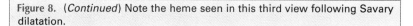

Figure 8. (*Continued*) Note the heme seen in this third view following Savary dilatation.

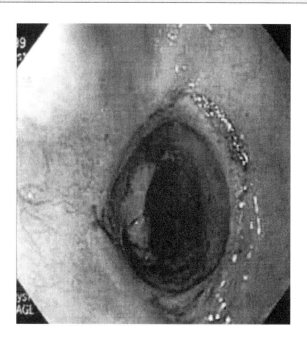

scopic evidence of esophagitis or Barrett's metaplasia, type of dilator or size used, aspirin or NSAID use, heavy alcohol abuse, or tobacco abuse have not been found to be predictive of stricture recurrence.

Stenting of Benign Esophageal Strictures

Esophageal stenting of strictures unresponsive to dilatation has been evaluated. This procedure is more suited to individuals who are elderly or whose multiple medical comorbidities makes them poor operative candidates. Reported experience with the placement of expandable metal stents describes high short-term patency rates.[91–93] However, cases of stent migration, tissue overgrowth, and exacerbation of reflux symptoms are described.[93,94] Such management is inadvisable in patients with a considerable life expectancy, and the clinician should be hesitant in general to stent patients with benign disease of the esophagus.

Surgical Management of Strictures

Ideally, severe esophageal strictures are averted by early and adequate medical therapy. Many reports confirm the benefit of conservative long-term management, making it unusual that surgery is necessary. The best candidates for antireflux surgery among patients with strictures are patients who obtain symptom relief with medication, require large doses of medicines to control their symptoms, and have poorly responding strictures.

In patients who have an esophagus of normal length with stricture, the indication for operative management is similar to the indication in the general GERD population. A standard antireflux procedure is best. Preoperative esophageal manometry demonstrating good motility is desirable, but some groups have reported that preoperative motility study results were not predictive of outcomes after surgery-resistant stricture.[95,96] The postoperative rate of dysphagia may be higher in patients with strictures managed operatively compared to the general GERD patient.[97] For this reason, some have advocated the Belsey partial fundoplication for this patient subset.[98] In general, results of surgical fundoplication in stricture patients are equivalent to results in the general GERD population.

An esophageal lengthening procedure coupled with an antireflux maneuver may give good relief of symptoms and control of GERD without esophageal resection. This is appropriate for the patient with a fibrotic shortened esophagus with stricture. Standard antireflux procedures often fail in these patients because the shortened esophagus must be pulled down into the abdominal cavity to perform the wrap, leaving the wrap under tension and susceptible to slippage or complete disruption. Two procedures, the Collis-Belsey gastroplasty and the Collis-Nissen gastroplasty have produced good results in this patient population.[99,100] In both procedures, the cardia and proximal fundus are tubularized and serve as an elongation of the esophagus. Fundoplication is then accomplished around this length of tubularized proximal stomach. Results are good in 50 to 80% of cases.

In patients with strictures unresponsive to recurrent dilatation, resection of the involved esophageal portion may be necessary. This is combined with interposition of other luminal organs such as the colon or jejunum,[101–103] or mobilization of the stomach, with esophagogastric anastomosis in the chest. Gastric pull-up with pyloroplasty is the more common procedure, largely because of the need for only one anastomosis. Good to excellent function is described in 70% of patients with an operative mortality rate less than 5%.[104] Left colonic interposition has been advocated for young patients because of reported superior long-term functionality relative to gastric or jejunal interposition.[105] However, this procedure is technically more demanding, with a higher operative morbidity rate.

Laparoscopic antireflux surgery in patients with medically refractory esophageal strictures generally results in a good clinical outcome with minimal complications. Approaches to management of peptic stricture such as laparoscopic Nissen fundoplication have shown a high rate of success.[106] Initial concern that the esophagus could not be mobilized or the stricture fully assessed using such techniques has not been realized as experience has accumulated. Laparoscopic experience with esophageal resection and lengthening is recorded, but definitive studies of their safety and efficacy in GERD patients are lacking.

A long-term follow-up study of a prospective randomized trial of medical and surgical antireflux treatments in patients with complicated GERD revealed that patients in the medical and surgical groups were equally likely to have developed strictures or to have subsequent antireflux surgery.[107] Sixty-two percent of the surgically treated patients and 92% of the medically treated patients reported ongoing use of medications for control of GERD symptoms. Overall, no significant difference was noted between the medical and the surgical groups in satisfaction with their antireflux therapy. Patients undergoing antireflux surgery should be advised that they may need to take antisecretory medications following the procedure.

Key Points: Esophageal Complications of Gastroesophageal Reflux Disease

- ❧ Esophageal complications of GERD, including stricture, ulceration, and bleeding, are commonly encountered.
- ❧ A rigorous antireflux program with PPIs is important for secondary prevention of these complications.
- ❧ Improvements in the management of stricture patients include over-the-wire and through-the-scope dilating systems.
- ❧ A series of carefully graduated dilatations is usually successful in resolving symptoms of dysphagia.
- ❧ Maintenance of patients with peptic strictures on chronic acid suppression with PPIs improves symptoms and decreases need for recurrent dilatation. Nonetheless, a small proportion of patients may go on to require surgery.
- ❧ The choice of surgical procedure is dependent on the characteristics of the patient and stricture, combined with the experience of the surgeon.

Suggested Readings

1. el-Serag HB, Sonnenberg A: Associations between forms of gastro-oesophageal reflux disease. Gut 41:594–599, 1997.

2. Monhemuller KE, Wilcox CM: Diagnosis of esophageal ulcers in acquired immun-odeficiency syndrome. Semin Gastrointest Dis 10:85–92, 1999.
3. Wilson CM, Straub RF, Schwartz DA: Prospective endoscopic characterization of cy-tomegalovirus esophagitis in AIDS. Gastrointest Endoscop 40:481–484, 1994.
4   Wilson CM, Schwartz DA: Endoscopic characterization of idiopathic esophageal ul-ceration associated with human immunodeficiency virus infection. J Clin Gastroen-terol 16:251–256, 1993.
5. Pearson FG, Cooper JD, Patterson GA, Prakash D: Peptic ulcer in acquired colum-nar-lined esophagus: Results of surgical treatment. Ann Thorac Surg 43:241–244, 1987.
6. Komorowski RA, Hogan WJ, Chausow DD: Barrett's ulcer: the clinical significance today. Am J Gastroenterol 91:2310–2313, 1996.
7. Altorki NK, Skinner DB, Segalin A, Stephens JK, Ferguson MK, et al: Indications for esophagectomy in nonmalignant Barrett's esophagus: A 10-year experience. Ann Thorac Surg 49:724–726, 1990.
8. Cappell MS, Sciales C, Biempica L: Esophageal perforation at a Barrett's ulcer. Clin Gastroenterol 11:663–666, 1989.
9. Kikendall JW: Pill-induced esophageal injury. Gastroenterol Clin North Am 20:835–846, 1991.
10. Spechler SJ: Epidemiology and natural history of gastro-oesophageal reflux disease. Digestion 51(suppl 1):24–29, 1992.
11. Voululainer M, Sipponen P Mecklin JP, et al: Gastroesophageal reflux diseases: Prevalence, clinical, endoscopic, and histopathological findings in 1,128 consecu-tive patients referred for endoscopy due to dyspeptic and reflux symptoms. Diges-tion 61:6–13, 2000.
12. Wara P: Incidence, diagnosis, and natural cause of upper gastrointestinal hemor-rhage: Prognostic value of clinical factors and endoscopy. Scand J Gastroenterol 137(suppl):26–27, 1987.
13. Sugawa C, Steffes CP, Nakamura R, et al: Upper GI bleeding in an urban hospital: Etiology, recurrence, and prognosis. Ann Surg 212:521–526, 1990.
14. Zimmerman J, Shohat V, Tsvang E, et al: Esophagitis is a major cause of upper gas-trointestinal hemorrhage in the elderly. Scand J Gastroenterol 32:906–909, 1997.
15. Orchard JL, Stromat J, Wolfgang M, Trumpey A: Upper gastrointestinal tract bleed-ing in institutionalized mentally retarded adults. Arch Fam Med 4:30–33, 1995.
16. Weston AP: Hiatal hernia with Cameron ulcers and erosions [review].Gastrointest Endosc Clin North Am 6:671–679, 1996.
17. Cameron AJ, Higgins JA: Linear gastric erosions: A lesion associated with large di-aphragmatic hernia and chronic blood loss anemia. Gastroenterology 91:338–342, 1986.
18. Cameron AJ: Incidence of iron deficiency anemia in patients with large diaphrag-matic hernia: A controlled study. Mayo Clin Proc 51:767–769, 1976.
19. DeVault KR: Lower esophageal (Schatzki's) ring: Pathogenesis, diagnosis, and ther-apy. Dig Dis 14:323–329, 1996.
20. Marshall JB, Kretschmar JM, Diaz-Arias AA: Gastroesophageal reflux as a pathogenic factor in the development of lower esophageal rings. Arch Intern Med 150:1669–1672, 1990.
21. Echardt VF, Kanzler G, Willems D: Single dilatation of symptomatic Schatzki's ring: A prospective evaluation of its effectiveness. Dig Dis Sci 37:557–582, 1992.
22. Groshreutz JL, Kim CH: Schatzki's ring: long-term results following dilatations. Gas-trointest Endosc 36:479–481, 1990.
23. Disaria JA, Pederson PJ, Bichi-Canoulus C, et al: Incision of distal esophageal (Schatzki) ring after dilatation. Gastrointest Endosc 56:244–248, 2002.

24. Marks RD, Shukla M: Diagnosis and management of peptic esophageal strictures. Gastroenterologist 4:223–227, 1996.

25. Sonnenberg A, Massy BT, Jacobsen SJ: Hospital discharges resulting form esophagitis among Medicare beneficiaries. Dig Dis Sci 39:183–188, 1994.

26. el-Serag HB, Sonnenberg A: Association of esophagitis and esophageal strictures with diseases treated with nonsteroidal anti-inflammatory drugs. Am J Gastroenterol 92:52–56, 1997.

27. Kim SL, Hunter JG, Wo JM, Davis LP, Waring JP: NSAIDS, aspirin, and esophageal strictures: Are over-the-counter medications harmful to the esophagus? J Clin Gastroenterol 29:32–34, 1999.

28. Richter JE: Gastroesophageal reflux disease in the older patient: Presentation, treatment, and complications. Am J Gastroenterol 95:368–373, 2000.

29. Cioffi U, Rosso L, de Simone M: Gastroesophageal reflux disease: Pathogenesis, symptoms, and complications. Panminerva Med 40:132–138, 1998.

30. Winwood PJ, Mavrogiannis CC, Smith CL: Reduced sensitivity to intra-oesophageal acid in patients with reflux-induced strictures. Scand J Gastroenterol 28:109–112, 1993.

31. Parkman HP, Fisher RS: Contributing role of motility abnormalities in the pathogenesis of Gastroesophageal reflux disease. Dig Dis 15(suppl 1):40–52, 1997.

32. Bell NJ, Burget D, Howden CW, et al: Appropriate acid suppression for the management of gastro-oesaphageal reflux disease. Digestion 51 (suppl):59–67, 1992.

33. Morrow JB, Vargo JJ, Golblum JR, Richter JE: The ringed esophagus: Histological features of GERD. Am J Gastroenterol 96:984–989, 2001.

34. Jasperson D, Schwacha H, Schoor W, et al: Omeprazole in the treatment of patients with complicated gastro-oesaphogeal. J Gastroenterol Hepatol 11:900–902, 1996.

35. Martinez-Serna T, Tercero F, Filipi CJ, et al: Symptom priority ranking in the case of gastroesophageal reflux: A review of 1850 cases. Dig Dis 17:219–224, 1999.

36. Longstreth GF, Longstreth KJ, Jao JK: Esophageal food impaction: Epidemiology and therapy—A retrospective, observational study. Gastrointest Endosc 53:193–198, 2001.

37. Wilcox CM, Alexander LN, Clark WS: Localization of an obstructing esophageal lesion: Is the patient accurate? Dig Dis Ser 11:2192–2196, 1995.

38. Kim SL, Wo JM, Hunter JG, et al: The prevelance of intestinal metaplasia in patients with and without peptic strictures. Am J Gastroenterol 93:53–55, 1998.

39. Halpert RD, Feczko PJ, Spickler EM, Ackerman LV: Radiologogical assessment of dysphagia with endoscopic correlation. Radiology 157:599–602, 1985.

40. Ghanremani GC, Weingardt JP, Curtin KR, Vaghmai V: Detection of occult esophageal narrowing with a barium tablet during chect radiography. Clin Imaging 20:184–190, 1996.

41. van Western D, Ekberg O: Solid bolus swallowing in the radiologic evaluation of dysphagia. Acta Radiol 34:372–375, 1993.

42. Castell DO, Katz PO: Approach to the patient with dysphagia and odynophagia. In Yamada T, ed. Textbook of Gastroenterology, 3rd ed. Philadelphia, JB Lippincott, 1999 pp 683–693.

43. Gupta SD, Petrus LV, Gibbins FJ, Delliapiani AW: Endoscopic evaluation of dysphagia in the elderly. Ageing 16:159–164, 1987.

44. Dakkak M, Hoare RC, Maslin SC, Benneett JR: Oesophagitis is as important as oesophageal stricture diameter in determining dysphagia. Gut 34:152–155, 1993.

45. Ferguson R, Dronfield MW, Atkinson M: Cimetidine in the treatment of reflux oesaphagitis with peptic stricture. Br Med J 25:472–474, 1979.

46. Starlinger M, Appel WH, Schemper M, Schiessel R: Long-term treatment of peptic esophageal stenosis with with dilatation and cimetidine: Factors that influnce clinical results. Eur Surg Res 17:207–214, 1985.

47. Smith PM, Kerr GD, Cockel R, et al: A comparison of omeprazole and ranitidine in the prevention of recurrence of benign esophageal stricture. Restore Investigator Group. Gastroenterology 107:1312–1318, 1994.

48. Colin-Jones DG: The role and limitations of H₂-receptor antagonists in the treatment of gastro-oesophageal reflux diseases. Aliment Pharmacol Ther 9(suppl 1):9–14, 1995.

49. Klinkenberg-Knol EC, Festen HP, Meuwissen SG: Pharmacological management of gastro-oesophageal reflux disease. Drugs 49:695–710, 1995.

50. Freston JW, Malagelada JR, Petersen H, McCLoy RF: Critical issues in the management of gastroesopahgeal reflux diseases. Eur J Gastroenterol Hepatol 7:577–586, 1995.

51. Swarbrick ET, Gough AL, Foster CS, et al: Prevention of recurrence of esophageal stricture, a comparison of lansoprazole and high-dose ranitidine. Eur J Gastroenterol Hepatol 8:431–438, 1996.

52. Barberzat GO, Schlup M, Lubike R: Omeprazole therapy decreases the need for dilation of peptic oesophageal strictures. Aliment Pharmacol Ther 13:1041–1048, 1999.

53. Marks RD, Richter JE, Rizzo J, et al: Omeprazole versus H₂-receptor antagonists in treating patients with peptic stricture and esophagitis. Gastroenterology 106:907–915, 1994.

54. Earlam R, Cunha-Melo JR: Benign oesophageal strictures: Historical and technical aspects of dilatation. Br J Surg 68:829–836, 1981.

55. Swaroop VS, Desai DC, Mohandeas KM, et al: Dilation of esophageal strictures induced by radiation. Gastrointest Endosc 40:311–315, 1994.

56. Saeed ZA, Ramirez FC, Hepps KS, et al: An objective end point for dilatation improves outcome of peptic esophageal strictures: A prospective randomized trial. Gastrointest Endosc 45:354–359, 1997.

57. Eckardt VF, Kanzler G, Willems D: Single dilation of symptomatic Schatzki rings: A prospective evaluation of its effectiveness. Dig Dis Sci 37:577–582, 1992.

58. Glick ME: Clinical course of esophageal stricture managed by bougienage. Dig Dis Sci 27:884–888, 1982.

59. Patterson DJ, Graham DY, Smith JL, et al: Natural history of benign esophageal stricture treated by dilatation. Gastroenterology 85:346–350, 1983.

60. Tucker LE: The importance of fluoroscopic guidance for Maloney dilatation. Am J Gastroenterol 87:1709–1711, 1992.

61. McClave SA, Brady PG, Wright RA, et al: Does fluoroscopic guidance for Maloney esophageal dilation impact on the clinical endpoint of therapy: Relief of dysphagia and achievement of luminal patency? Gastrointest Endosc 43:93–97, 1996.

62. Ho SB, Cass O, Katsman RJ, et al: Fluoroscopy is not necessary for Maloney dilation of chronic esophageal strictures. Gastrointest Endosc 41:11–14, 1995.

63. Bozymski EM, Shaheen NJ: Wire-guided dilation and fluoroscopy: Is seeing believing. Am J Gastroenterol 91:1486–1487, 1996.

64. Grobe JL, Kozarek RA, Sanowski RA: Self-bougienage in the treatment of benign esophageal stricture. J Clin Gastroenterol 6:109–112, 1984.

65. Bapat RD, Bakhshi GD, Kanthasia CV, et al: Self-bougienage: Long-term relief of corrosive esophageal stricture. Indian J Gastroenterol 20:180–182, 2001.

66. Heiser MC: Esophageal self-dilatation: Interdisciplinary responsibilities for a comprehensive treatment plan. Gastroenterol Nurs 12:246–249, 1990.

67. Saeed ZA, Winchester CB, Ferro PS, et al: Prospective randomized comparison of polyvinyl bougies and through-the-scope balloons for dilatation of peptic strictures of the esophagus. Gastrointest Endosc 41:189–195, 1995.

68. Cox JG, Winter RK, Maslin SC, et al: Balloon or bougie for dilatation of benign esophageal stricture? Dig Dis Sci 39:776–781, 1994.

69. McLean GK, Leveen RF: Shear stress in the performance of esophageal dilation: Comparison of balloon dilation and bougienage. Radiology 172:983–986, 1989.

70. Kozarek RA: Hydrostatic balloon dilatation of gastrointestinal stenoses: A national survey. Gastrointest Endosc 32:15–19, 1986.

71. O'Sullivan GC, O'Brien MG: Successful retrograde dilatation and oesophageal conservation after failed antegrade management of a reflux stricture. Endoscopy 29:141, 1997.

72. Bueno R, Swanson SJ, Jaklitsch MT, et al: Combined antegrade and retrograde dilation: A new endoscopic technique in the management of complex esophageal obstruction. Gastrointest Endosc 45:368–372, 2001.

73. Kubuk CM, Polhamus CD, Clement DJ: Endoscopic steroid injection therapy for refractory esophageal strictures. Am J Gastroenterology 89:A1621, 1994.

74. Silvis SE, Nebel O, Rogers, et al: Endoscopic complications: Results of the 1974 American Society for Gastrointestinal Endoscopy Survey. JAMA 235:928–930, 1976.

75. Marks RD, Richter JE: Peptic strictures of the esophagus. Am J Gastroenterol 88:1160–1173, 1993.

76. Dumon JF, Meric B, Sivak MVJ, Fleischer D: A new method of esophageal dilation using Savary-Gilliard bougies. Gastrointest Endosc 31:379–382, 1985.

77. Clouse RE: Complications of endoscopic gastrointestinal dilation techniques. Gastrointest Endosc Clin North Am 6:323–341, 1996.

78. Marchall JB, Afridi SA, King PD, et al: Esophageal dilation with polyvinyl (American) dilators over a marked guidewire: practice and safety at one center over a 5-yr period. Am J Gastroenterol 91:1503–1506, 1996.

79. Hernandez LJ, Jacobsen JW, Harris MS: Comparison among the perforation rates of Maloney, balloon, and Savary dilation of esophageal strictures. Gastrointest Endosc 51:460–462, 2000.

80. Kozarek RA: Esophageal dilatation and prostheses. Endosc Rev 4:9–14, 1987.

81. Nelson DB, Sanderson SJ, Azar MM: Bacteremia with esophageal dilation. Gastrointest Endosc 48:563–567, 1999.

82. Coles EF, Reed WW, Tighe JF Jr: Bacterial meningitis occurring after esophageal dilation in an otherwise healthy patient. Gastrointest Endosc 38:384–385, 1992.

83. Ersahin Y, Mutluer S, Cakir Y: Multiple brain abscesses following esophageal dilation. Child Nerv Syst 11:351–353, 1995.

84. Harp DL, Schlitt M, Williams JP, Shamoun JM: Brain abscess following dilation of esophageal stricture. Clin Imaging 13:140–141, 1989.

85. ASGE: Infection control during gastrointestinal endoscopy 1999; 49:836–841.

86. Yamamoto H, Hughes RWJ, Schroeder KW, Viggiano TR, DiMagno EP: Treatment of benign esophageal stricture by Eder-Puestow or balloon dilators: A comparison between randomized and prospective nonrandomized trials. Mayo Clin Proc 67: 228–236, 1992.

87. Ogilvie AL, Ferguson R, Atkinson M: Outlook with conservative treatment of peptic oesophageal stricture. Gut 56:23–25, 1980.

88. Hands LG, Dennison AR, Paparramides S, McIntyre RL, Bishop H, et al: The natural history of peptic oesophageal stricture treated by dilation and antirflux therapy alone. Ann R Coll Surg Engl 371:306–309, 1989.

89. Wesdorp IC, Bartelsman JF, den Hartog J, et al: Results of conservative treatment of benign esophageal strictures: a follow-up study in 100 patients. Gastroenterology 82:487–493, 1982.

90. Agnew SR, Panya SP, Reynolds RP, Preiksaitis HG: Predictors for frequent esophageal dilations of benign peptic strictures. Dig Dis Sci 41:931–936, 1996.

91. Moores DW, Ilves R: Treatment of esophageal obstruction with covered, self-expanding esophageal wallstents. Ann Thorac Surg 62:963–967, 1996.

92. Sheikh RA, Trudeau WL: Expandable metallic stent placement in patients with benign esophageal strictures: Results of long-term follow-up. Gastrointest Endosc 48:227–229, 1998.

93. Song HY, Park SI, Do YS, Yoon HK, Sung KB, et al: Expandable metallic stent placement in patients with benign esophageal strictures: Results of long-term follow-up. Radiology 203:131–136, 1997.

94. Hramiec JE, O'Shea MA, Quinlan RM: Expandable metallic esophageal stents in benign disease: A cause for concern. Surg Laparosc Endoc 8:40–43, 1998.

95. Booth M, Stratfordt J, Dehn TC: Preoperative esophageal body motility does not influence the outcome of laparoscopic Nissen fundoplication for gastroesophageal reflux disease. Dis Esophagus 15:57–60, 2002.

96. Beckingham IJ, Couem AK, Bornman PC, et al: Oesophageal dysmotility is not associated with poor outcome after laparoscopic Nissen fundoplication. Br J Surg 86:969, 1999.

97. Ellis FHJ, Garabedian M, Gibb SP: Fundoplication for gastroesophageal reflux: Indications, surgical technique, and manometric results. Arch Surg 103:186–192, 1973.

98. Skinner DB: Benign esophageal strictures. Adv Surg 10:177–196, 1976.

99. Richardson JD, Richardson RL: Collis-Nissen gastroplasty for shortened esophagus: Long-term evaluation. Ann Surg 227:735–740, 1998.

100. Beggs FD, Salama FD, Knowles KR: Management of benign oesophageal stricture by total fundoplication gastroplasty. J R Coll Surg Edinburgh 40:305–307, 1995.

101. Mansour KA, Bryan FC, Carlson GW: Bowel interposition for esophageal replacement: Twenty-five year experience. Ann Thorac Surg 64:752–756, 1997.

102. Picchio M, Lomabardi A, Zolovkins A, et al: Jejunal interposition for peptic stenosis of the esophagus following esophagomyotomy for achalasia. Int Surg 82:198–200, 1997.

103. Thomas P, Fuentes P, Guideiceelli R, Reboud E: Colon interposition for esophageal replacement: Current indications and long-term function. Ann Thorac Surg 64:757–764, 1997.

104. Orringer MB, Marshall B, Stirling MC: Tranhiatal esophagectomy for benign and malignant disease. J Thorac Cardiovasc Surg 105:265–276, 1993.

105. Ahmad SA, Sylvester KG, Hebra A, et al: Esophageal replacement using the colon: Is it a good choice? J Ped Surg 31:1026–1030, 1996.

106. Spivak H, Farrell TM, Trus TL, et al: Laparoscopic fundoplication for dysphagia and peptic esophageal stricture. J Gastrointest Surg 2:550–560, 1998.

107. Spechler SJ, Lee F, Ahnen D, et al: Long-term outcome of medical and surgical therapies for gastroesophageal reflux disease: Follow-up of a randomized controlled trial. JAMA 285:2331–2338, 2001.

Erosive Esophagitis

Jaime A. Oviedo, M.D., and
M. Michael Wolfe, M.D.

chapter
5

The concept of *peptic esophagitis* dates back to 1935, when Winkelstein suggested that gastric secretions were the cause of the damage observed in the esophageal mucosal lining of some patients.[1] The term *reflux esophagitis* was introduced in 1946 to describe esophageal mucosal injury resulting from irritant gastric juices refluxed from the stomach into the esophagus.[2] Today, the terms *peptic, reflux,* and *erosive esophagitis* are used interchangeably to describe a condition experienced by a subset of patients with gastroesophageal reflux disease (GERD) in whom histopathologically demonstrable changes in esophageal mucosa usually correlate with symptoms of acid reflux.[3] Esophageal mucosal damage is thought to be caused by the reflux of gastric contents, principally acid and pepsin, into the esophagus. The severity of the epithelial injury is generally assessed by the presence of symptoms or endoscopic signs.

Gastroesophageal reflux disease is widely reported to be one of the most prevalent clinical conditions affecting the gastrointestinal tract; however, figures on the incidence and prevalence of GERD and esophagitis are based more on estimates than on actual data. Estimates of the prevalence of GERD in the adult population range from 21 to 44%.[4,5] When ambulatory esophageal pH measurements are used to define the presence of gastroesophageal reflux, 48% to 79% of patients with GERD have esophagitis,[6,7] which suggests a 3% to 4% prevalence of esophagitis in the general population, and about 5% in individuals 55 years of age or older.[8,9]

Although little information is available regarding the incidence of the different stages of esophagitis, existing data suggest that most patients suffer mild or moderate forms of the disease. With the exception of pregnant women, in whom the incidence of heartburn is as high as 79%, the analysis of the sex ratio of GERD shows equal proportions of affected males and females but a male preponderance of esophagitis (2:1 to 3:1).[8,3]

In addition to GERD, a variety of infectious agents, systemic illness, medications, and environmental agents have been associated with the

TABLE 1. Possible Causes of Erosive Esophagitis
Gastroesophageal reflux disease
Infections
Fungal (candida)
Viral (cytomegalovirus, herpes virus, human immunodeficiency virus)
Bacterial (*Nocardia,* syphilis)
Mycobacterium (tuberculosis, avium)
Parasitic (Chagas' disease, leishmania)
Systemic illness
Skin disorder (epidermolysis bullosa, pemphigus, drug-induced)
Behçet's disease
Graft-versus-host disease
Inflammatory bowel disease
Sarcoidosis
Metastatic cancer
Collagen vascular disease
Medications
Pill esophagitis (antibiotics, potassium chloride, bisphosphonates)
Chemotherapy esophagitis
Radiation esophagitis
Sclerosant therapy for varices
Trauma
Nasogastric tube injury

development of erosive esophagitis (Table 1). This chapter focuses on the current knowledge and management issues pertaining to erosive esophagitis caused by GERD, also known as *reflux esophagitis.*

Pathophysiology

Although intra-abdominal (gastric) pressure exceeds intrathoracic (esophageal) pressure by approximately 10 mm Hg throughout most of the day, the intraesophageal pH of normal volunteers drops below 4.0 for less than 5% of the total time, as a result of an effective antireflux barrier at the esophagogastric junction.[10] In addition to the mechanical barrier formed by the lower esophageal sphincter (LES), efficient esophageal clearance mechanisms, as well as salivary and epithelial buffering mechanisms, maintain the integrity of the distal esophageal mucosa. When this barrier fails, gastric refluxate bathes the esophageal mucosa for extended periods, and symptoms and inflammation occur.[11] GERD is thus a primarily a motor disorder caused by abnormal LES function, a gastric emptying disorder, or failed esophageal peristalsis.[12]

The mechanisms of LES malfunction that have been identified in the literature include transient LES relaxations, hypotensive or incompetent LES, and anatomic disruption of the esophagogastric junction (i.e., hiatal hernia). Excessive acid exposure in the distal esophagus and a reduction of the esophageal pH below 4.0 can be detected in 75% to 90% of patients with erosive esophagitis.[13,14] Repeated events of acid reflux are associated with the continued presence of esophageal erosions, and a greater duration of abnormal acid exposure correlates with increased severity of inflammation.[15]

Although reflux caused by transient LES relaxations is common under physiologic conditions, patients with symptomatic GERD have a higher likelihood of experiencing significant acid reflux during transient relaxations. More severe GERD, or GERD combined with erosive esophagitis, esophageal stricture, or Barrett's epithelium, may be associated with a hypotensive or incompetent sphincter. LES hypotension may be aggravated by a number of external factors, including foods such as fat, chocolate, and mint; medications such as oral contraceptives, narcotic analgesics, oral β_2 agonists, anticholinergics, and calcium-channel blockers; smoking; and pregnancy.[16]

Hiatal hernias can also compromise the LES[17–19] and are commonly associated with GERD. Patients with GERD and hiatal hernias have greater esophageal acid exposure than patients without them.[20,21] Whether hiatal hernia is a causal factor or a consequence of esophagitis remains unclear.

Recent studies have suggested that impaired esophageal clearance of refluxed material during sleep contributes to the development of reflux esophagitis. Patients with erosive esophagitis demonstrated abnormal nocturnal reflux on 24-hour esophageal pH monitoring.[22] There is also evidence suggesting that patients with severe esophagitis have more frequent episodes of nocturnal acid reflux and longer mucosal acid exposure during sleep than patients with milder forms of GERD.[23] The number of nocturnal reflux episodes lasting greater than 5 minutes, as documented on 24-hour pH monitoring, can thus be used to discriminate between patients with erosive and those with nonerosive GERD.[24] The factors involved in the pathogenesis of GERD are summarized in Table 2.

Clinical Presentation

Although clinical history is the cornerstone of the diagnosis of GERD and esophagitis, the symptoms do not always correlate with the degree of acid exposure or with the presence or absence of esophagitis. Heartburn (pyrosis), a burning sensation beginning in the retrosternal area and radiating under the sternum toward the neck, is widely recognized as the key clinical symptom. However, because "heartburn" is a commonly used lay term with variable meaning among patients, physicians

TABLE 2.	Pathogenesis of Gastroesophageal Reflux Disease

- Motility factors
  - Lower esophageal sphincter
    - Decreased resting pressure
    - Excessive spontaneous relaxations
  - Hiatal hernia
  - Esophageal dysmotility
    - Decrease amplitude of peristaltic contractions
    - Aperistalsis
  - Gastroparesis
  - Antropyloriduodenal dysmotility
    - Excessive bile reflux
- Nonmotility factors
  - Acid hypersecretion
  - Bile reflux

must take time to determine precisely whether the patient is truly describing acid reflux and not dyspepsia (abdominal discomfort) or abdominal pain. Heartburn may be exacerbated by eating certain foods, bending, or lying down, and it may be relieved, at least transiently, by the ingestion of antacids.

Regurgitation, another symptom classically associated with GERD, is defined as the passive movement of chyme across the esophagogastric junction into the esophagus, often extending into the mouth and resulting in a bitter or acidic taste.[25] Regurgitation may be aggravated by recumbency during sleep or by increased intra-abdominal pressure during straining at defecation, coughing, exercise, or bending over. Water brash, an infrequent symptom of GERD, describes a sensation of increased warm liquid in the mouth that may occur simultaneously with heartburn. Although this symptom is often attributed to regurgitation of chyme extending up to the oropharynx, in fact, water brash is due to an esophagosalivary reflex triggered by acidification or distention of the distal end of the esophagus.[11] Nighttime symptoms are common in patients with GERD and may be related, at least in part, to a nocturnal reduction in esophageal protective mechanisms, including esophageal acid clearance, peristaltic activity, and saliva production.[12] Nocturnal heartburn is also associated with a higher incidence of esophagitis and an increased risk of stricture formation.[24]

Untreated erosive esophagitis may lead to the development of a benign distal esophageal stricture.[26] Patients with strictures initially complain of dysphagia (difficulty swallowing) for solids but eventually may also experience difficulty with soft foods and even liquids. Patients who experience dysphagia in the absence of stricture should be investigated for possible esophageal dysmotility syndromes such as scleroderma. Rarely, decreased salivation, when extreme, as in the case of patients with Sjögren's syndrome, may also result in increased resistance to the movement of a food bolus out of the oropharynx and through the esophagus.

Patients with erosive esophagitis may present with acute or chronic bleeding from inflamed esophageal mucosa. Esophagitis is one of the more common causes of upper gastrointenstinal bleeding in critically ill patients in intensive care units. The cause of this problem remains unclear, since most patients in this setting are treated with antisecretory agents. Esophageal acid irritation caused by a nasogastric tube and the presence of nonacid refluxed materials, with irritants such as bile salts from duodenogastric reflux. have been postulated as possible explanations.[27,28] Chronic bleeding is usually mild but may lead to iron deficiency anemia with consequent symptoms of fatigue, weakness, and shortness of breath.[11] Although, as stated earlier, the severity of symptoms does not reliably predict the presence or absence of esophageal mucosal injury, patients with erosive esophagitis commonly demonstrate complete or marked resolution of symptoms in association with healing of erosions.[15,29,30]

Diagnosis

In patients with uncomplicated GERD, additional testing to establish the diagnosis is typically unnecessary. It is reasonable to consider an empiric trial of antisecretory therapy in a patient with classic symptoms of GERD (acid regurgitation, heartburn) in the absence of "alarm signs." Such an approach is appealing based on simplicity, cost, and lack of invasive testing. "Alarm signs," such as weight loss, dysphagia, odynophagia, hematemesis, melena, or iron deficiency anemia, should immediately prompt further testing for complications of GERD, including esophagitis, esophageal stricture, and adenocarcinoma. Endoscopy is usually indicated to evaluate those patients with alarm signs, those who do not respond to empiric therapy, and as a one–time screening tool to evaluate for the presence of Barrett's esophagus.

Although a double contrast barium esophagogram may be more sensitive for detecting a subtle esophageal ring, most cases of low-grade esophagitis will be missed by this modality. Therefore, a normal radiograph will rarely preclude the need for a subsequent endoscopic examination. Conversely, once an endoscopic examination has been done, it is unusual to require any other testing before appropriate therapy is instituted.[3]

Endoscopy is diagnostic of erosive GERD, with a specificity of 90% to 95% if esophagitis is present. Most false-positive diagnoses are attributable to either infectious or pill-induced mucosal injury. Although symptoms and mucosal injury do not necessarily correlate with one another, patients with erosive esophagitis tend to show a better correlation between symptoms and endoscopic findings, as well as a more predictable response to therapy, than patients with nonerosive (endoscopy-negative) reflux disease.[15,31] Additional diagnostic techniques, such as ambulatory 24-hour esophageal pH monitoring, are thus less useful in cases in which esophagitis has been documented by endoscopy.

Esophageal pH testing is a useful test to document esophageal acid exposure in patients with atypical symptoms not responding to therapy. In general, pH testing should take place after discontinuation of antisecretory agents, unless the purpose of the test is to determine the adequacy of therapy.[12]

Esophageal manometry has little, if any, role in the routine evaluation of patients with esophagitis. Although a variety of manometric abnormalities have been described in cases of GERD, including a hypotensive LES and ineffective esophageal peristalsis, such findings are not helpful in diagnosis. Manometry is, however, essential for accurate probe placement during pH monitoring and is often recommended for those individuals in whom surgical or endoscopic therapy is being considered.

An accurate description of endoscopic findings is essential in cases of GERD. The term *esophagitis* is nonspecific and should no longer be used in endoscopy reports without a detailed description of the findings. Numerous systems are available for the endoscopic grading of esophagitis (Table 3),[32–34] but none is universally accepted, and questions regarding interobserver consistency describing the severity of esophagitis have been raised, especially in mild cases (low-grade).[35] Most recent studies have, however, reported good reproducibility in grading esophagitis by endoscopy and an adequate correlation between the Los Angeles classification and the clinical severity of esophagitis.[36]

The diagnostic tests commonly used in the evaluation of patients with GERD and esophagitis are summarized in Table 4.

Treatment

Complete symptom relief and mucosal healing should be the goal in all individuals with GERD, although it is now clear that the majority of individuals with acid reflux disease have mild-to-moderate, intermittent symptoms, usually in the absence of esophageal mucosal injury. This section focuses on the treatment of erosive esophagitis, including strategies to achieve mucosal healing, symptom relief, prevention and treat-

TABLE 3. Grading Systems for Erosive Esophagitis

Los Angeles Classification	Hetzel-Dent Classification	
A One (or more) mucosal break no longer than 5 mm that does not extend between the tops of two mucosal folds	Grade 0	No mucosal abnormalities
	Grade 1	Erythema, hyperemia or mucosal friability
B One (or more) mucosal break more than 5 mm long that does not extend between the tops of two mucosal folds	Grade 2	Superficial erosions involving <10% of mucosal surface of the last 5 cm of esophageal mucosa
C One (or more) mucosal break that is continuous between the tops of two or more mucosal folds but involves <75% of the circumference	Grade 3	Superficial erosions or ulceration involving 105 to 50% of the mucosal surface of the last 5 cm of esophageal squamous mucosa
D One (or more) mucosal break that involves at least 75% of the esophageal circumference	Grade 4	Deep ulceration anywhere in the esophagus or confluent erosion of >50% of the mucosal surface of the last 5 cm of esophageal squamous mucosa.

ment of complications of erosive GERD (i.e., esophageal strictures), and maintenance of remission. The management of nonerosive GERD is discussed elsewhere in this textbook.

Therapy for GERD can be approached in two different fashions. The correction of the mechanisms involved in the pathogenesis of GERD includes a reduction in the frequency of transient LES relaxations and an improvement of esophageal clearance to minimize the exposure of the esophagus to acidic gastric contents. The more commonly used ap-

TABLE 4. Diagnostic Tests in the Evaluation of Gastroesophageal Reflux Disease

Endoscopy
    Alarm signs or symptoms
    Evaluation of esophagitis or strictures
    Screening of Barrett's esophagus
24-hour esophageal pH monitoring
    Gastroesophageal reflux disease symptoms not responding to therapy
    Prior to antireflux surgery
Barium swallow
    Evaluation of subtle anatomic anomalies (rings)
    Evaluation of short esophagus or fixed hiatal hernia
Esophageal manometry
    Assessment of dysmotility syndromes
    Prior to antireflux surgery

proach, however, employs the neutralization or suppression of gastric acid, whereby, despite the continued reflux of gastric contents into the esophagus, the refluxate is rendered nonirritating to the esophageal mucosa. This approach not only provides symptomatic relief but also treats and prevents mucosal injury.[37] In general, the physician should establish the severity and frequency of symptoms. Patients with mild and infrequent symptoms may need only reassurance, education regarding lifestyle modifications, and nonprescription medications. Those with more frequent and severe symptoms will probably benefit from prescription drug therapy.[12]

Pharmacologic Therapy

Relieving Symptoms and Healing Esophagitis

Antacids. Most antacid preparations contain different combinations of aluminum hydroxide magnesium hydroxide, and calcium salts. Gastric acidity is reduced by a chemical reaction between antacid constituents and hydrochloric acid. Antacids have a relatively brief duration of action (30 to 60 minutes) and thus need to be taken frequently. Although some clinical trials[38–40] did not demonstrate a statistically significant benefit of antacids in reducing the severity or frequency of heartburn or promoting healing of erosive esophagitis, others[41,42] have shown that antacids are associated with reductions in pain scores and global symptomatic relief. In a recent, large randomized study comparing an histamine$_2$-receptor antagonist (H$_2$RA)/antacid combination with antacid or famotidine alone, the antacid arm showed better symptom relief than the placebo arm.[43,44]

Antacids offer the advantage of prompt, although unsustained, relief and are now used exclusively as over-the-counter preparations to treat mild episodic heartburn. Alginic acid has been added to antacids in an attempt to improve efficacy. Antacid/alginate combinations produce a hydrophobic viscous layer that floats on the liquid meniscus within the stomach. Whether this viscous layer selectively delivers antacid into the esophagus during reflux episodes, acts as a mechanical barrier to diminish reflux quantitatively, or both, has not been clearly determined.[11] Most studies evaluating the effectiveness of alginate/antacid combination did not demonstrate any benefit of this agents when compared to antacid alone or to placebo.[43] One randomized, double-blind trial compared alginate/antacid with sucralfate. Sucralfate resulted in a higher rate of complete esophageal healing when compared with the antacid/alginate combination (53% vs 34%, respectively), but the difference was not statistically significant.[45]

Histamine$_2$-Receptor Antagonists. These agents are specific antagonists that inhibit gastric acid secretion competitively and reversibly by blocking the histamine receptor on the parietal cell basolateral membrane. H_2RAs have shown to be effective in relieving mild to moderate GERD symptoms, as well as in preventing postprandial symptoms, when taken 30 to 60 minutes before meals.[46] H_2RAs are also effective in healing erosive esophagitis. The rates of mucosal healing are clearly related to the initial severity of esophagitis, with rates approaching 80% for grade I-II esophagitis, and rates of only 30% to 50% for grade III-IV disease.[47] In patients with erosive esophagitis, most reflux episodes occur between the evening meal and midnight. However, although nocturnal administration of H_2RAs after dinner or at bedtime may be sufficient in patients with mild disease, patients with severe (grade II and IV) erosive esophagitis will require multiple doses per day.[37]

The H_2RAs are useful both in relieving symptoms and in healing esophagitis in individuals with mild-to-moderate acid reflux disease with intermittent symptoms, usually in the absence of esophageal mucosal injury. H_2RAs are often effective in patients with nocturnal breakthrough symptoms who are treated with proton pump inhibitors. The onset of action of H_2RAs is approximately 60 minutes, and thus combinations of antacids and H_2RAs have been formulated to provide both prompt and sustained symptom relief.

A variety of H_2RAs are available (e.g., nizatidine, famotidine, ranitidine, and cimetidine), both over-the-counter and in prescription dosages. There are some differences in potency and onset of action, but they are generally considered interchangeable. All four H_2RAs have a strong safety record, although cytochrome P_{450} interactions may be a problem, particularly when cimetidine is used in patients taking theophylline, warfarin, or phenytoin.[12]

Proton Pump Inhibitors (PPI). PPIs are the most potent inhibitors of gastric acid secretion available and are considered the drug class of choice for the treatment of patients with serious or refractory GERD. PPIs act by selectively inhibiting H^+, K^+-ATPase in the secretory canaliculus of the stimulated parietal cell. Because PPIs are most effective when the parietal cell is stimulated to secrete acid after a prolonged fast and in response to a meal, these agents are most effective when taken before the initial meal of the day (i.e., breakfast). PPIs inhibit only stimulated *active* proton pumps, with the potential to provide antisecretory activity for 24 hours, which allows once-daily dosing. Over time, inactive pumps are stimulated to become active, and new pumps are continually being synthesized by the parietal cells. Therefore, several days of PPI therapy are required to achieve a steady-state reduction in acid secretion, which explains why PPI therapy is generally ineffective when used "on demand." When therapy is discontinued, the pumps are fully regenerated in 3 to 7 days. Although rebound hyperacidity may occur following abrupt discontinuation of PPI therapy, the clinical significance of this phenomenon remains unclear.

Numerous studies have documented the efficacy of PPIs in controlling reflux symptoms and healing erosive esophagitis.[37] Pooled data from three studies including 653 patients treated with lansoprazole, 30 mg daily, in patients with grade II or worse esophagitis showed 80% to 90% healing at 4 weeks and 92% healing at 8 weeks.[48–50] When analyzed in comparative trials, the healing rates of erosive esophagitis in patients receiving PPIs are far superior to those treated with H_2RAs.[51] One trial comparing lansoprazole, 30 mg daily, and ranitidine, 300 mg twice daily, in patients with moderate-to-severe erosive GERD showed 91% healing in 8 weeks with lansoprazole compared with 66% healing for ranitidine.[52] PPIs are also effective in patients with GERD and esophagitis unresponsive to high dose H_2RA therapy. In patients refractory to cimetidine, 800 mg four times daily, or ranitidine, 300 mg three times daily, therapy with 40 mg of omeprazole in the morning healed esophagitis in 91% of patients studied.[53] In general, standard doses of PPIs (20 mg omeprazole, 30 mg lansoprazole, 20 mg rabeprazole, 40 mg pantoprazole, or 40 mg esomeprazole, all administered before breakfast) will heal esophagitis in approximately 85% to 90% of cases.[37]

Comparative studies have shown different PPIs to have similar efficacy in the treatment of GERD. A recent study comparing esomeprazole, the S-isomer of omeprazole, with lansoprazole for the healing of erosive esophagitis, randomized 5241 patients with endoscopically documented erosive esophagitis to receive 40 mg of esomeprazole ($n = 2624$) or 30 mg of lansoprazole ($n = 2617$) once daily before breakfast for up to 8 weeks. Esophagitis was healed in 92.6% of the patients in the esomeprazole group and 88.8% in the lansoprazole group.[54] The small difference found in such large group of patients highlights the clinical equivalence of these agents. Other studies comparing omeprazole with the newer PPIs in the treatment of GERD have reported similar efficacy in terms of heartburn control, healing rates, and relapse rates.[55] Clinical differences among the PPIs are small, and available data provide little justification for generally recommending one agent over another. However, as in all classes of medication, clinical responses may vary among individuals, with one PPI favored over the others.

The PPIs are remarkably effective in the treatment of esophageal strictures, a well-known complication of erosive esophagitis. The management of peptic strictures consists of endoscopic dilatation and antisecretory therapy to heal esophagitis. Comparative studies have shown that PPIs are more effective than H_2RAs in healing esophagitis, decreasing the number of esophageal dilatations required to relieve dysphagia, and preventing recurrent stricture development.[26,56]

Despite the efficacy of PPIs in controlling esophageal reflux, 25% of patients need more than the standard dosing to eliminate their symptoms or to heal their esophagitis.[57] In nonresponders, a careful history regarding the timing of PPI administration should be obtained. As stated previously, the optimal time is immediately before breakfast. Once the correct timing is established, a second dose of the PPI (before the evening meal) should be attempted initially before substituting with another PPI. If symptoms persist, patients should undergo an endoscopic evaluation, if not already done, and pH testing while on medication should be considered to confirm the presence of acid reflux and to assess the ability of the medications in effectively suppressing acid secretion. The use of H_2RAs at bedtime has been advocated for these patients,[58] but caution must be exercised because of the inhibitory effects of H_2antagonists on PPI prodrug activation. Recently, concerns about the development of tolerance to the effects of H_2-blockers after prolonged use have been raised. In a small prospective study,[59] evaluating the use of bedtime H_2RAs in addition to PPI therapy to control nocturnal acid breakthrough, 23 healthy volunteers and 20 GERD patients underwent ambulatory pH monitoring at baseline and after 2 weeks on PPI twice daily before meals (omeprazole 20 mg). Subsequently, all subjects received 28 days of PPI plus H_2RA at bedtime (ranitidine 300 mg), with repeat pH testing on days 1, 7, and 28. The administration of PPI plus 1 day of H_2RA was the only therapy that significantly decreased the percentage of time with gastric pH < 4 for the supine period compared with PPI twice daily alone ($P < 0.001$). There was no difference in the percentage of time with supine gastric pH < 4 between 2 weeks of PPI twice daily alone and either 1 week or 1 month of PPI plus bedtime H_2RA. The combination of H_2RA and PPI therapy reduced nocturnal acid breakthrough only with the introduction of therapy. Because of H_2RA tolerance, there is no difference in acid suppression between PPI twice daily and PPI twice daily plus H_2RA after 1 week of combination therapy.

Maintaining Remission

Because GERD is a chronic disorder, and since most patients with erosive esophagitis, especially those with severe cases, will relapse once therapy is discontinued,[60] maintenance therapy has emerged as an important management issue. Maintenance of remission usually requires the same type and dose of medication that healed the initial esophagitis. For many patients with reflux esophagitis, however, the prescribed PPI dose may be reduced after the initial 8 weeks of treatment, provided they continue to be asymptomatic.

H_2RA. Although H_2RAs are approved for short-term use, there is evidence suggesting that chronic maintenance therapy with these agents may be beneficial in preventing recurrence of erosive esophagitis.[61] However, chronic use of H_2RAs has been associated to the development of tolerance, with subsequent reduction in antisecretory response. The mechanism of this tolerance appears to be multifactorial and is related to, among other things, an increase in circulating gastrin and subsequent stimulation of the parietal cell. Tolerance occurs within 72 hours of oral therapy and is more marked with multiple daily doses than with a single evening dose regimen.[62–65]

Proton Pump Inhibitors. PPIs have produced significantly better rates of remission than H_2RAs or prokinetic agents.[66,67] A landmark study of maintenance therapy compared five regimens: ranitidine, cisapride, ranitidine plus cisapride, omeprazole, and omeprazole plus cisapride. All patients ($n = 175$) had esophagitis on initial endoscopic examination and were treated with 40 mg omeprazole daily for 8 weeks before starting one of the maintenance regimens ($n = 35$ for each group). After 12 months of treatment, remission was maintained in 80% of the omeprazole group versus 54% in the cisapride and 49% in the ranitidine groups. Ranitidine plus cisapride was significantly better than ranitidine alone (66% remission), and the combination of omeprazole plus cisapride was best of all, with an 89% remission rate; however, the latter combination was not significantly better than omeprazole alone (80%).[68] Because of an increased incidence of serious cardiac arrythmias, cisapride is no longer available in the United States and other nations. In long-term follow-up trials, individuals with erosive esophagitis on PPI therapy have been maintained in remission for up to 11 years, with episodes of recurrent esophagitis managed by transiently increasing the dose of omeprazole.[69]

Antireflux Surgery. Numerous surgical techniques have been developed to attempt to restore LES competence and decrease acid reflux. Partial or complete fundoplication may be performed with a laparoscopic or an open approach. The basic premise is that wrapping the gastric fundus around the abdominal portion of the esophagus promotes distal esophageal contraction, increases LES pressure, and reduces the amount of refluxate into the esophagus.[12] When performed appropriately, fundoplication heals erosive esophagitis and may lead to reversal of peptic strictures.

Several trials have demonstrated the efficacy of both PPI therapy and conventional fundoplication in healing erosive esophagitis. Because GERD is a chronic condition, however, erosive esophagitis is likely to recur, especially in severe cases, and the more relevant issue is thus the need for maintenance therapy. Randomized trials comparing the outcomes of PPI therapy with antireflux surgery in patients with erosive esophagitis have reported comparable rates of maintenance of remission and quality of life in both groups.[70,71]

There are no long-term controlled data available on the efficacy of laparoscopic fundoplication for maintaining esophagitis healing. Follow-up data on open fundoplication show that the outcomes are substantially better when the procedure is performed in referral centers by skilled surgeons.[72,73] There is no evidence to suggest any increased efficacy or durability of the laparoscopic method when compared to the conventional open technique.

Surgery has also been considered as an alternative to lifelong medical therapy. Available data indicate that approximately 40% of patients undergoing fundoplication are free of heartburn and do not require medical therapy after prolonged follow-up. The proportion of patients returning to medical therapy is substantial (11% to 32% in studies extending to 5 years and >60% at 10 years).[43] Although the mortality rate of antireflux surgery is low (<1%), many patients develop new symptoms after surgery. Dysphagia is a common complaint that is usually transient but can become persistent. Other less common symptoms include abdominal bloating, flatulence, diarrhea, and nausea.[12] Surgery may be offered as a treatment alternative to certain patients with complicated GERD.

Endoscopic Therapy. Several endoscopic techniques have been developed for the treatment of GERD. Radiofrequency energy delivery (Stretta) and endoscopic suturing are currently used in clinical trials. Both procedures are approved by the Food and Drug Administration for safety but not for efficacy. The Stretta procedure delivers energy to the distal esophagus and the LES to create a thermal lesion, which, upon healing, will result in fibrosis and increased LES competence. The same effect is sought with endoscopic suturing, which creates a plication by intraluminally suturing the distal esophagus.

Endoscopic procedures have largely been examined in patients without erosive esophagitis. It is currently unclear whether these techniques will be of therapeutic value for the management of erosive esophagitis, as the central pathogenic mechanism for this condition is acid clearance rather than reflux.

Key Points: Erosive Esophagitis

- ☞ Erosive esophagitis is a condition experienced by a subset of GERD patients in whom changes in esophageal mucosa correlate with symptoms of acid reflux.
- ☞ Excessive acid exposure in the distal esophagus and a reduction of the esophageal pH can be detected in most patients with erosive esophagitis.

Key Points (*Continued*)

ᗡ Untreated esophagitis may lead to the development of a benign distal esophageal stricture.

ᗡ In patients with classic GERD who have "alarm signs," endoscopy is indicated and is diagnostic of erosive GERD.

ᗡ Treatment involves relieving symptoms and healing the esophagitis as well as maintaining remission.

ᗡ Initial treatment modalities include antacids, H_2RAs, and PPIs. Maintenance also makes use of H_2RAs and PPIs as well as surgery and endoscopic therapy.

Suggested Reading

1. Winkelstein A: Peptic esophagitis: A new clinical entity. JAMA 1935; 104:906.
2. Allison PR: Peptic ulcer of the esophagus. J Thorac Surg 15:308, 1946.
3. Kahrilas PJ: Gastroesophageal reflux disease and its complications. In Feldman M, Sleisenger MH, (eds): Sleisenger & Fordtran's. Gastrointestinal and Liver Disease, Vol 1. Philadelphia, W.B. Saunders, 1998: pp 498–517.
4. Gallup: A Gallup organization national survey: Heartburn across America. Princeton, NJ, Gallup Organization, 1988.
5. Locke GR 3rd, Talley NJ, Fett SL, et al: Prevalence and clinical spectrum of gastroesophageal reflux: A population-based study in Olmsted County, Minnesota. Gastroenterology 112:1448–1456, 1997.
6. Johnsson F, Joelsson B, Gudmundsson K, Greiff L: Symptoms and endoscopic findings in the diagnosis of gastroesophageal reflux disease. Scand J Gastroenterol 22:714–718, 1987.
7. DeMeester TR, Wang CI, Wernly JA, et al: Technique, indications, and clinical use of 24 hour esophageal pH monitoring. J Thorac Cardiovasc Surg 79:656–670, 1980.
8. Tibbling L: Epidemiology of gastro-oesophageal reflux disease. Scand J Gastroenterol 19:14, 1984.
9. Harris RA, Kuppermann M, Richter JE: Prevention of recurrences of erosive reflux esophagitis: A cost- effectiveness analysis of maintenance proton pump inhibition. Am J Med 102:78–88, 1997.
10. Johnson LF: 24-hour pH monitoring in the study of gastroesophageal reflux. J Clin Gastroenterol 2:387–399, 1980.
11. Fisher RS: Treatment of gastroesophageal reflux disease. In Wolfe MM (ed): Therapy of Digestive Disorders. Philadelphia, W.B. Saunders, 2000, pp 3–13.
12. American Medical Association: New considerations in the evaluation and management of GERD. Chicago, AMA, 2002.
13. Kahrilas PJ, Dodds WJ, Hogan WJ, et al: Esophageal peristaltic dysfunction in peptic esophagitis. Gastroenterology 91:897–904, 1986.
14. Ott DJ, McManus CM, Ledbetter MS, et al: Heartburn correlated to 24-hour pH monitoring and radiographic examination of the esophagus. Am J Gastroenterol 92:1827–1830, 1997.
15. Fass R, Ofman JJ: Gastroesophageal reflux disease: Should we adopt a new conceptual framework? Am J Gastroenterol 97:1901–1909, 2002.
16. Castell DO: Medical therapy for reflux esophagitis: 1986 and beyond. Ann Intern Med 104:112–114, 1986.

17. Mittal RK: Hiatal hernia: Myth or reality? Am J Med 103:33S-39S, 1997.
18. Mittal RK: Hiatal hernia and gastroesophageal reflux: Another attempt to resolve the controversy. Gastroenterology 105:941–943, 1993.
19. Sloan S, Rademaker AW, Kahrilas PJ: Determinants of gastroesophageal junction incompetence: Hiatal hernia, lower esophageal sphincter, or both? Ann Intern Med 117:977–982, 1992.
20. Van Herwaarden MA, Samsom M, Smout AJ: Excess gastroesophageal reflux in patients with hiatus hernia is caused by mechanisms other than transient LES relaxations. Gastroenterology 119:1439–1446, 2000.
21. Katzka DA: Motility abnormalities in gastroesophageal reflux disease. Gastroenterol Clin North Am 28:905–915, 1999.
22. Adachi K, Fujishiro H, Katsube T, et al: Predominant nocturnal acid reflux in patients with Los Angeles grade C and D reflux esophagitis. J Gastroenterol Hepatol 16: 1191–1196, 2001.
23. Timmer R, Breumelhof R, Nadorp JH, Smout AJ: Ambulatory esophageal pressure and pH monitoring in patients with high- grade reflux esophagitis. Dig Dis Sci 39:2084–2089, 1994.
24. Orr WC, Allen ML, Robinson M: The pattern of nocturnal and diurnal esophageal acid exposure in the pathogenesis of erosive mucosal damage. Am J Gastroenterol 89:509–512, 1994.
25. Klauser AG, Schindlbeck NE, Muller-Lissner SA: Symptoms in gastro-oesophageal reflux disease. Lancet 335:205–208, 1990.
26. Marks RD, Richter JE, Rizzo J, et al: Omeprazole versus H2-receptor antagonists in treating patients with peptic stricture and esophagitis. Gastroenterology 106:907–915, 1994.
27. Wilmer A, Tack J, Frans E, et al: Duodenogastroesophageal reflux and esophageal mucosal injury in mechanically ventilated patients. Gastroenterology 116:1293–1299, 1999.
28. Orlando RC: Overview of the mechanisms of gastroesophageal reflux. Am J Med 111(Suppl 8A):174S–177S, 2001.
29. Johnson DA, Benjamin SB, Vakil NB, et al: Esomeprazole once daily for 6 months is effective therapy for maintaining healed erosive esophagitis and for controlling gastroesophageal reflux disease symptoms: A randomized, double-blind, placebo-controlled study of efficacy and safety. Am J Gastroenterol 96:27–34, 2001.
30. Castell DO, Richter JE, Robinson M, et al: Efficacy and safety of lansoprazole in the treatment of erosive reflux esophagitis. The Lansoprazole Group. Am J Gastroenterol 91:1749–1757, 1996.
31. Martinez SD, Malagon IB, Garewal H, et al: Non-erosive reflux disease (NERD). Is it really just a mild form of gastroesophageal reflux disease (GERD)? [abstract]. Gastroenterology 120:2163, 2001.
32. Armstrong D, Bennett JR, Blum AL, et al: The endoscopic assessment of esophagitis: A progress report on observer agreement. Gastroenterology 111:85–92, 1996.
33. Lundell LR, Dent J, Bennett JR, et al: Endoscopic assessment of oesophagitis: Clinical and functional correlates and further validation of the Los Angeles classification. Gut 45:172–180, 1999.
34. Hetzel DJ, Dent J, Reed WD, et al: Healing and relapse of severe peptic esophagitis after treatment with omeprazole. Gastroenterology 95:903–912,1988.
35. Bytzer P, Havelund T, Hansen JM: Interobserver variation in the endoscopic diagnosis of reflux esophagitis. Scand J Gastroenterol 28:119–125, 1993.
36. Pandolfino JE, Vakil NB, Kahrilas PJ: Comparison of inter- and intraobserver consistency for grading of esophagitis by expert and trainee endoscopists. Gastrointest Endosc 56:639–643, 2002.

37. Wolfe MM, Sachs G: Acid suppression: Optimizing therapy for gastroduodenal ulcer healing, gastroesophageal reflux disease, and stress-related erosive syndrome. Gastroenterology 118:S9–31, 2000.
38. Petrokubi RJ, Jeffries GH: Cimetidine versus antacid in scleroderma with reflux esophagitis: A randomized double-blind controlled study. Gastroenterology 77: 691–695, 1979.
39. Graham DY, Patterson DJ: Double-blind comparison of liquid antacid and placebo in the treatment of symptomatic reflux esophagitis. Dig Dis Sci 28:559–563, 1983.
40. Grove O, Bekker C, Jeppe-Hansen MG, et al: Ranitidine and high-dose antacid in reflux oesophagitis: A randomized, placebo-controlled trial. Scand J Gastroenterol 20:457–461, 1985.
41. Weberg R, Berstad A: Symptomatic effect of a low-dose antacid regimen in reflux oesophagitis. Scand J Gastroenterol 24:401–406, 1989.
42. Farup PG, Weberg R, Berstad A, et al: Low-dose antacids versus 400 mg cimetidine twice daily for reflux oesophagitis: A comparative, placebo-controlled, multicentre study. Scand J Gastroenterol 25:315–320, 1990.
43. Peterson W: Improving the management of GERD. Evidence-based therapeutic strategies. In Consensus Opinion in Gastroenterology. American Gastroenterological Association, 2002.
44. Johnson & Johnson Merck consumer pharmaceuticals. Data on file.
45. Chevrel B: A comparative crossover study on the treatment of heartburn and epigastric pain: Liquid Gaviscon and a magnesium—aluminium antacid gel. J Int Med Res 8:300–302, 1980.
46. Wolfe MM: H_2receptor antagonists vs OTC medications: How beneficial have they been? Pract Gastroenterol 20:10–16, 1996.
47. Sontag SJ: The medical management of reflux esophagitis: Role of antacids and acid inhibition. Gastroenterol Clin North Am 19:683–712, 1990.
48. Dobrilla G, Di Fede F: Treatment of gastroesophageal (acid) reflux with lansoprazole: An overview. Clin Ther 15:2–13, 1993.
49. Robinson M, Sahba B, Avner D, et al: A comparison of lansoprazole and ranitidine in the treatment of erosive oesophagitis. Multicentre Investigational Group. Aliment Pharmacol Ther 9:25–31, 1995.
50. Bardhan KD, Hawkey CJ, Long RG, et al: Lansoprazole versus ranitidine for the treatment of reflux oesophagitis. UK Lansoprazole Clinical Research Group. Aliment Pharmacol Ther 9:145–151, 1995.
51. Kaspari S, Biedermann A, Mey J: Comparison of pantoprazole 20 mg to ranitidine 150 mg b.i.d. in the treatment of mild gastroesophageal reflux disease. Digestion 63:163–170, 2001.
52. Jansen JB, Van Oene JC: Standard-dose lansoprazole is more effective than high-dose ranitidine in achieving endoscopic healing and symptom relief in patients with moderately severe reflux oesophagitis. The Dutch Lansoprazole Study Group. Aliment Pharmacol Ther 13:1611–1620, 1999.
53. Bardhan KD, Morris P, Thompson M, et al: Omeprazole in the treatment of erosive oesophagitis refractory to high dose cimetidine and ranitidine. Gut 31:745–749, 1990.
54. Castell DO, Kahrilas PJ, Richter JE, et al: Esomeprazole (40 mg) compared with lansoprazole (30 mg) in the treatment of erosive esophagitis. Am J Gastroenterol 97:575–583, 2002.
55. Caro JJ, Salas M, Ward A: Healing and relapse rates in gastroesophageal reflux disease treated with the newer proton-pump inhibitors lansoprazole, rabeprazole, and

pantoprazole compared with omeprazole, ranitidine, and placebo: Evidence from randomized clinical trials. Clin Ther 23:998–1017, 2001.

56. Swarbrick ET, Gough AL, Foster CS,et al: Prevention of recurrence of oesophageal stricture, a comparison of lansoprazole and high-dose ranitidine. Eur J Gastroenterol Hepatol 8:431–438, 1996.

57. Hendel J, Hendel L, Hage E,et al: Monitoring of omeprazole treatment in gastro-oesophageal reflux disease. Eur J Gastroenterol Hepatol 8:417–420, 1996.

58. Peghini PL, Katz PO, Castell DO: Ranitidine controls nocturnal gastric acid breakthrough on omeprazole: a controlled study in normal subjects. Gastroenterology 115:1335–1339, 1998.

59. Fackler WK, Ours TM, Vaezi MF, Richter JE: Long-term effect of H_2RA therapy on nocturnal gastric acid breakthrough. Gastroenterology 122:625–632, 2002.

60. Chiba N: Proton pump inhibitors in acute healing and maintenance of erosive or worse esophagitis: A systematic overview. Can J Gastroenterol 11(Suppl B):66B–73B, 1997.

61. Simon TJ, Roberts WG, Berlin RG, et al: Acid suppression by famotidine 20 mg twice daily or 40 mg twice daily in preventing relapse of endoscopic recurrence of erosive esophagitis. Clin Ther 17:1147–1156, 1995.

62. Nwokolo CU, Smith JTL, Gavey C, et al: Tolerance during 29 days of conventional dosing with cimetidine, ranitidine, famotidine or nizatidine. Aliment Pharmacol Ther 4:15–27, 1990.

63. Smith JTL, Gavey C, Nwokolo CU, et al: Tolerance during 8 days of high-dose H2-blockade: Placebo-controlled study of 24-hour acidity and gastrin. Aliment Pharmacol Ther 4:15–27,47–63, 1990.

64. Wilder-Smith CH, Ernst T, Genonni M, et al: Tolerance to oral H2-receptor antagonists. 8:976–983, 1990.

65. Wilder-Smith CH, Halter F, Ernst T, et al: Loss of acid suppression during dosing with H_2receptor antagonists. Aliment Pharmacol Ther 4:15–27, 1990.

66. Vigneri S, Termini R, Leandro G, et al: A comparison of five maintenance therapies for reflux esophagitis. N Engl J Med 333:1106–1110, 1995.

67. Klinkenberg-Knol EC, Festen HP, Jansen JB, et al: Long-term treatment with omeprazole for refractory reflux esophagitis: Efficacy and safety. Ann Intern Med 121:161–167, 1994.

68. Vigneri S, Termini R, Leandro G, et al: A comparison of five maintenance therapies for reflux esophagitis. N Engl J Med 333:1106–1110, 1995.

69. Klinkenberg-Knol EC, Nelis F, Dent J, et al: Long-term omeprazole treatment in resistant gastroesophageal reflux disease: Efficacy, safety, and influence on gastric mucosa. Gastroenterology 118:661–669, 2000.

70. Lundell L, Miettinen P, Myrvold HE, et al: Long-term management of gastro-oesophageal reflux disease with omeprazole or open antireflux surgery: Results of a prospective, randomized clinical trial. The Nordic GORD Study Group. Eur J Gastroenterol Hepatol 12:879–887, 2000.

71. Lundell L, Miettinen P, Myrvold HE, et al: Continued (5-year) followup of a randomized clinical study comparing antireflux surgery and omeprazole in gastro-esophageal reflux disease. J Am Coll Surg 192:172–179; discussion 179–181, 2001.

72. Lundell L, Abrahamsson H, Ruth M, et al: Long-term results of a prospective randomized comparison of total fundic wrap (Nissen-Rossetti) or semifundoplication (Toupet) for gastro-oesophageal reflux. Br J Surg 83:830–835, 1996.

73. Rantanen TK, Halme TV, Luostarinen ME, et al: The long term results of open antireflux surgery in a community-based health care center. Am J Gastroenterol 94:1777–1781, 1999.

Nonerosive Reflux Disease

chapter

6

Roy Dekel, M.D.,
and Ronnie Fass, M.D.

Symptoms of gastroesophageal reflux disease (GERD) are very common in the United States and are reported to occur monthly by 44% and weekly by 20% of the adult population.[1,2] Our current therapeutic approach is based on the concept that GERD represents a spectrum of tissue damage. On one end are patients with classic symptoms of GERD (heartburn, acid regurgitation) but without any evidence of esophageal mucosal injury, and on the other end are patients with erosive esophagitis and GERD complications such as stricture, Barrett's esophagus, and even adenocarcinoma of the esophagus.[3] Thus, it has been assumed that those patients with GERD symptoms—but normal esophageal mucosa—represent a mild form of the disease. Consequently, a much more conservative therapeutic approach has been suggested to be adequate for these patients. This approach was quickly adopted by health plans and third-party payers.[4] Interesting to note is that there are very few data to support such a strategy, because most of the well-designed therapeutic trials in GERD during the last two decades have focused primarily on mucosal healing and symptom improvement in patients with erosive esophagitis.

In recent years, two important developments have emerged in the field of GERD that have shifted our attention back to those patients with a normal esophagus and typical symptoms of reflux disease. The first was the observation that most patients with GERD appear to have no evidence of esophageal mucosal injury. The second development, which was a great surprise to many investigators, originated from recent therapeutic trials in patients with GERD symptoms and absence or presence of esophageal mucosal injury: patients with normal esophageal mucosa demonstrated lower rates of symptom improvement during potent antireflux treatment (proton pump inhibitors [PPIs]) than did patients with erosive esophagitis. Additional evaluation of treatment response in individuals with GERD symptoms and normal esophageal mucosa revealed other unexpected results, leading to a reassessment of our current understanding of this group of patients.

101

Epidemiology

The prevalence of nonerosive reflux disease (NERD) is primarily dependent on the definition of the disorder that has been used in each study. This is compounded by lack of a generally accepted definition for NERD.

In most studies, diagnosis of nonerosive reflux disease (symptomatic GERD or endoscopically negative reflux disease) was solely dependent on the absence of esophageal mucosal injury on upper endoscopy. Consequently, the recently proposed definition of NERD by a group of experts suggested that "these are individuals who satisfy the definition of GERD but who do not have either Barrett's esophagus or definite endoscopic esophageal breaks."[4] A similar definition has been proposed by Waring[5]: "burning retrosternal discomfort for at least 3 months, but with normal esophageal mucosa on upper endoscopy." Both of these definitions assume that all patients who present with heartburn, regardless of the presence or absence of esophageal mucosal injury, have GERD.[6] Currently, however, there is sufficient data to suggest that acid is not the only intraesophageal stimulus that can lead to heartburn sensation. In fact, heartburn appears to be the "common pathway" of a variety of intra-esophageal events, of which acid reflux is just one.[7] Hence, Fass et al.[8] proposed a different definition for NERD that underscores the close relationship between symptoms and gastric content reflux. NERD was defined as the presence of typical symptoms of GERD caused by intraesophageal gastric content, in the absence of visible esophageal mucosal injury at endoscopic examination.

Early studies have reported that approximately 50% of the patients with heartburn will demonstrate normal esophageal mucosa during endoscopy.[9] However, several recent European studies have explored the prevalence of NERD in community-based patients, finding a much higher prevalence that reached 70%.[8–10] Galmiche et al.[11] assessed the efficacy of on-demand H_2-blockers in patients with GERD symptoms who were recruited from general practice clinics. A total of 423 patients completed the study; of those, 71% met the definition of NERD. In another study, Carlsson et al.[12] evaluated different treatment strategies in patients with GERD from 36 primary care centers in Europe and Australia. This study enrolled 538 patients and of those, 49% demonstrated lack of esophageal mucosal breaks. In a study that was conducted in the United States, Robinson et al.[13] evaluated only subjects who used antacids for symptomatic relief of heartburn. Of the 165 patients who were enrolled in this study, 53% were found to have normal esophageal mucosa on upper endoscopy.

Overall, these studies and others have suggested that the prevalence of NERD is between 50% and 70% of the general GERD population. However, we have to recall that most patients with GERD symptoms never seek medical attention. It is still unknown what percentage of these non-consulters are NERD patients. There are very few studies that can shed light on the clinical characteristics of NERD patients, particularly in comparison with patients with erosive esophagitis. In a large study that involved 25 centers in Denmark and Sweden, 424 patients with troublesome heartburn were identified as having NERD. Mean age was 50, 58% were female, only 21% were smokers, 45% were active alcohol users, 53% had more than 5 years' history of heartburn, and in only 37% was hiatal hernia documented during upper endoscopy.[14] Carlsson et al.[12] provided a comparison of the clinical characteristics between patients with NERD and those with erosive esophagitis. In the NERD group, 62% were female, mean age was 48, mean weight for male subjects was 79 kg and for female subjects 69 kg, 24% were smokers, 58% were alcohol consumers, 75% had symptom duration that was longer than 12 months, 24% had hiatal hernia, and 30% were infected with *Helicobacter pylori*. In comparison, of the patients with erosive esophagitis, 42% were female, mean age was 50, mean weight for male subjects was 86 kg and for female subjects 76 kg, 23% were smokers, 64% were alcohol consumers, 81% had symptom duration longer than 12 months, 56% had hiatal hernia, and 26% were positive for *H. pylori*.

Table 1 summarizes the clinical characteristics of patients with NERD. Although not clearly demonstrated in the studies above, pooled data from two other studies have revealed that patients with erosive esophagitis were significantly older than those with NERD.[15]

TABLE 1. Clinical Characteristics of Patients with Nonerosive Reflux Disease as Compared to Those with Erosive Esophagitis	
Characteristic	**NERD Patients Compared with Erosive Esophagitis Patients**
Gender	↑ Female
Mean age	ND
Mean weight (M/F)	↓
Smoking	ND
Alcohol consumption	ND
Symptoms duration	↓
Hiatal hernia	↓
Helicobacter pylori infection	ND

NERD = nonerosive reflux disease, ND = no difference
Adapted from Fass R: Epidemiology and pathophysiology of symptomatic gastroesophageal reflux disease. Am J Gastroenterol 98 (3 Suppl): S2–S7, 2003.

Natural History

Information is lacking about the natural course of NERD patients. This is an important question that can determine the likelihood of these patients to develop esophageal mucosal injury in the form of erosive esophagitis or GERD complications over time. Additionally, it may determine whether these patients are at increased risk of developing Barrett's esophagus and thus adenocarcinoma of the esophagus. The very few studies that are available in the literature about the natural course of NERD are rich with flaws and primarily demonstrate the difficulties and the shortcomings in studying the natural history of this disease. In all of these studies, there is very limited control over the patients' consumption of antireflux medications. Overall, very few NERD patients develop erosive esophagitis or even GERD complications over time (Fig. 1).[16,17] The vast majority remain NERD patients throughout their lifetime. Currently, there are no data to demonstrate that these patients are at increased risk of developing Barrett's esophagus, let alone adenocarcinoma of the esophagus over a longer period of time.

Pathophysiology

Intriguing findings have recently emerged from clinical studies in NERD patients. Heartburn severity or intensity was found to be similar in both patients with erosive esophagitis and those with NERD.[15] Addi-

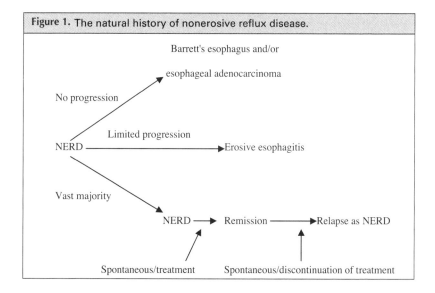

Figure 1. The natural history of nonerosive reflux disease.

tionally, the impact of heartburn severity on patients' quality of life was similar in both groups.[12,18] Furthermore, PPIs and antireflux surgery have demonstrated lower efficacy in controlling symptoms in patients with NERD as compared to those with erosive esophagitis. The response rate to potent medical therapy in NERD patients has consistently been 10% to 30% less than in subjects with erosive esophagitis.[19,20] Additionally, the lag time to complete symptom relief is longer in NERD patients. Patients with NERD undergoing laparoscopic fundoplication were less likely to achieve symptom improvement or resolution and were more likely to develop postoperative dysphagia and report dissatisfaction with surgery.[21]

These findings regarding the severity of the disease and the unpredictable response to potent medical or surgical therapy required reassessment of our knowledge about the pathophysiology of NERD.

Physiology

Physiologic studies in patients with NERD have revealed minimal abnormalities. These patients have a slightly higher rate of primary peristalsis failure, defined by nontransmitted contractions or peristaltic contractions that do not traverse the entire esophageal body.[22] Distal amplitude contractions as well as mean lower esophageal resting pressure are mildly reduced as compared with normal subjects. Resting lower esophageal sphincter pressure is rarely lower than 10 mm Hg.[22] Only in the minority of NERD patients is hiatal hernia found on upper endoscopic examination. Cameron et al.[23] demonstrated that 29% of the NERD patients had hiatal hernia, as compared with 71% of patients with erosive esophagitis, 72% with short-segment Barrett's esophagus, and 96% with long-segment Barrett's esophagus. The absence of diaphragmatic hernia suggests that transient lower esophageal sphincter relaxation is likely the sole mechanism for acid reflux in most of these patients.[24] The extent of esophageal acid exposure in NERD patients as compared to those with erosive esophagitis or Barrett's esophagus hs been recently reported. Martinez et al.[25] demonstrated that NERD patients had the lowest total, supine, and erect percentage of time at pH less than 4 (6%, 4.9%, and 6.2%, respectively), as compared with patients with erosive esophagitis (11.4%, 9.3%, and 13.4%, respectively) and those with Barrett's esophagus (18.8%, 19.4%, and 18.2%, respectively).

Very limited data are available about the role of bile reflux in symptom generation of patients with NERD. The mean fasting gastric bile acid concentration in these patients is similar to that in healthy control subjects. Additionally, combined acid and duodenogastroesophageal reflux, which correlates with severity of mucosal involvement in GERD, has been documented in only 50% of the NERD patients, as compared with 79% of the erosive esophagitis and 95% of the Barrett's esophagus patients. Table 2 summarizes the physiologic characteristics of patients with NERD.

Nonerosive Reflux Disease Subgroups

Further studies in NERD patients suggest that this is a much more complex group of patients, with potentially multiple underlying mechanisms for their symptoms (Fig. 2). Studies that evaluated NERD patients with ambulatory 24-hour esophageal pH monitoring have consistently demonstrated that 33% to 51% of these patients have esophageal acid exposure within the normal range.[26–29] In a recent study, Martinez et al.[25], demonstrated that 50% of the NERD patients had a normal pH test result, as compared with 25% of the patients with erosive esophagitis and 7% of those with Barrett's esophagus. This study suggests that the likelihood that a pH probe will detect an abnormal pH is dependent on the duration of esophageal acid exposure. Consequently, patients with Barrett's esophagus, who display the highest esophageal acid exposure, are less likely to have a normal pH test result than NERD patients, who display the lowest esophageal acid exposure and thus are more likely to have a normal pH test result.

Other investigators have also demonstrated that approximately half of the patients with NERD appear to have acid exposure within the physiologic range.[15] This group of patients has been termed by the Rome II committee for functional bowel disorders as having "functional heart-

TABLE 2. Physiological Characteristics of Patients With Symptomatic Gastroesophageal Reflux Disease Compared with Healthy Control Subjects	
Physiologic Characteristic	Symptomatic GERD Patients Compared with Healthy Control Subjects
Resting LES pressure	Normal
LES resting pressure < 10 mm Hg	Rare
Distal amplitude contractions	Slightly reduced
Motility abnormalities	Slightly increased
Time pH < 4(%)	
Total	Slightly increased
Supine	Slightly increased
Erect	Slightly increased
Mean gastric bile acid concentration	Normal

GERD = gastroesophageal reflux disease, LES = lower esophageal sphincter.
Adapted from Fass R: Epidemiology and pathophysiology of symptomatic gastroesophageal reflux disease. Am J Gastroenterol 98 (3 Suppl): S2–S7, 2003.

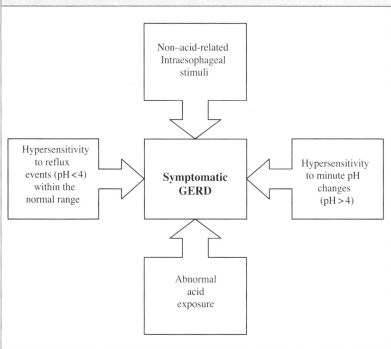

Figure 2. The proposed underlying mechanisms for symptoms in patients with nonerosive reflux disease. (Adapted from Fass R: Epidemiology and pathophysiology of symptomatic gastroesophageal reflux disease. Am J Gastroenterol 98 (3 Suppl): S2–S7, 2003.)

burn," defined as at least 12 weeks, which need not be consecutive, in the preceding 12 months of burning retrosternal discomfort or pain and absence of pathologic gastroesophageal reflux, achalasia, or other motility disorders with a recognized pathologic basis.[20] This definition is vague and provides no clues about the underlying mechanisms responsible for these patients' symptoms. Additionally, it may suggest that this is a homogeneous group of patients with no known cause for their symptoms.

Several mechanisms for heartburn symptoms in patients with normal endoscopy and pH testing findings (functional heartburn) have been recently proposed. Martinez et al.[25] evaluated 71 patients with NERD and found that 50% of them had a negative pH test result. Of those, 37% demonstrated a close relationship between heartburn symptoms and acid reflux events, suggesting a hypersensitivity to physiologic amounts of acid exposure. This group of patients, whose condition is termed the *hyper-*

sensitive esophagus, demonstrates a limited response to PPI treatment that markedly improves if higher doses are used.[20,30] Another subgroup includes patients with heartburn due to non–acid related intraesophageal stimuli. Nonacidic reflux, motor events, and other intraesophageal stimuli may trigger heartburn in a subset of patients.[31–33] Knowing the limited repertoire of esophageal symptoms, it is presently clear that esophageal symptoms are not stimulus specific. Thus, heartburn serves as the "common pathway" for different intraesophageal events.[34]

Diagnostic Approach

In patients who present with alarm symptoms, such as dysphagia, weight loss, anorexia, and anemia, among others, upper endoscopy should be favored as the first-line diagnostic approach. However, patients who present with typical symptoms of GERD, but without alarm symptoms, will most likely be treated empirically, without the patient or the physician knowing whether there is esophageal mucosal injury. The focus of our therapeutic approach in NERD is symptom relief or improvement, rather than healing of erosive esophagitis.

Currently, there are no adequate clinical factors to help us predict whether esophageal mucosal injury is present or absent. Several studies evaluated the specific use of the PPI therapeutic trial in patients who presented with NERD.[28,35,36] The purpose of these investigations was primarily to detect those patients with classic heartburn due to non–acid related intraesophageal stimuli. The assumption was that most patients with acid-related symptoms would demonstrate some level of response to high-dose PPI therapy given during a short period (7–14 days) (Table 3).

TABLE 3. Therapeutic Trials in Nonerosive Reflux Disease Patients						
First Author	Reference	Patients	Dose	% Symptom Improvement	Duration (days)	Sensitivity (%)
Schindlbeck	43	11	40 mg/day	75	7	27
		10	40 mg twice daily	75	7	83
Johnson	13	160	20 mg twice daily	At least 1 grade improvement in symptom score	7	75
Schenk	12	85	40 mg/day	50	14	66

Adapted from Fass R: Epidemiology and pathophysiology of symptomatic gastroesophageal reflux disease. Am J Gastroenterol 98 (3 Suppl): S2–S7, 2003.

In one study, the symptom response rate in NERD patients improved from 27.2% to 83.3% when the omeprazole dose was increased from 40 mg/day to 40 mg twice daily.[36] Although these studies are limited by the lack of a "gold standard" for diagnosing GERD, it appears that in NERD patients, a high dose of PPI will be required to achieve a maximal symptom response. The latter is essential for improved sensitivity of the therapeutic trial.

Biopsy of the distal esophagus in patients with heartburn and normal endoscopic findings remains a common practice. Despite the lack of data to support such a strategy, many gastroenterologists hope to use biopsy to detect histopathologic changes in the esophagus that are consistent with GERD. These changes include the presence of neutrophils and eosinophils, epithelial hyperplasia (basal cell hyperplasia and elongated papillae), and dilated vessels in the papillae.[37] However, assessments of the diagnostic accuracy of distal esophageal biopsy are hampered by the lack of "gold standard" for diagnosing GERD. In one study, typical GERD symptoms were used as the comparative tool in patients without esophageal inflammation, revealing GERD-related histopathologic changes in only 47.8% of patients, in addition to 21.6% of healthy control subjects.[38,40] In this study, biopsy specimens were obtained at 4 cm above the esophagogastric junction.

In yet another study in which samples were obtained at 2 and 5 cm above the esophagogastric junction, the results of esophageal biopsies in NERD patients did not fare any better.[39] For those patients with NERD who had a positive pH test result, most histopathologic changes were in biopsy specimens taken at the 2 cm mark, and the sensitivity ranged from 15.4% to 46.2%. By contrast, for NERD patients with a negative pH test result, histopathologic changes were documented only in biopsy specimens taken at the 5 cm mark, with a sensitivity of 9.1%. Interesting to note was that 28.6% of healthy control subjects had positive esophageal biopsy results as well, mainly from specimens taken at the 2 cm location.

For NERD patients in whom standard-dose PPI therapy fails, further evaluation by 24-hour esophageal pH monitoring has been suggested by an American Gastroenterological Association medical position statement.[40] However, a recent study revealed that more than 60% of patients who continued to be symptomatic while taking standard-dose PPIs actually demonstrated acid exposure values that were within normal limits.[41] This suggests that these patients may demonstrate increased esophageal chemosensitivity to acid (which may require additional elimination of acid) or experience non–acid related intra-esophageal stimuli. A clue to the solution to this dilemma derives from a recent study showing a lack of increased esophageal chemosensitivity to acid in most of these patients.[42]

Treatment

Due to a lack of esophageal mucosal injury in patients with NERD, the general assumption is that this population represents just a mild form of GERD. Consequently, a step-up approach is considered appropriate for NERD patients, starting with over-the-counter histamine$_2$-receptor antagonists (H$_2$RAs) or standard-dose H$_2$RAs.[43] Despite the absence of any data to support such a therapeutic approach in these patients, it appeared a logical strategy to many clinicians who accepted the concept that the severity of disease in GERD is solely determined by the extent of esophageal mucosal injury.

For decades, the focus of many therapeutic trials was on the healing of erosive esophagitis, which was considered a more accurate, reliable, and reproducible clinical endpoint. However, when assessing treatment response in patients with NERD, symptom relief or improvement became the primary clinical endpoint. As more validated tools were developed to assess symptom response in GERD, data began to accumulate regarding the clinical efficacy of various therapeutic modalities in NERD patients.

Overall, therapeutic trials in patients with NERD have demonstrated a lower efficacy for PPIs in symptom control than had been previously reported for patients with erosive esophagitis. At 4 weeks of therapy with omeprazole 20 mg/day, only 57% of NERD patients reported complete symptom relief.[19] In another study, NERD patients were randomized to omeprazole 20 mg/day; omeprazole 10 mg/day; or placebo.[20] The study authors found that at 4 weeks 46% of patients treated with omeprazole 20 mg/day, 31% treated with omeprazole 10 mg/day, and 13% of those who received placebo reported complete relief of heartburn.

It is apparent from the results of these and other large, multicenter studies that the symptom response rate of NERD patients to PPI therapy is surprisingly low; in fact, it is almost 10% to 30% less than the rate observed in patients with erosive esophagitis who are taking similar doses.[44] Unexpectedly, the proportion of NERD patients with complete control of heartburn after 4 weeks of therapy was found to be in accordance with their pretreatment level of esophageal acid exposure.[20] That is, the higher the acid exposure in the distal esophagus is, the greater the number of patients who achieved complete control of their heartburn symptoms. Furthermore, comparative studies randomizing NERD patients to either standard-dose PPI or H$_2$RA therapy clearly demonstrated that the former was significantly more efficacious in symptom control.[18,29] In one study, approximately 60% of NERD patients receiving omeprazole 20 mg/day, reported symptom relief versus only 40% of those receiving ranitidine, 150 mg twice daily.[18] The PPIs were also shown to be more effective in achieving symptom control in NERD patients when compared with promotility drugs, such as cisapride.[45]

When maintenance therapy was assessed in patients with NERD, again PPIs appeared to be more effective than any other antireflux treatment. More than 50% of NERD patients remained heartburn free while taking omeprazole 20 mg/day compared with less than 30% of those who received ranitidine 150 mg twice daily.[18] Similar results were achieved when omeprazole was compared with cisapride: at 4 weeks of therapy, 63% versus 46% remained heartburn free, respectively.[11]

Only 25% of those NERD patients who initially achieved complete symptom resolution while taking PPIs remain symptom free after 6 months of not undergoing any antireflux therapy.[11] This finding suggests that most patients with NERD will require long-term maintenance therapy, regardless of the therapeutic regimen that initially induced the symptom remission. While taking placebo, however, NERD patients who achieved symptom resolution initially on PPI therapy demonstrated a higher remission rate at 6 months than did patients not undergoing any therapy (56%).[14] This fact may suggest a short-term placebo effect, which may not necessarily translate into any long-term effect. Predictive factors for relapse while undergoing maintenance therapy in NERD patients who have achieved complete remission initially included duration of symptom history and duration of treatment required to gain control of symptoms before beginning maintenance therapy.[46]

Large trials assessing symptom response in NERD patients have not attempted to determine the specific response of different subgroups. In a small study that included 18 endoscopy-negative patients with a normal pH test result, omeprazole 20 mg twice daily improved symptoms of heartburn in 61% of subjects at 4 weeks.[30] Most responders also had a positive correlation between their symptoms and their acid reflux events. Although long-term follow-up is lacking, symptom improvement while undergoing high-dose PPI therapy was achieved by this subgroup of NERD patients with the hypersensitive esophagus.

The role of antireflux surgery in patients with NERD has scarcely been evaluated. One study showed that NERD patients had significantly less symptom improvement or resolution than did patients with erosive esophagitis and reported more postoperative dysphagia.[21] In this study, only patients with negative endoscopic findings and abnormal pH test results were included. A predictive factor for favorable outcome was a positive preoperative response to PPI therapy.

The results of these therapeutic trials can be explained by acknowledging the fact that NERD comprises different subgroups, each with different response patterns to antireflux treatment. The symptom response rate among NERD patients to potent antireflux therapy has been disappointingly lower than that observed in patients with erosive esophagitis. This phenomenon may also explain recent data that have revealed a lack of improvement in symptom response rate, even when more potent or higher doses of PPIs have been used in NERD patients.[47]

Treatment for Functional Heartburn

The functional heartburn group is likely the main reason for the limited clinical response to PPI therapy in NERD patients. More than 45% of the patients with functional heartburn reported insufficient control of heartburn after 4 weeks of treatment with omeprazole 20 mg once daily.[20] Interestingly, in the same study, the authors demonstrated that in patients with NERD receiving omeprazole 20 mg daily, the higher the acid exposure in the distal esophagus was, the greater the symptom response was. Thus, duration of distal esophageal acid exposure appears to be a reliable predictive factor for response to PPI therapy.

In patients with functional heartburn who failed to respond to standard-dose PPI, the hypersensitive esophagus subgroup may potentially respond to higher doses of PPI. Further suppression of gastric acid and thus minimization of esophageal acid exposure may eventually result in symptom improvement or possibly complete symptom relief. While using omeprazole 40 mg daily over a period of 14 days, Schenk et al.[28] demonstrated a 37% symptom response rate in patients with heartburn. In another study, omeprazole 40 mg in the morning and 20 mg in the evening were administered for a period of 7 days to patients with functional heartburn.[48] More than 40% of the patients reported a greater than 50% reduction in symptom intensity. Watson et al.[30] performed a double-blind, crossover, placebo-controlled trial of omeprazole 20 mg twice daily for 4 weeks in the treatment of patients with functional heartburn.[30] Omeprazole twice daily improved symptoms in 61% of the subjects. As expected, almost all responders also had a positive correlation between their symptoms and acid reflux events (the hypersensitive esophagus group). This study, although lacking long-term follow-up, further cements the notion that the hypersensitive esophagus subgroup will likely respond to higher doses of PPI. It has yet to be elucidated how high one can raise the PPI dose and still improve symptoms or increase the number of responders.

Pain modulators have not been systematically studied in patients with functional heartburn but may ultimately become an essential component of the therapeutic armamentarium for this disorder. The pain modulators may be effective on their own in certain subsets of patients with functional heartburn, or in combination with a PPI in others. Low doses of tricyclic antidepressants, trazodone, or selective serotonin reuptake inhibitors have been shown to reduce pain in other functional esophageal disorders, such as noncardiac chest pain.[49,50] The 5-HT$_3$ antagonists may also have a certain pain-modulatory effect, probably by altering initiation, transmission, or processing of extrinsic sensory information from the gastrointestinal tract.[51] The effect of 5-HT$_4$ agonists may prove to be efficacious in patients with functional heartburn by reducing acid reflux events and potentially modulating esophageal pain perception,[52] but clinical studies are needed to support these possibilities. Other agents with visceral analgesic effect, currently under investigation, may eventually become important additions to our treatment of functional bowel disorders as well as functional heartburn. These include κ agonists, neurokinin receptor antagonists (NK$_1$ and NK$_2$), and N-methyl-D-aspartate receptor antagonists.[21]

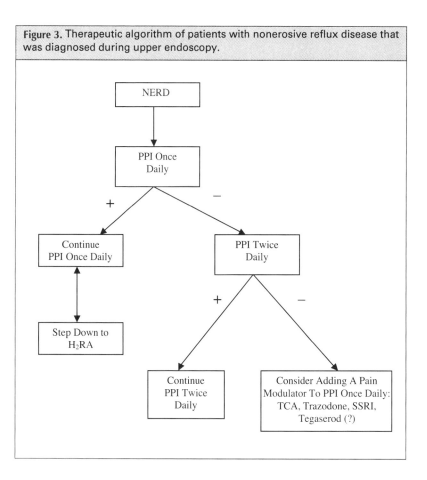

Figure 3. Therapeutic algorithm of patients with nonerosive reflux disease that was diagnosed during upper endoscopy.

The role of antireflux surgery in functional heartburn has not been assessed. Studies that evaluated the efficacy of antireflux surgery in patients with NERD specifically excluded subjects with normal pH testing results.[21] It is currently believed that functional heartburn patients will not benefit from this type of therapeutic intervention.

In summary, patients with functional heartburn should be approached as patients with NERD and treated with anti-reflux medications. Due to the need for profound acid suppression in this group of patients, PPIs should be considered relatively early in their care. Failure to respond to standard dose of PPI will require doubling the dose. If patients continue to report heartburn symptoms while receiving PPI twice daily (am – before breakfast and pm – before dinner), then adding or switching to pain modulators may be appropriate (see Fig. 3).

Key Points: Nonerosive Reflux Disease

∽ Most patients with GERD appear to have no evidence of esophageal mucosal injury.
∽ In patients with GERD, those with normal esophageal mucosa demonstrate lower rates of symptom improvement with PPIs.
∽ NERD is defined as the presence of typical symptoms of GERD caused by intraesophageal gastric content, in the absence of visible esophageal mucosal injury at endoscopic examination.
∽ NERD patients represent a complex group, with many subgroups, each with it's own features and underlying mechanisms.
∽ The therapeutic approach to NERD is symptom relief or improvement. Most NERD patients will have NERD all their lives.

Suggested Reading

1. Locke GR 3rd, Talley NJ, Fett SL, et al: Prevalence and clinical spectrum of gastroesophageal reflux: A population-based study in Olmsted County, Minnesota. Gastroenterology 112:1448–1456, 1997.
2. A Gallup Organization National Survey: Heartburn Across America. Princeton, NJ, Gallup Organization, 1988.
3. Richter JE: Long-term management of gastroesophageal reflux disease and its complications. Am J Gastroenterol 92(4 Suppl):30S–34S, 1997.
4. Dent J, Brun J, Fendrick AM, et al: An evidence-based appraisal of reflux disease management: The Genval Workshop Report. Gut 44(Suppl 2):S1–S16, 1999.
5. Waring JP: Nonerosive reflux disease. Semin Gastrointest Dis 12:33–37, 2001.
6. Fass R: Focused clinical review: nonerosive reflux disease. Medscape Gastroenterology 3:1–13, 2001.
7. Fass R, Tougas G: Functional heartburn: The stimulus, the pain, and the brain. Gut 51:885–895, 2002.

8. Fass R, Fennerty MB, Vakil N: Nonerosive reflux disease: Current concepts and dilemmas. Am J Gastroenterol 96:303–314, 2002.

9. Winters C Jr, Spurling TJ, Chobanian SJ, et al: Barrett's esophagus: A prevalent, occult complication of gastroesophageal reflux disease. Gastroenterology 92:118–124, 1987.

10. Jones RH, Hungin ADS, Phillips J, et al: Gastroesophageal reflux disease in primary care in Europe: Clinical presentation and endoscopic findings. Eur J Gen Pract 1:149–154, 1995.

11. Galmiche JP, Barthelemy P, Hamelin B: Treating the symptoms of gastro-oesophageal reflux disease: A double-blind comparison of omeprazole and cisapride. Aliment Pharmacol Ther 11:765–773, 1997.

12. Carlsson R, Dent J, Watts R, et al: Gastro-oesophageal reflux disease in primary care: An international study of different treatment strategies with omeprazole. International GORD Study Group. Eur J Gastroenterol Hepatol 10:119–124, 1998.

13. Robinson M, Earnest D, Rodriguez-Stanley S, et al: Heartburn requiring frequent antacid use may indicate significant illness. Arch Intern Med 158:2373–2376, 1998.

14. Lind T, Havelund T, Lundell L, et al: On demand therapy with omeprazole for the long-term management of patients with heartburn without oesophagitis: A placebo-controlled randomized trial. Aliment Pharmacol Ther 13:907–914, 1999.

15. Smout AJPM: Endoscopy-negative acid reflux disease. Aliment Pharmacol Ther 11(Suppl 2):81–85, 1997.

16. Pace F, Sasntalucia F, Bianchi Porro G: Natural history of gastro-oesophageal reflux disease without oesophagitis. Gut 32:845–848, 1991.

17. Isolauri J, Luostarinen M, Isolauri E, et al: Natural course of gastroesophageal reflux disease: 17–22 year follow-up of 60 patients. Am J Gastroenterol 92:37–41, 1997.

18. Venables TL, Newland RD, Patel AC, et al: Omeprazole 10 milligrams once daily, omeprazole 20 milligrams once daily, or ranitidine 150 milligrams twice daily, evaluated as initial therapy for the relief of symptoms of gastro-oesophageal reflux disease in general practice. Scand J Gastroenterol 320:965–973, 1997.

19. Bate CM, Griffin SM, Keeling PW, et al: Reflux symptom relief with omeprazole in patients without unequivocal oesophagitis. Aliment Pharmacol Ther 10:547–555, 1996.

20. Lind T, Havelund T, Carlsson R, et al: Heartburn without oesophagitis: Efficacy of omeprazole therapy and features determining therapeutic response. Scand J Gastroenterol 32:974–979, 1997.

21. Fenton P, Terry ML, Galloway KD, et al: Is there a role for laparoscopic fundoplication in patients with non-erosive reflux disease (NERD)? Gastroenterology 118(Suppl 2):A481, #2600, 2000.

22. Kahrilas PJ, Dodds WJ, Hogan WJ, et al: Esophageal peristaltic dysfunction in peptic esophagitis. Gastroenterology 91:897–904, 1986.

23. Cameron AJ: Barrett's esophagus: Prevalence and size of hiatal hernia. Am J Gastroenterol 94:2054–2059, 1999.

24. van Herwaarden MA, Samsom M, Smout AJ: Excess gastroesophageal reflux in patients with hiatus hernia is caused by mechanisms other than transient LES relaxations. Gastroenterology 119:1439–1446, 2000.

25. Martinez SD, Malagon I, Garewal HS, Fass R: Non-erosive reflux disease (NERD): Is it really just a mild form of gastroesophageal reflux disease (GERD)? Gastroenterology 120(Suppl 1):A-424, #2163, 2001.

26. DeMeester TR, Wang CI, Wernly JA, et al: Technique, indications, and clinical use of 24 hour esophageal pH monitoring. J Thorac Cardiovasc Surg 79:656–670, 1980.

27. Johnsson F, Weywadt L, Solhaug JH, et al: One-week omeprazole treatment in the

diagnosis of gastro-oesophageal reflux disease. Scand J Gastroenterol 33:15–20, 1998.

28. Schenk BE, Kuipers EJ, Klinkenberg-Knol EC, et al: Omeprazole as a diagnostic tool in gastroesophageal reflux disease. Am J Gastroenterol 92:1997–2000, 1997.

29. Richter JE, Campbell DR, Kahrilas PJ, et al: Lansoprazole compared with ranitidine for the treatment of nonerosive gastroesophageal reflux disease. Arch Intern Med 160:1803–1809, 2000.

30. Watson RG, Tham TC, Johnston BT, McDougall NI: Double blind cross-over placebo controlled study of omeprazole in the treatment of patients with reflux symptoms and physiological levels of acid reflux: the "sensitive oesophagus". Gut 40(5):587–590, 1997.

31. Pehlivanov ND, Liu J, Mittal R: Sustained esophageal contraction: A motor correlate of heartburn symptom. Gastroenterology 116:A1062, #G4613, 1999.

32. Sifrim D, Holloway R, Silny J, et al: Acid, nonacid, and gas reflux in patients with gastroesophageal reflux disease during ambulatory 24-hour pH-impedance recordings. Gastroenterology 120:1588–1598, 2001.

33. Vela MF, Camacho-Lobato L, Srinivasan R, et al: Simultaneous intraesophageal impedance and pH measurement of acid and nonacid gastroesophageal reflux: Effect of omeprazole. Gastroenterology 120:1599–1606, 2001.

34. Fass R, Ofman JJ: Gastroesophageal reflux disease: Should we adopt a new conceptual framework? Am J Gastroenterol 97:1901–1909, 2002.

35. Fass R, Fennerty MB, Ofman JJ, et al: The clinical and economic value of a short course of omeprazole in patients with noncardiac chest pain. Gastroenterology 115:42–49, 1998.

36. Schindlbeck NE, Klauser AG, Voderholzer WA, Muller-Lissner SA: Empiric therapy for gastroesophageal reflux disease. Arch Intern Med 155:1808–1812, 1995.

37. Lewin KJ, Riddel RH, Weinstein WM: Inflammatory disorders of the esophagus: Reflux and nonreflux types. In Gastrointestinal Pathology and Its Clinical Implications. New York, Igaku-Shoin, 1992, pp 401–439.

38. Funch-Jensen P, Kock K, Christensen LA, et al: Microscopic appearance of the esophageal mucosa in a consecutive series of patients submitted to upper endoscopy: Correlation with gastroesophageal reflux symptoms and macroscopic findings. Scand J Gastroenterol 21:65–69, 1986.

39. Schindlbeck NE, Wiebecke B, Klauser AG, et al: Diagnostic value of histology in non-erosive gastro-oesophageal reflux disease. Gut 39:151–154, 1996.

40. Kahrilas PJ, Quigley EM: Clinical esophageal pH recording: A technical review for practice guideline development. Gastroenterology 110:1982–1986, 1996.

41. Fass R, Ofman JJ, Pulliam G, Lembo A: Persistent symptoms of heartburn in patients on standard doses of proton pump inhibitors (PPI) are not due to acid reflux in most patients. Gastroenterology 116(Part 2):A160, #G0694, 1999.

42. Fass R, Pulliam G: Chemosensitivity to acid in patients with persistent heartburn (HB) on standard doses of proton pump inhibitor (PPI) and normal 24-hour esophageal pH (24-H pH) monitoring. Gastroenterology 166(Part 2):A159, #G0691, 1999.

43. de Boer WA, Tytgat GN: Review article: Drug therapy for reflux oesophagitis. Aliment Pharmacol Ther 8:147–157, 1994.

44. DeVault KR, Castell DO: Guidelines for the diagnosis and treatment of gastroesophageal reflux disease. Practice Parameters Committee of the American College of Gastroenterology. Arch Intern Med 155:2165–2173, 1995.

45. Hatlebakk JG, Hyggen A, Madsen PH, et al: Heartburn treatment in primary care: Randomised, double-blind study for 8 weeks. BMJ 319 (7209): 550–553.

46. Venables TL, Newland RD, Patel AC, et al: Maintenance treatment for gastro-

oesophageal reflux disease: A placebo-controlled evaluation of 10 milligrams omeprazole once daily in general practice. Scand J Gastroenterol 32:627–632, 1997.

47. Talley NJ, Venables TL, Green JR, et al: Esomeprazole 40 mg and 20 mg is efficacious in the long-term management of patients with endoscopy-negative GERD: A placebo-controlled trial of on-demand therapy for 6 months. Gastroenterology 118(Suppl 2):A658, #3608, 2000.

48. Fass R, Ofman JJ, Gralnek IM, et al: Clinical and economic assessment of the omeprazole test in patients with symptoms suggestive of gastroesophageal reflux disease. Arch Intern Med 159:2161–2168, 1999.

49. Clouse RE, Lustman PJ, Eckert TC, et al: Low-dose trazodone for symptomatic patients with esophageal contraction abnormalities: A double-blind, placebo-controlled trial. Gastroenterology 92:1027–1036, 1987.

50. Cannon RO 3rd, Quyyumi AA, Mincemoyer R, et al: Imipramine in patients with chest pain despite normal coronary angiograms. N Engl J Med 330:1411–1417, 1994.

51. Camilleri M, Mayer EA, Drossman D, et al: Improvement in pain and bowel function in female irritable bowel patients with alosetron, a 5-HT3 receptor antagonist. Aliment Pharmacol Ther 13:1149–1159, 1999.

52. Kahrilas PJ, Quigley EM, Castell DO, Spechler SJ: The effects of tegaserod (HTF 919) on oesophageal acid exposure in gastro-oesophageal reflux disease. Aliment Pharmacol Ther 14:1503–1509, 2000.

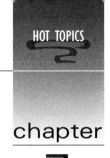

Extraesophageal Manifestations of Gastroesophageal Reflux Disease

chapter 7

*Howard Hampel, M.D., Ph.D., and
Hashem B. El-Serag, M.D., M.P.H.*

Gastroesophageal reflux disease (GERD) has been implicated in causing several supraesophageal or extraesophageal disorders involving the respiratory tract, the larynx, and the oropharynx. A list of these disease associations is presented in Table 1. Asthma and laryngitis are the two diseases for which there are the strongest epidemiologic associations with GERD. Dental erosions are the predominant oral lesions associated with GERD. A number of other disease states have been associated with acid reflux disease, although the data are less compelling. In this chapter, we review and summarize the available data on the epidemiology, pathogenesis, and treatment of these disorders and conclude with a suggested plan of management.

Epidemiology

Pulmonary Disorders

A variety of acute and chronic pulmonary diseases have been linked to GERD. Several epidemiologic studies have reported the strength of these associations. For example, El-Serag et al[1] evaluated the prevalence of various pulmonary diseases among 101,366 veterans with erosive esophagitis or esophageal strictures compared to control patients without these conditions. They found that those patients with GERD-related erosive esophagitis were at a significantly higher risk for asthma, chronic obstructive pulmonary disease bronchiectasis, pneumonia, and pulmonary fibrosis. These results are shown in Figure 1. On the other hand, GERD symptoms are also more common among patients with asthma. Field et al[2] found that 77% of asthma patients had at least weekly heartburn, and that pulmonary symptoms were more severe among those with GERD

119

Disease	Strong Association w/GERD	Weak Association w/GERD
TABLE 1.	**Extraesophageal Diseases Associated with Gastroesophageal Reflux Disease**	
Pulmonary disease	Asthma	Pneumonia Chronic obstructive pulmonary disease Bronchiectasis Pulmonary fibrosis Obstructive sleep apnea
Ear, nose, and throat disease	Reflux laryngitis	Larynogospasm Leukoplakia Laryngomalacia Laryngeal cancer Tracheal stenosis Chronic sinusitis
Dental disease	Erosions	—

symptoms. Evidence of abnormal acid reflux has been demonstrated in asthmatic patients even in the absence of heartburn symptoms. Harding et al[3] prospectively evaluated 26 asthmatic patients without symptoms of acid reflux and found that 65% had abnormal 24-hour esophageal pH study findings showing increased esophageal acid contact times. The increased prevalence of GERD symptoms and esophageal acid exposure

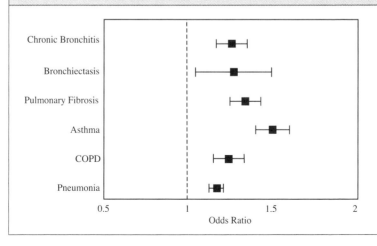

Figure 1. Pulmonary disorders associated with erosive esophagitis or esophageal stricture. Each box represents an odds ratio and each line a 95% confidence interval. COPD = chronic obstructive pulmonary disease. (Data from El-Serag HB, Sonnenberg A: Comorbid occurrence of laryngeal or pulmonary disease with esophagitis in United States military veterans. Gastroenterology 113:755–760, 1997.)

has been shown to be independent of the use of medications that are used by asthmatic patients, such as beta-receptor agonist inhalers and aminophylline, which may increase GERD by decreasing the lower esophageal sphincter pressure. Sontag et al[4] also found that among 104 adult patients with asthma, at least 80% had reflux, which was frequently nocturnal but which was independent of bronchodilator use.

Ear, Nose, and Throat Disorders

There is a rising tendency among ear, nose, and throat specialists to implicate GERD in various laryngopharyngeal ailments. The prevalence of ear, nose, and throat signs and symptoms related to GERD is not well defined because of the difficulty in establishing these diagnoses. For example, there is a relatively high prevalence of both laryngitis and GERD in the general population, a broad differential diagnosis of laryngitis, and no acceptable "gold standard" test for diagnosing GERD. Estimates of the prevalence of heartburn symptoms among patients with reflux laryngitis vary widely in the literature from 6% to 43%. However, using 24-hour esophageal pH monitoring, it has been estimated that 20% to 70% of patients with chronic hoarseness have abnormal acid reflux in the distal or proximal esophagus or in the pharynx.[5–8] In a case-control study of patients with erosive esophagitis, concurrent diagnoses of sinusitis, pharyngitis, laryngitis, and laryngeal stenosis were 1.5 to 2 times more likely in the patients with GERD as compared with control subjects.[1] GERD has also been shown to be a risk factor for laryngeal cancer, being two times more common among patients with laryngeal cancer than among control subjects.[9]

Chronic cough deserves special attention, as it may be a manifestation of irritation of either the respiratory or the laryngeal mucosa. The prevalence of typical GERD-related symptoms, such as heartburn, among patients with chronic cough is 10%. However, up to 40% of patients with chronic cough have abnormal findings on 24-hour esophageal pH studies.[10–12] Irwin et al[13] studied patients with chronic cough who: (1) were nonsmokers, (2) had a normal chest x-ray; and (3) did not take angiotensin-converting enzyme inhibitors. They found that cough in virtually all of these patients could be attributed to one or a combination of three disorders: asthma, postnasal drip, and GERD. GERD was the sole cause of cough in 20% of patients.

Dental

The prevalence of dental erosions among patients with GERD has been estimated at 25% to 70%.[14–16] This compares to a prevalence of 2% to 18% in the general population.[17] Conversely, other studies have found a prevalence of GERD of 25% to 83% among patients with dental erosions.[15,17–18] Dental erosions are defined as loss of tooth enamel by a chemical process that does not involve bacteria. Dental erosions are not detectable until the dentin (yellow) is exposed; they are smooth and are seen on the buccal surface of teeth (i.e., facing the outside). Dental erosion are not to be confused with dental caries (not associated with reflux) in which bacteria are involved in plaque formation. Caries are jagged and uneven on the dental and lingual surfaces of teeth (i.e., facing inside and facing other teeth respectively).

Most extraesophageal conditions associated with reflux in adults have also been documented with infants and children with GERD. In infants and children, gastroesophageal reflux has been reported to cause apnea and sudden infant death syndrome.

Pathogenesis

There are two general theories concerning the pathogenesis of GERD-related extraesophageal disease. The first hypothesis suggests *reflex*-mediated mechanisms, whereby esophageal acid stimulates vagally mediated reflexes such as bronchospasm, laryngospasm, and cough. The second hypothesis implicates a *reflux* mechanism involving direct exposure of refluxed gastroduodenal contents, resulting in injury to oropharyngeal and respiratory tract mucosa. These two mechanisms are by no means mutually exclusive (Fig. 2).

Reflex

Reflex-mediated mechanisms are the primary explanation for GERD-related asthma, based on the shared innervation related to common embryologic origin between the esophagus and the pulmonary tree. In animal studies, it has been shown that esophageal acid perfusion increases airway resistance, and this effect can be overcome by bilateral vagotomy.[19,20] In human volunteers, esophageal acid perfusion resulted in significant deterioration in pulmonary function as measured by peak expiratory flow rates.[21,22] In these studies, clearance of acid from the esophagus did not result in improved airway resistance. However, bronchoconstrictive effects of esophageal acid perfusion were abolished by pretreatment with atropine. These results have led to the proposal that esophageal reflux stimulates esophageal vagal afferent nerves, which can trigger a reflex stimulation of pulmonary vagal efferent nerves, causing bronchial smooth muscle constriction and mucus production.

Reflux

Reflux of gastroduodenal contents into the larynx and hypopharynx is the primary explanation for reflux laryngitis and its associated symptoms. Microaspiration of refluxed gastric contents, and hence pul-

Figure 2. The proposed mechanism of reflux-related extraesophageal disorders. **A,** Vagal model "reflex"; **B,** direct contact model "reflux."

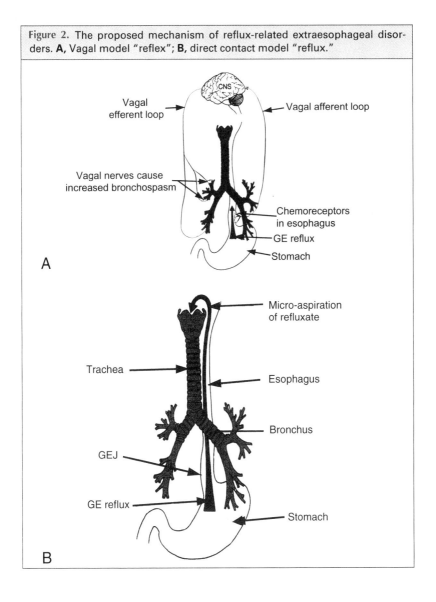

monary disorders, has been difficult to document in humans. Animal studies have shown that direct infusion of even minute amounts of gastric acid and pepsin onto laryngeal mucosa results in significant inflammation and edema;[23,24] when there is preexisting laryngeal mucosal injury, the inflammatory effects of acid exposure are potentiated, and delayed healing may result. These findings have not been replicated in human studies. Another means to relate laryngeal symptoms to direct acid exposure is by performing 24-hour pH testing with a probe at the upper esophageal sphincter or at the level of the hypopharynx. Proximal acid reflux events, which approximate exposure to the larynx, can thus be ascertained. Although a few reported studies show that patients with reflux laryngitis have significantly more proximal esophageal or hypopharyngeal reflux events than control subjects,[5–6,25] others have found that proximal esophageal reflux has no predictive value in identifying patients with suspected reflux laryngitis.[26,27] Up to 30% of patients with suspected reflux laryngitis have normal pharyngeal pH study findings, and 20% of asymptomatic control subjects have abnormal pH testing findings. It has been observed that reflux laryngitis has the highest prevalence, 45%, in professional voice users, including singers and public speakers.[28] It has been suggested that mucosal injury such as that incurred during voice overuse is a necessary precursor to acid-induced injury. However, the exact mechanisms are not fully understood.

Diagnosis

An accurate diagnosis of an extraesophageal manifestation of GERD is often difficult to make. There is no gold standard diagnostic test. There is a large degree of overlap in signs and symptoms between GERD-related and non-GERD-related extraesophageal disorders. Paradoxically, in some asthmatic patients, asthma may actually cause or worsen gastroesophageal reflux because the increase in transdiaphragmatic pressure during airflow obstruction may "suck" the gastric contents into the esophagus.

The diagnosis is usually made on the basis of a suggestive history and physical examination, and directed testing to exclude other disorders. A common theme to most potential extraesophageal manifestations of GERD is that the most accurate and cost-effective diagnostic strategy consists of therapeutic trials of maximum gastric acid suppression with medications such as proton pump inhibitors (PPIs) alone or in combination with histamine-2 receptor antagonists (H$_2$RAs). At this time, apart from a favorable response of laryngitis or asthma to acid suppressive therapy, there is no accepted test used to confirm the clinical diagnosis of GERD-related laryngitis or asthma. More expensive and invasive diagnostic testing such as endoscopy or 24-hour pH-metry is reserved for complicated cases or when the diagnosis remains unclear after therapeutic trials.

Evaluation of the Patient with Suspected Laryngeal Manifestations

Symptoms that help diagnose reflux laryngitis include morning hoarseness or concomitant pulmonary symptoms, including chronic cough and asthma. Other symptoms include excessive phlegm, halitosis, globus sensation, frequent throat clearing and sore throat. Hoarseness is the most commonly reported symptom of reflux laryngitis, occurring in up to 90% of patients.[29] Classic symptoms of GERD are absent in more than half of the patients with suspected GERD-related laryngitis. Features on laryngoscopic examination that are specific for reflux laryngitis include edema or erythema on the posterior cricoid wall, vocal cords, and medial wall of the arytenoids (Fig. 3). Less specific features, include granularity with or without cobblestoning or interarytenoid bar. Infrequently ulcers, polyps, or granulomas are seen. Some of these signs are also seen in association with smoking, viral illness, and voice abuse. Overall, only 50% of patients with laryngoscopic signs suggestive of GERD have abnormal esophageal acid exposure on ambulatory pH testing.[30] Adding a pharyngeal probe increases the yield of positive results. However, ability of pH testing to distinguish healthy persons from those with GERD, or from patients with laryngitis is generally poor. Moreover, pH measurement does not predict the response to antisecretory therapy. We do not recommend this test in the initial evaluation of suspected GERD-related laryngitis.

Evaluation of the Patient with Suspected Pulmonary Manifestations

Heartburn, which immediately precedes wheezing in asthma patients, is somewhat predictive of a response to antireflux treatment.[31] Heartburn symptoms at any time and the presence of predominantly nocturnal asthma also predict good response to antireflux therapy. GERD-related cough is often long-standing, with a mean duration of at least 1 year. Heartburn and regurgitation are present in less than 50% of cases and, when present, usually precede the cough symptoms. Concurrent laryngeal complaints of hoarseness or sore throat also support a GERD-related origin of cough.

Management

Asthma

At least six studies have evaluated the effects of PPI therapy on asthma symptoms. Kiljander et al[32] performed a randomized controlled crossover trial of 52 asthma patients with abnormal 24-hour pH study findings to evaluate the effects of omeprazole 40 mg daily for 8 weeks on asthma symptoms and pulmonary function test results. They found that 35% of patients had significant improvement in nighttime but not daytime asthma symptoms. There was no significant improvement in pulmonary function

Figure 3. **A,** Normal larynx. (TVF = true vocal fold, FVF = false vocal fold, AMW = arytenoids medial wall, AC = arytenoids complex, PCW = posterior cricoid wall, PPW = posterior pharyngeal wall.) **B,** Vocal cord granuloma. (*continued*)

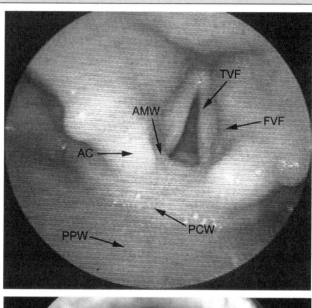

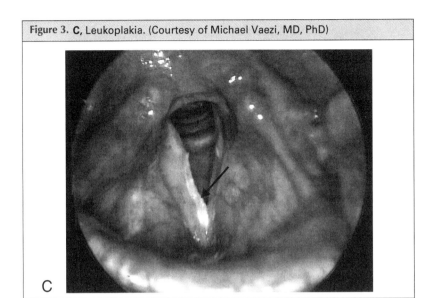

Figure 3. **C**, Leukoplakia. (Courtesy of Michael Vaezi, MD, PhD)

test results. Teichtahl et al[33] reported on a randomized controlled trial of 20 patients with asthma and GERD to evaluate the effects of omeprazole 40 mg twice daily for 4 weeks on asthma symptoms and peak expiratory flow rates. Although there was small improvement in evening peak expiratory flow in the treatment group, there was no difference in reported asthma symptoms, bronchodilator use, or 1- second forced expiratory volumes between the two groups. Ford et al[34] reported on a randomized controlled trial of 14 adult asthmatic patients with GERD documented by endoscopy or 24-hour pH monitoring comparing the effects of omeprazole 20 mg daily on asthma control assessed by symptoms, peak expiratory flow rate, and bronchodilator usage. Omeprazole treatment did not improve asthma symptoms during the day or night, bronchodilator usage, or peak expiratory flow rate readings. In a randomized controlled trial by Boeree et al,[35] 36 patients with either asthma or chronic obstructive pulmonary disease received omeprazole 40 mg PO twice daily for 3 months to evaluate the effects of therapy on airway reactivity measured by methacholine inhalation challenge test. They found that omeprazole had no benefit on any of the measured parameters. Harding et al[31] performed an uncontrolled evaluation of 30 asthmatic patients using graduated doses of omeprazole for 3 months. The starting dose of omeprazole was 20 mg per day and doses were increased 20 mg per day until acid suppression was documented using 24-hour pH monitoring. The average required dose was 27 mg per day. The authors found that 73% of patients had improved peak expiratory flow or a decrease in asthma symptoms. In sum, the evidence that acid suppression therapy significantly improves asthma symptoms by subjective or objective criteria is rather weak. Certain subsets of patients with asthma have been identified that are more likely to respond to acid suppression therapy. These include patients with classic GERD symptoms, such as frequent heartburn or acid regurgitation those with nocturnal predominant asthma; those with heartburn symptoms that precede the onset of asthma; and those who are found to have proximal reflux on pH testing.

Trials of surgical treatment, with one exception, are uncontrolled. The only randomized controlled trial of fundoplication versus medical therapy was done in the era before the use of PPIs (90 patients with pulmonary symptoms who were randomly assigned to antireflux surgery or cimetidine 300 mg four times daily, or placebo). This trial showed some improvement in asthma symptoms and asthma medication use in the surgically treated group. H_2RAs are of limited or no benefit for pulmonary complaints related to GERD.[36]

Asthma patients who have GERD symptoms or who have difficult to control asthma should be considered for trials of acid suppression therapy. We recommend a twice-daily dose of a PPI, which gives the best chance to normalize gastric acid pH. Currently available PPIs and their doses are shown in Table 2. A therapeutic trial, which frequently serves as a diagnostic test, should continue for at least 3 months. No or minimal response usually indicates the absence of GERD-related symptoms. Ambulatory esophageal pH testing (with simultaneous gastric pH testing) should be reserved for patients with continued respiratory and esophageal symptoms while on PPI.

Chronic Cough

There is only one small randomized controlled trial of acid suppression therapy for cough. Ours et al[37] performed a double-blind placebo-controlled trial of omeprazole 40 mg PO twice daily for 3 months in 23

TABLE 2. Available Proton Pump Inhibitors*		
Generic Name	Trade Name	Capsule Strength
Omeprazole	Prilosec	20 mg
Lansoprazole	Prevacid	30 mg
Pantoprazole	Protonix	40 mg
Rabeprazole	Aciphex	20 mg
Esomeprazole	Nexium	40 mg

* For the treatment of a potential GERD-related extra esophageal disorder, all are recommended in twice-daily dosing 30 minutes before meals.

patients with cough. Among six patients who had normal pH study findings prior to testing, none had improvement of symptoms with PPI. Of 17 patients with an abnormal pH study finding, 35% had subjective improvement in cough with therapy, which was significantly better than among control subjects. Of the patients who responded, all did so within 2 weeks. Several small uncontrolled trials of H_2RAs showed response rates of 80% to 100%, with the full effect taking up to 6 months to achieve.[12,27,38]

A treatment algorithm for chronic cough is shown in Figure 4. The cause of chronic cough is multifactorial in up to 30% of patients.[39] All patients should undergo chest radiography. A laryngoscopic examination should be considered in those patients with concomitant laryngeal symptoms. If the chest radiograph is normal, and the patient has classi-

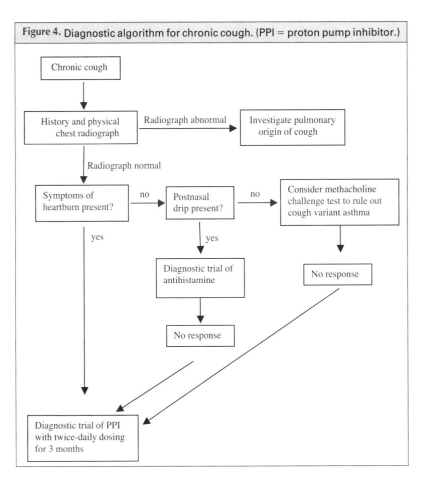

Figure 4. Diagnostic algorithm for chronic cough. (PPI = proton pump inhibitor.)

cal reflux symptoms such as heartburn and regurgitation, then a trial of PPI twice-daily dosing should be considered. If GERD symptoms are absent, cough-variant asthma should be ruled out with a methacholine inhalation challenge or a trial of bronchodilators. Postnasal drip syndrome, commonly due to allergic rhinitis, should be considered and tackled with a trial of antihistamines and/or inhaled steroids.

Reflux Laryngitis

Only two small randomized placebo-controlled trials evaluated PPI therapy for suspected reflux laryngitis. El-Serag et al[40] randomized 22 patients with suspected reflux laryngitis to receive 3 months of either lansoprazole 30 mg PO twice daily or matching placebo. The authors found a complete symptomatic response in 50% of the lansoprazole group, as compared with 10% of the placebo group ($P = 0.04$). Among complete symptomatic responders, none of the initial diagnostic tests results and symptoms were predictive of eventual response; these tests results and symptoms included GERD symptoms, ambulatory distal or proximal 24-hour esophageal pH monitoring findings, laryngeal examination findings, and gastrointestinal endoscopic findings. Noordzij et al[41] randomized 30 patients with suspected reflux laryngitis to receive 2 months of omeprazole 40 mg PO twice daily or placebo. They reported significant improvement in symptoms of hoarseness and throat clearing in the omeprazole group as compared with the placebo group. Five uncontrolled studies have evaluated laryngeal symptom response to PPI therapy[42–45] and reported varying response rates, from 60% to 100% with a weighted average of 67%.

An algorithm for diagnosis and treatment of suspected reflux laryngitis is shown in Figure 5. Because of the broad differential diagnosis of chronic hoarseness, all patients should undergo laryngoscopic examination. If patients have symptoms and laryngoscopic examination findings suspicious for reflux laryngitis, then a trial of acid suppression with PPI twice-daily dosing should be started and continued for at least 3 months. If there is incomplete symptomatic response at 3 months, 24-hour esophageal pH metry should be performed while the patients is on acid suppression therapy to document adequate medical treatment, which is absence of esophageal acid exposure. We recommend performing the pH-metry using gastric, distal, and proximal esophageal sensors, while the patient is on antireflux therapy. The absence of evidence of an abnormal increase in acid in all three sensors, coupled with the absence of symptomatic response, virtually eliminates the possibility of GERD-related disorders.

If acid reflux is not controlled, then increasing the dose of PPI (double dose twice daily) and/or adding a nocturnal H_2RA can be attempted;

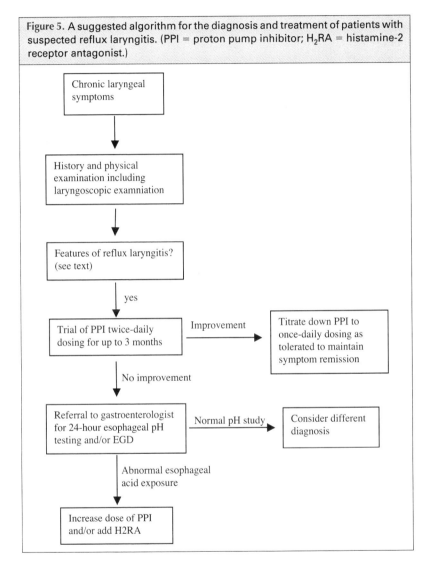

Figure 5. A suggested algorithm for the diagnosis and treatment of patients with suspected reflux laryngitis. (PPI = proton pump inhibitor; H₂RA = histamine-2 receptor antagonist.)

for example, ranitidine 150 mg PO daily at bedtime. It should be noted that laryngoscopic findings usually lag behind symptomatic improvement. If symptoms persist despite adequate acid suppression, a different diagnosis should be considered. For patients who respond well to antisecretory therapy, PPI therapy should be maintained, but the dosing should titrated down to once daily as symptoms allow. In case of multiple recurrence or relapse, or concomitant episodes of aspiration-related pneumonia, surgical therapy of GERD (fundoplication) should be considered. Conversely, we do not recommend surgical therapy of GERD for patients with poor response to medical therapy; these patients typically have poor surgical outcomes. In other words, antireflux surgery should not be an acceptable diagnostic test for suspected reflux-related laryngitis.

Dental Erosions

Although there are no therapeutic trials evaluating the effects of acid suppression therapy on dental erosions, it makes sense to ask and examine patients with multiple dental erosions about reflux symptoms. If a patient complains of heartburn or regurgitation, aggressive acid-lowering therapy should be started. Also, it is important for GERD patients to have regular dental care, as they might be at higher risk of tooth decay.

Suggested Reading

1. El-Serag HB, Sonnenberg A: Comorbid occurrence of laryngeal or pulmonary disease with esophagitis in United States military veterans. Gastroenterology 113:755–760, 1997.
2. Field SK, Underwood M, Brant R, Cowie RL: Prevalence of gastroesophageal reflux symptoms in asthma. Chest 109:316–322, 1996.
3. Harding SM, Guzzo MR, Richter JE: The prevalence of gastroesophageal reflux in asthma patients without reflux symptoms. Am J Respir Crit Care Med 162:34–39, 2000.
4. Sontag SJ, O'Connell S, Khandelwal S, et al: Most asthmatics have gastroesophageal reflux with or without bronchodilator therapy. Gastroenterology 99:613–620, 1990.
5. Shaker R, Milbrath M, Ren J, et al: Esophagopharyngeal distribution of refluxed gastric acid in patients with reflux laryngitis. Gastroenterology 109:1575–1582, 1995.
6. Jacob P, Kahrilas PJ, Herzon G: Proximal esophageal pH-metry in patients with 'reflux laryngitis'. Gastroenterology 100:305–310, 1991.
7. Katz PO: Ambulatory esophageal and hypopharyngeal pH monitoring in patients with hoarseness. Am J Gastroenterol 85:38–40, 1990.
8. Wilson JA, White A, von Haacke NP, et al: Gastroesophageal reflux and posterior laryngitis. Ann Otol Rhinol Laryngol 98:405–410, 1989.
9. El-Serag HB, Hepworth EJ, Lee P, Sonnenberg A: Gastroesophageal reflux disease is a risk factor for laryngeal and pharyngeal cancer. Am J Gastroenterol 96:2013–2018, 2001.
10. Irwin RS, French CL, Curley FJ, et al: Chronic cough due to gastroesophageal reflux: Clinical, diagnostic, and pathogenetic aspects. Chest 104:1511–1517, 1993.
11. Ing AJ, Ngu MC, Breslin AB: Chronic persistent cough and clearance of esophageal acid. Chest 102:1668–1671, 1992.
12. Vaezi MF, Richter JE: Twenty-four-hour ambulatory esophageal pH monitoring in the diagnosis of acid reflux-related chronic cough. South Med J 90:305–311, 1997.
13. Irwin RS, Madison JM: The diagnosis and treatment of cough. N Engl J Med 343:1715–1721, 2000.
14. Loffeld RJ: Incisor teeth status in patients with reflux oesophagitis. Digestion 57:388–390, 1996.
15. Schroeder PL, Filler SJ, Ramirez B, et al: Dental erosion and acid reflux disease. Ann Intern Med 122:809–815, 1995.

16. Meurman JH, Toskala J, Nuutinen P, Klemetti E: Oral and dental manifestations in gastroesophageal reflux disease. Oral Surg Oral Med Oral Pathol 78:583–589, 1994.

17. Lazarchik DA, Filler SJ: Dental erosion: Predominant oral lesion in gastroesophageal reflux disease. Am J Gastroenterol 95(Suppl):S33–38, 2000.

18. Jarvinen V, Rytomaa I, Meurman JH: Location of dental erosion in a referred population. Caries Res 26:391–396, 1992.

19. Mansfield LE, Stein MR: Gastroesophageal reflux and asthma: A possible reflex mechanism. Ann Allergy 41:224–226, 1978.

20. Tuchman DN, Boyle JT, Pack AI, et al: Comparison of airway responses following tracheal or esophageal acidification in the cat. Gastroenterology 87:872–881, 1984.

21. Wright RA, Miller SA, Corsello BF: Acid-induced esophagobronchial-cardiac reflexes in humans. Gastroenterology 99:71–73, 1990.

22. Schan CA, Harding SM, Haile JM, et al: Gastroesophageal reflux-induced bronchoconstriction: An intraesophageal acid infusion study using state-of-the-art technology. Chest 106:731–737, 1994.

23. Little FB, Koufman JA, Kohut RI, Marshall RB: Effect of gastric acid on the pathogenesis of subglottic stenosis. Ann Otol Rhinol Laryngol 94:516–519, 1985.

24. Ludemann JP, Manoukian J, Shaw K, et al: Effects of simulated gastroesophageal reflux on the untraumatized rabbit larynx. J Otolaryngol 27:127–131, 1998.

25. Ylitalo R, Lindestad PA, Ramel S: Symptoms, laryngeal findings, and 24-hour pH monitoring in patients with suspected gastroesophago-pharyngeal reflux. Laryngoscope 111:1735–1741, 2001.

26. Wo JM, Hunter JG, Waring JP: Dual-channel ambulatory esophageal pH monitoring: A useful diagnostic tool? Dig Dis Sci 42:2222–2226, 1997.

27. Waring JP, Lacayo L, Hunter J, et al: Chronic cough and hoarseness in patients with severe gastroesophageal reflux disease: Diagnosis and response to therapy. Dig Dis Sci 40:1093–1097, 1995.

28. Sataloff RT, Speigel JR, Hawkshaw M, Rosen DC: Gastroesophageal reflux laryngitis. Ear Nose Throat J 72:113–134, 1993.

29. Toohill RJ, Kuhn JC: Role of refluxed acid in pathogenesis of laryngeal disorders. Am J Med 103:100S–106S, 1997.

30. Richter JE, Hicks DM: Unresolved issues in gastroesophageal reflux-related ear, nose, and throat problems. Am J Gastroenterol 92:2143–2144, 1997.

31. Harding SM, Richter JE, Guzzo MR, et al: Asthma and gastroesophageal reflux: Acid suppressive therapy improves asthma outcome. Am J Med 100:395–405, 1996.

32. Kiljander TO, Salomaa ER, Hietanen EK, Terho EO: Gastroesophageal reflux in asthmatics: A double-blind, placebo-controlled crossover study with omeprazole. Chest 116:1257–1264, 1999.

33. Teichtahl H, Kronborg IJ, Yeomans ND, Robinson P: Adult asthma and gastro-oesophageal reflux: The effects of omeprazole therapy on asthma. Aust N Z J Med 26:671–676, 1996.

34. Ford GA, Oliver PS, Prior JS, et al: Omeprazole in the treatment of asthmatics with nocturnal symptoms and gastro-oesophageal reflux: A placebo-controlled crossover study. Postgrad Med J 70:350–354, 1994.

35. Boeree MJ, Peters FT, Postma DS, Kleibeuker JH: No effects of high-dose omeprazole in patients with severe airway hyperresponsiveness and (a)symptomatic gastro-oesophageal reflux. Eur Respir J 11:1070–1074, 1998.

36. Larrain A, Carrasco E, Galleguillos F, et al: Medical and surgical treatment of nonallergic asthma associated with gastroesophageal reflux. Chest 99:1330–1335, 1991.

37. Ours TM, Kavuru MS, Schilz RJ, Richter JE: A prospective evaluation of esophageal testing and a double-blind, randomized study of omeprazole in a diagnostic and therapeutic algorithm for chronic cough. Am J Gastroenterol 94:3131–3138, 1999.

38. Smyrnios NA, Irwin RS, Curley FJ: Chronic cough with a history of excessive sputum production: The spectrum and frequency of causes, key components of the diagnostic evaluation, and outcome of specific therapy. Chest 108:991–997, 1995.

39. Irwin RS, Richter JE: Gastroesophageal reflux and chronic cough. Am J Gastroenterol 95(Suppl):S9–14 2000.

40. El-Serag HB, Lee P, Buchner A, et al: Lansoprazole treatment of patients with chronic idiopathic laryngitis: A placebo-controlled trial. Am J Gastroenterol 96:979–983, 2001.

41. Noordzij JP, Khidr A, Evans BA, et al: Evaluation of omeprazole in the treatment of reflux laryngitis: A prospective, placebo-controlled, randomized, double-blind study. Laryngoscope 111:2147–2151, 2001.

42. Wo JM, Grist WJ, Gussack G, et al: Empiric trial of high-dose omeprazole in patients with posterior laryngitis: A prospective study. Am J Gastroenterol 92:2160–2165, 1997.

43. Shaw GY, Searl JP: Laryngeal manifestations of gastroesophageal reflux before and after treatment with omeprazole. South Med J 90:1115–1122, 1997.

44. Metz DC, Childs ML, Ruiz C, Weinstein GS: Pilot study of the oral omeprazole test for reflux laryngitis. Otolaryngol Head Neck Surg 116:41–46, 1997.

45. Jaspersen D, Weber R, Hammar CH, Draf W: Effect of omeprazole on the course of associated esophagitis and laryngitis. J Gastroenterol 31:765–767, 1996.

Barrett's Esophagus

Richard E. Sampliner, M.D.

What is Barrett's Esophagus?

Barrett's esophagus is a change in the lining of the distal end of the esophagus that is recognizable as abnormal mucosa at the time of endoscopic examination and is documented to have intestinal metaplasia with goblet cells by biopsy.[1] The normal distal esophagus is lined with squamous epithelium; in a patient with Barrett's esophagus, however, it is lined by a columnar-appearing mucosa (Fig. 1) that visually resembles the color of the stomach and histologically resembles the small intestines but is located in a different site, hence the term *intestinal metaplasia.*

Barrett's esophagus is thought to be a complication of chronic gastroesophageal reflux disease (GERD). Refluxate damages the distal esophagus, and, in a subgroup of patients, a unique lining replaces the squamous epithelium. The importance of Barrett's esophagus is that it is the premalignant lesion for adenocarcinoma of the esophagus. Adenocarcinoma of the esophagus has been the cancer with the most rapidly rising incidence in the United States and western Europe over the last two decades.[2] As a result, Barrett's esophagus has received the attention of gastroenterologists, oncologists, and ultimately the lay public. The publication of a population-based study from Sweden highlighting the increased risk of adenocarcinoma of the esophagus in patients with chronic and severe symptoms of gastroesophageal reflux disease was widely discussed in the lay press.[3]

When to Look for Barrett's Esophagus

Whether physicians should screen for Barrett's esophagus in patients with gastroesophageal reflux disease is controversial. In practice, however, many patients are referred to a gastroenterologist with symptoms of GERD. The primary rationale for endoscopy in patients with reflux

Figure 1. Endoscopic view of Barrett's esophagus.

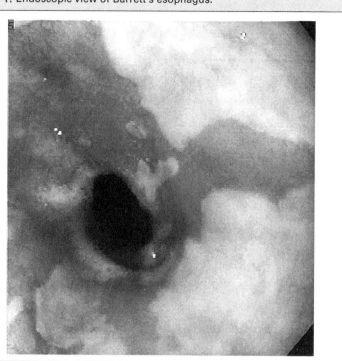

symptoms is the detection of Barrett's esophagus. Unfortunately, we do not yet have evidence-based criteria to utilize in assessing patients for Barrett's esophagus. It is clear, however, from patients we currently identify as having Barrett's esophagus, that on average they are older, have an onset of reflux symptoms at a younger age, have reflux symptoms for a longer duration of time, are more likely male, and are predominantly white.

Esophageal reflux symptoms are very common in the adult population in the United States. Twenty percent of people have weekly heartburn and as many as 10% may have daily heartburn.[5] Many of these patients have not sought medical attention and therefore have not been assessed or treated with prescription drugs. Screening for Barrett's esophagus will not be cost-effective unless we can identify the criteria to select patients at highest risk of having Barrett's esophagus. With the increasing understanding of gastroesophageal reflux disease and Barrett's esophagus, and with an increasingly informed public, many patients do in fact, seek to have an endoscopic evaluation.

Treatment of Barrett's Esophagus

The mainstay of therapy of Barrett's esophagus is proton pump inhibitor therapy.[1] This class of potent acid blockers is usually effective in controlling the reflux symptoms of patients with Barrett's esophagus. It is controversial whether the end point of medical therapy should be control of reflux symptoms or control of intraesophageal pH. As a clinical approach, reducing esophageal acid exposure to normal would be difficult and would require repeat 24-hour pH testing in some patients.

In a patient who still has symptoms on proton pump inhibitor therapy, twice-daily dosing should be used. It is important that the dose be given approximately 30 minutes before breakfast and before dinner to achieve optimal symptom control (Fig. 2). Some patients continue to have so-called volume reflux—that is, they will have regurgitation of material, even into their oral cavity or nasopharynx, but the material will no longer cause heartburn. This patient should be considered for antireflux surgery for control of regurgitation. Currently antireflux surgery can be performed with laparoscopic fundoplication with minimal morbidity and hospitalization time.[6] Furthermore, some patients would rather have antireflux surgery even given its small risk of operative mortality than take medications for the rest of their lives.

Unfortunately, there are no data in the medical literature to document that any form of current therapy prevents the development of adeno-

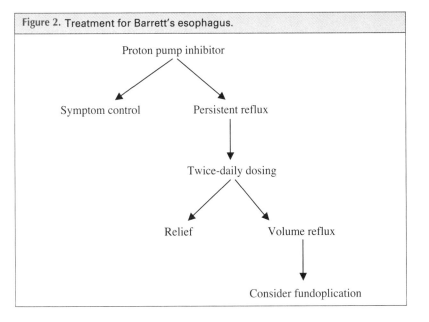

Figure 2. Treatment for Barrett's esophagus.

carcinoma of the esophagus. Even patients with Barrett's esophagus who have had antireflux surgery have been documented to go on to develop adenocarcinoma of the esophagus.[7] It is unlikely for medical therapy to prevent cancer if antireflux surgery, which theoretically prevents all gastric contents from going up into the esophagus, does not result in a reduction of progression to cancer.

Cancer Prevention in Barrett's Esophagus

As mentioned previously, it is not clear that any current intervention will prevent the development of adenocarcinoma of the esophagus short of esophagectomy. However, as part of routine practice, almost all gastroenterologists in the United States perform surveillance endoscopy.[8] This involves upper endoscopy with systematic biopsies of the Barrett's segment of the esophagus, looking for dysplasia. Dysplasia is the first step in the neoplastic process and is recognized pathologically as both cytologic and architectural change in the glands of Barrett's mucosa. Again, the appropriate intervals and methods of endoscopic surveillance are not evidence based. Recommendations have been made that if no dysplasia is recognized after two endoscopic evaluations with biopsy, a patient can undergo endoscopy at 3- to 4-year intervals (Fig. 3).[1] If low-grade dysplasia is found, a repeat endoscopy is necessary to confirm that only low-grade dysplasia is present in the esophagus. If low-grade dysplasia is once again documented, then the patient can undergo two more endoscopic examination at 6-month intervals and then yearly examinations until low-grade dysplasia is no longer recognized. If a patient has high-grade dysplasia, a change that has the highest risk for progressing to cancer, a repeat endoscopic examination needs to confirm that in fact cancer is not yet present in the esophagus.

Unfortunately, in cases of Barrett's esophagus, high-grade dysplasia or even frank adenocarcinoma can be detected on biopsy when the Barrett's mucosa lacks any irregularity. At the time of endoscopy, special attention is focused on biopsying nodular areas, erosions, and strictures. If a nodule is present that shows high-grade dysplasia, an endoscopic resection is an appropriate technique that can identify whether in fact there is an underlying cancer.

Any time cancer is detected on biopsy in an appropriate surgical candidate, esophageal resection is the next step. If a patient has documented high-grade dysplasia that is confirmed by an expert gastrointestinal pathologist, and the patient is young and a reasonable operative candidate, resection may be appropriate. However, many patients with high-grade dysplasia or early cancer with Barrett's esophagus are elderly and have major comorbidities. For these patients, endoscopic therapy

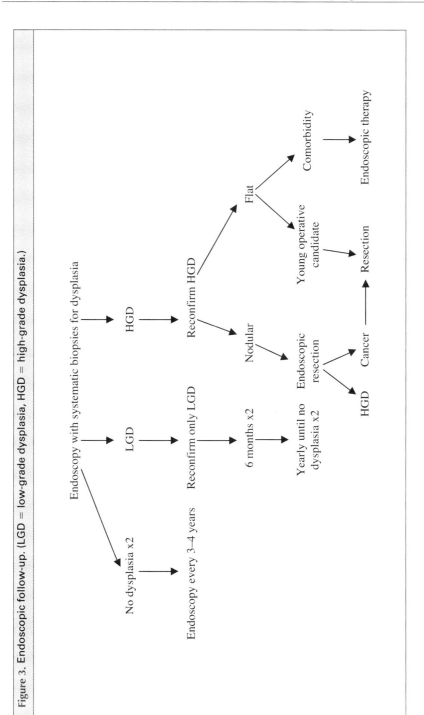

Figure 3. Endoscopic follow-up. (LGD = low-grade dysplasia, HGD = high-grade dysplasia.)

aimed at ablating the dysplasia, cancer, and Barrett's esophagus may be an alternative approach.

Patients with Barrett's Esophagus at Highest Risk of Cancer

More effective risk stratification of patients with Barrett's esophagus would allow more focused endoscopic surveillance and therapeutic intervention. Although risk factors are not evidence based, there is suggestive evidence that male gender, white race, older age, dysplasia, smoking, obesity, and long segment Barrett's esophagus represent greater risk for adenocarcinoma of the esophagus.[9–11] In the future, an index of criteria will be available to estimate the risk of cancer in individual patients. Accumulating all the demographic and endoscopic criteria will enable better assessment of cancer risk for individual patients. In the last decade, much research has been done to identify biomarkers of cancer risk. Unfortunately, these studies have not been validated in multicenter trials. Validated genetic mutations or epigenetic changes could help develop much more specific risk stratification of patients with Barrett's esophagus.

Key Points: Barrett's Esophagus

- ∞ Barrett's esophagus is a complication of chronic gastroesophageal reflux disease.
- ∞ It is an important clinical issue because of the risk for patients with Barrett's esophagus progressing to cancer.
- ∞ The primary mode of therapy for patients with Barrett's esophagus is proton pump inhibition.
- ∞ Prevention or early detection of cancer is possible with interval endoscopy and biopsy.
- ∞ The future offers a number of exciting possibilities that will allow more effective risk stratification of patients to screen for Barrett's esophagus and to survey for adenocarcinoma of the esophagus.
- ∞ Endoscopic therapy offers the opportunity for treatment of high-grade dysplasia or early cancers in a nonoperable patient and also retains the function of the esophagus.
- ∞ The task of detecting and appropriately referring patients with Barrett's esophagus is that of the primary care physician, who sees most of the patients who have chronic reflux disease.

Suggested Reading

1. Sampliner RE, Practice Parameters Committee ACG: Updated guidelines for the diagnosis, surveillance, and therapy of Barrett's esophagus. Am J Gastroenterol 97:1888–1895, 2002.

2. Devesa SS, Blot WJ, Fraumeni JF: Changing patterns in the incidence of esophageal and gastric carcinoma in the United States. Cancer 83:2049–2053, 1998.

3. Lagergren J, Bergstrom R, Lindgren A, Nyren O: Symptomatic gastroesophageal reflux as a risk factor for esophageal adenocarcinoma. N Engl J Med 340:825–831, 1999.

4. Lieberman DA, Oehlke M, Helfand M, G.O.R.E: Risk factors for Barrett's esophagus in community-based practice. Am J Gastroenterol 92:1293–1297, 1997.

5. Locke GR, Talley NJ, Fett SL, Zinsmeister AR, Melton LJ: Prevalence and clinical spectrum of gastroesophageal reflux: A population-based study in Olmsted County, Minnesota. Gastroenterology 112:1448–1456, 1997.

6. Farrell TM, Smith CD, Metreveli RE, et al: Fundoplication provides effective and durable symptom relief in patients with Barrett's esophaugs. Am J Surg 178:18–21, 1999.

7. Ye W, Chow WH, Lagergren J, et al: Risk of adenocarcinomas of the esophagus and gastric cardia in patients with gastroesophageal reflux disease and after antireflux surgery. Gastroenterology 121:1286–1293, 2001.

8. Falk GW, Ours TM, Richter J: Practice patterns for surveillance of Barrett's esophagus in the United States. Gastrointest Endosc 52:197–203, 2000.

9. Blot W, Devesa SS, Kneller RW, Fraumeni JF: Rising incidence of adenocarcinoma of the esophagus and gastric cardia. JAMA 265:1287–1289, 1991.

10. Gammon MD, Schoenbeg JB, Ahsan H, et al: Tobacco, alcohol, and socioeconomic status and adenocarcinomas of the esophagus and gastric cardia. J Natl Cancer Inst 89:1277–1284, 1997.

11. Lagergren J, Bergstrom R, Nyren O: Association between body mass and adenocarcinoma of the esophagus and gastric cardia. Ann Intern Med 130:883–890, 1999.

GERD in the Elderly

Mai-Sie Chan, M.D.,
Ronald W. Yeh, M.D., and
George Triadafilopoulos, M.D.

chapter

9

Gastroesophageal reflux disease (GERD) in the elderly presents physicians with certain challenges in diagnosis and management. Older patients more often present with atypical symptoms, suffer greater complication rates, and have higher mortality. Treatment decisions are also more complex. It is estimated that 21% of the U.S. population will be over the age of 65 by 2030. As the population ages, physicians will encounter more elderly patients, and it will be important to become familiar with the evaluation and treatment of older patients with GERD.

Epidemiology

GERD is the most common esophageal mucosal disorder in the elderly, and is more common in the elderly than in the general population.[4,19,65] Although the prevalence of GERD in younger adults ranges from 13% to 35%,[36] it is estimated to be 20% to 35% in the elderly. This latter figure is likely even higher because older patients with GERD experience fewer symptoms[43] and are more likely to have other co-morbid conditions, such as cardiac or pulmonary disease, which make it more difficult for physicians to recognize symptoms of GERD.

Pathophysiology

Factors that promote reflux of gastric contents (gastric acid, pepsin, bile acids, and trypsin) into the esophagus, cause symptoms, and perpetuate mucosal injury include transient lower esophageal sphincter relaxations, presence of hiatal hernia, impaired motility, and poor esophageal clearance.

Lower Esophageal Sphincter Pressure. Lower esophageal sphincter (LES) incompetence has been historically recognized as the primary mechanism for GERD,[8] but more recent evidence suggests that it plays a relatively minor role in its pathogenesis.[56] Instead, studies now show

143

that the majority of patients with GERD have a normal basal LES pressure and that the reflux is caused by neurogenically mediated, transient LES relaxations that are not associated with swallowing.[35] The presence of acid in the esophagus subsequently causes esophagitis, which in turn reduces LES pressure and impairs esophageal contractility. It is unclear whether the elderly have altered basal LES pressure or a different rate of transient LES relaxation as compared to the general population.[41,47] However, the elderly often are on multiple medications that can reduce LES pressure (Table 1), thereby worsening GERD.

Hiatal Hernia. Sliding hiatal hernia is a major cause of symptomatic and complicated GERD,[56] especially in the elderly. The prevalence of hiatal hernia increases with age[59] and is greater than 60% in the population aged 65 and older.[13, 23] Such high prevalence in the elderly results from degeneration of the phreno-esophageal ligament[14,32,52] and from acid-induced fibrosis and scarring of the esophagus due to prolonged GERD. The presence of hiatal hernia is often associated with low LES pressures[21] and with erosive esophagitis.[18] Over time, the presence of acid in the esophagus causes acid-induced fibrosis, esophageal foreshortening, and lengthening of the hernia. The presence of sliding hiatal hernia further impairs LES function by dissociating the intrinsic LES tone from the support of the diaphragm. This vicious self-perpetuating cycle leads to worsening of GERD (Fig. 1).

Impaired Motility. In the normal esophagus, secondary peristalsis helps to clear refluxed gastric contents from the esophageal lumen. The amplitude of esophageal peristalsis decreases with age,[16] and abnormal peristalsis—which is more common in the elderly—delays clearing of the gastric refluxate.[5] Although the frequency of reflux episodes may be

TABLE 1. Common Drugs that Reduce Lower Esophageal Sphincter Pressure
Alpha-adrenergic antagonists
Beta-adrenergic agonists
Anticholinergics
Benzodiazepines
Calcium antagonists
Levodopa
Nicotine (transdermal)
Nitrates
Opioid analgesics
Progestogens
Theophylline

From Ouatu-Lascar R, Triadafilopoulos G: Esophageal mucosal diseases in the elderly. Drugs Aging 12: 261–276, 1998; with permission.

Figure 1. Sliding hiatal hernia contributing to gastroesophageal reflux. This is a retroflexed endoscopic view of the proximal stomach herniating into the chest through the diaphragmatic hiatus.

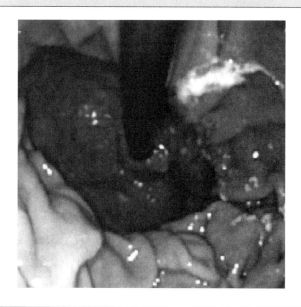

unchanged, the duration of individual episodes becomes longer, leading to an increased likelihood of esophageal mucosal damage.[11] Decreased motility causing delayed gastric emptying has also been observed in the elderly, usually in those older than 80 or 90.[3,33] Because of this, accumulation of stomach contents leads to an increased likelihood of reflux. It is unclear, however, whether the decreased gastric or esophageal motility observed in older patients is due to other systemic diseases such as diabetes mellitus or rheumatologic disorders, or the aging process itself.[25]

The Role of Saliva. Saliva helps to flush refluxate from the esophagus back into the stomach. Bicarbonate in saliva also neutralizes acid in refluxed contents. Although aging has not been shown to affect the quantity or quality of saliva consistently,[26,55] elderly patients are more likely to suffer salivary gland hypofunction secondary to other systemic disorders or the use of medications.

Medications. Medications may contribute to the development of GERD or aggravate existing esophagitis. The mechanisms involved include decreased LES pressure (see Table 1), decreased saliva, and direct injury to the esophageal mucosa (Table 2).

TABLE 2.   Commonly Used Drugs that May Induce Esophageal Injury in the Elderly
Alendronic acid
Aspirin
Doxycycline and other tetracyclines
Emepronium bromide
Ferrous sulfate or succinate
Mexiletine
NSAIDs
Potassium chloride
Quinidine
Theophylline

From Ouatu-Lascar R, Triadafilopoulos G: Esophageal mucosal diseases in the elderly. Drugs Aging 12: 261–276, 1998; with permission.

Clinical Presentation

The most common symptom of GERD is heartburn, described as a burning chest sensation, often occurring after large meals, exercise, or reclining. Other symptoms include regurgitation, belching, water brash, nausea, chest pain, dysphagia, and odynophagia. Extra-esophageal symptoms or complications (Table 3) that may mimic other conditions are more common in the elderly.[44] The higher prevalence of coronary artery disease and pulmonary disease, such as chronic obstructive pulmonary disease (COPD) and chronic bronchitis, also makes the diagnosis of GERD especially difficult in older patients. Older patients are less likely to perceive symptoms like heartburn and acid regurgitation.[43] They have diminished chemo-sensitivity to acid and decreased visceral pain sensation.[9,29,39] Diseases of the central nervous system (CNS), such as dementia or depression, may also impair the ability of elderly patients

TABLE 3. Complications of Gastroesophageal Reflux Disease in the Elderly	
Esophageal	Extra-esophageal
Barrett's esophagus	Angina-like chest pain
Esophageal adenocarcinoma	Asthma
Esophageal ulcer	Chronic cough
Peptic stricture	Chronic hiccups
	Dental erosions
	Laryngitis
	Recurrent pneumonia

From Ouatu-Lascar R, Triadafilopoulos G: Esophageal mucosal diseases in the elderly. Drugs Aging 12: 261–276, 1998; with permission.

to perceive or describe symptoms.[29] Perhaps in part because of such decreased symptom perception, elderly people are more likely to present with serious symptoms such as dysphagia, vomiting, bleeding, or weight loss.[43] Upper GI bleeding is seen more often in elderly patients with esophagitis [51,66] (Fig. 2) and may reflect underlying peptic stricture, Barrett's esophagus, or cancer, possibly resulting from an increased duration of undetected GERD.[19,44] Therefore, clinicians caring for elderly patients must be more aggressive in screening and evaluating for GERD.

Differential Diagnosis

When evaluating an elderly patient presenting with possible reflux symptoms, physicians must distinguish GERD from coronary artery disease, pulmonary disease, gastritis, peptic ulcer disease, esophageal motor disorders, and other causes of esophagitis. GERD-related chest pain can closely mimic cardiac angina, and an electrocardiogram and exercise stress test should be considered prior to gastrointestinal evaluation. Pulmonary symptoms secondary to GERD may be difficult to distinguish

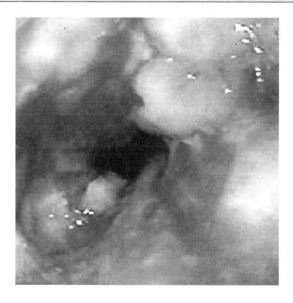

Figure 2. Endoscopic appearance of erosive esophagitis. The distal esophagus is edematous, ulcerated, and friable.

from COPD, asthma, or pulmonary fibrosis. Achalasia is an idiopathic motor disorder of the esophagus characterized by incomplete or absent LES relaxation and absent esophageal peristalsis associated with deglutination. The prevalence of achalasia increases with age.[54] Patients typically present with dysphagia to both liquids and solids, but may also experience chest discomfort, burning, and regurgitation that can be confused with GERD.[34] Elderly patients are more likely to receive multiple medications and thus are at higher risk for pill-induced esophagitis. Infectious esophagitis, caused by candida, herpes simplex virus, cytomegalovirus, or human immunodeficiency virus, is less common in the elderly and is usually seen in those who are immuno-compromised, and/or those who are treated with corticosteroids or chemotherapy.

Another important condition to be considered is pseudo-membranous esophagitis (Fig. 3). It is characterized by thin, concentric membranes and/or thick layers of sloughing of exudates and necrotic debris and occurs predominantly in the elderly with systemic illness and dehydration. The condition clears rapidly with supportive care and acid suppression, and recurrences are rare.[37]

Figure 3. Endoscopic appearance of pseudomebranous esophagitis. The esophagus is covered with thin, whitish membranes coating underlying friable mucosa.

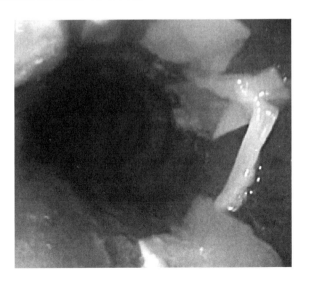

Significance of Barrett's Esophagus in the Elderly

Barrett's esophagus implies the replacement of esophageal squamous epithelium by metaplastic intestinal epithelium as a result of reflux injury and is associated with up to a thirty-fold increase in risk of esophageal adenocarcinoma (Fig. 4).[49,58] The incidence of Barrett's esophagus increases with age, with most patients presenting in their 60s or 70s. The incidence of esophageal adenocarcinoma and its associated mortality is also highest after age 60, making Barrett's esophagus a condition of particular significance in the elderly population.[31] Older patients with GERD tend to experience fewer or less severe symptoms, but are more likely to have complications such as esophagitis, strictures, and Barrett's metaplasia.[4,6,43,65] Elderly patients with Barrett's esophagus also tend to have fewer symptoms when compared with younger patients.[62] Esophageal sensitivity to acid is further reduced in patients with Barrett's esophagus.

Figure 4. Barrett's esophagus. This is an endoscopic view of the distal esophagus exhibiting salmon-colored mucosa. Histologically, the squamous esophageal epithelium has been replaced by columnar metaplasia containing goblet cells (specialized intestinal metaplasia).

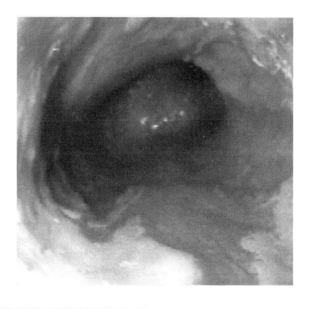

The presence of high-grade dysplasia or early adenocarcinoma in an elderly patient with Barrett's esophagus portends a poor prognosis, since the only potentially curative therapy is esophagectomy. Since most elderly patients are at increased surgical risk, palliative treatments intended to preserve quality of life are generally pursued. Such treatments include mucosal ablation using photodynamic therapy, esophageal mucosal resection, stricture dilation, or palliative stent placement.

Diagnosis and Therapy

Heartburn is such a common complaint in adults that it would be impractical to pursue a diagnostic evaluation in every symptomatic patient. Younger patients typically receive empiric therapy, while invasive diagnostic testing is reserved for patients with symptoms refractory to medications or suggestive of complications. Because the elderly tend to have fewer symptoms and are at increased risk for complications, they should undergo early diagnostic evaluation regardless of the duration or severity of their symptoms—even if they are asymptomatic but give a history of previous symptoms.

Empiric therapy, especially with proton pump inhibitors, can be very effective at relieving symptoms and facilitating the diagnosis of GERD, but it does not detect potential complications.[9,50] Depending on the clinical situation, useful diagnostic studies may include endoscopy, ambulatory esophageal pH monitoring (Fig. 5), esophageal manometry, or barium swallow examination. A stepwise approach to the management of patients with GERD is shown in Figure 6.

Endoscopy

The gold standard for the diagnosis of GERD is upper endoscopy. Endoscopy is both sensitive and specific for detecting esophageal mucosal disease (i.e., erosive esophagitis, Barrett's esophagus) but it may miss 36–50% of patients with pathologic acid exposure detected by esophageal pH monitoring.[37] Endoscopy is especially important for patients who present with "warning" or "alarm" symptoms, such as dysphagia, bleeding, or weight loss. Direct visualization of the esophageal mucosa can detect causes of esophagitis, such as erythema, erosions, and ulcerations, as well as complications of erosive disease, such as strictures or cancer. Endoscopic biopsies and brushings can distinguish reflux from infectious esophagitis and histologically prove Barrett's esophagus with or without dysplasia or cancer. Endoscopy also allows therapeutic interventions, such as stricture dilation, stent placement, and laser ablation of malignant or dysplastic lesions.

Figure 5. Ambulatory 24-hr pH monitoring of the distal esophagus (*thin [top] black line*) and proximal stomach (*thick [bottom] black line*) demonstrating pathologic intraesophageal acid exposure. During the 24-hr study period, there are many episodes during which the intraesophageal pH falls below 4.0.

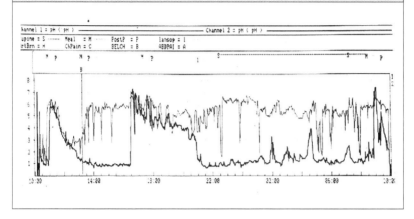

Figure 6. A stepwise approach to the management of patients with GERD.

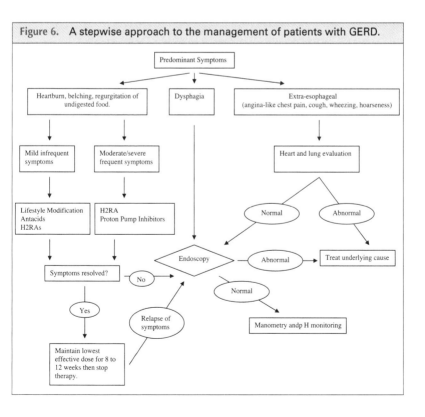

Ambulatory Twenty-Four Hour Esophageal pH Monitoring

Twenty-four hour esophageal pH monitoring can be particularly useful in elderly patients presenting with atypical symptoms and in those with unremarkable endoscopy. The sensitivity and specificity of the test are reported to be 80–90%. A thin, flexible esophageal pH probe is attached to a portable recorder and worn by the patient for 24 hours. In cases where endoscopy demonstrates no esophagitis, a normal esophageal pH may help the detection of non-erosive GERD. Esophageal pH monitoring can also help identify reflux as the underlying etiology for patients who present with extra-esophageal symptoms, such as chronic cough, wheezing, or chest pain, by demonstrating a temporal relationship between acid reflux episodes and such symptoms.

Esophageal Manometry

Esophageal manometry assesses LES tone, relaxation, and esophageal contractile strength and coordination. It is particularly important in the differential diagnosis of elderly patients presenting with atypical symptoms since it may identify an esophageal motility disorder (e.g., achalasia) as the cause of the patients' symptoms. It is also important in the preoperative evaluation in patients considering surgical therapy.

Barium Swallow Radiography

Barium studies actually have poor sensitivity and specificity for GERD. Although reflux of barium into the esophagus can often be visualized, this sign is not specific for GERD. Reflux can occur in healthy individuals, or as a result of other disorders.[48] However, a barium swallow can be helpful in *differentiating* GERD from other disorders, by detecting strictures, ulcerations, or masses. Barium studies also allow observation of esophageal motility. Barium tablet radiography, which involves the administration of a radio-opaque tablet followed by fluoroscopy, may be particularly useful in the evaluation of an elderly patient presenting with dysphagia but with normal endoscopy and motility studies. Typically in such cases, the tablet is temporarily arrested or delayed behind a distal esophageal (Schatzki's) ring or a peptic stricture.

Pharmacologic Therapy

The goals of therapy for GERD in the elderly are: symptom relief, healing of esophagitis, prevention and management of complications, and maintenance of remission. A typical approach to therapy for GERD begins with **lifestyle modification** (Table 4) and over-the-counter antacids or histamine H2 receptor antagonists, followed by a trial of proton pump inhibitors if symptoms still are not controlled. While over-the-counter antacids may provide symptomatic relief in mild GERD, they are ineffec-

TABLE 4. Lifestyle Modifications for GERD
• Avoid tobacco products.
• Elevate head of bed.
• Lose weight.
• Modify diet to avoid fatty foods, citrus juices, coffee, tomato products, and alcohol.
• Stop eating 2–3 hours prior to bedtime.

tive at healing existing esophagitis. Histamine H2 antagonists and proton pump inhibitors are the most common medications used to treat reflux esophagitis or symptomatic GERD. They work by reducing gastric acid secretion, thus decreasing the caustic elements of the refluxate. They do not, however, prevent reflux from occurring, and regurgitation may persist. The effects of the antisecretory drugs are dose-dependent, and their doses can be adjusted to the severity of disease for each individual patient.

The goal of lifestyle changes is to decrease the frequency of gastroesophageal reflux events post-prandially and during the supine position and to enhance esophageal acid clearance of refluxed material. This alone may be effective for elderly patients with mild symptoms of GERD, or with non-erosive or mild esophagitis.

H2 Blockers

The H2 blockers include cimetidine, ranitidine, famotidine, and nizatidine. All are equally effective when taken in equivalent doses, and have been found to decrease gastric acid secretion by 60–70%. As a class they are relatively safe and are less expensive than the newer proton pump inhibitors. However, they are less effective at treating severe esophagitis. Much higher doses are often necessary in these cases, increasing the risk of adverse effects and reducing the cost benefit.[65] Additionally, dose adjustment for renal failure is necessary. Cimetidine has been found to cause confusion in older patients. H2 antagonists also inhibit the cytochrome P450 system, thereby decreasing the metabolism of drugs such as theophylline, warfarin, phenytoin, and benzodiazepines. Therefore, physicians need to carefully monitor elderly patients for potential side effects and drug-drug interactions while on H2 blockers.

Proton Pump Inhibitors

Proton pump inhibitors (PPIs) specifically inhibit the gastric parietal cell enzyme $H+/K+$ ATPase, which regulates the final common pathway of acid secretion. The current available PPIs are omeprazole, lansoprazole, pantoprazole, rabeprazole, and esomeprazole. As with H2 blockers, most studies have demonstrated that the different proton pump inhibitors have similar efficacy when given in equivalent doses.[17]

Older patients may require greater degree of acid suppression to heal their esophagitis.[6,20] As a class, PPIs are more effective then other medications at acid inhibition, enabling more rapid and complete mucosal healing and providing faster symptom relief. They have been shown to be very effective in the elderly, with 80–100% healing rate within 8 weeks.[42] PPIs have also been shown to decrease the need for dilatation in patients with strictures.[53]

Overall, PPIs have an excellent safety profile. No dose adjustment is necessary for elderly patients, even in renal or hepatic impairment.[15] There is a variable degree of P450 metabolism. Symptoms such as abdominal pain, nausea, diarrhea, headache, and weight gain are rare. Theoretically, the profound acid suppression from PPIs may have a pro-carcinogenic effect by inducing hypergastrinemia, but this has not been observed.[27] The acid suppression also has the potential for decreasing vitamin B_{12} metabolism. Although this also has not been demonstrated to occur to a significant degree, it is important to consider and to test patients who may be at increased risk for B_{12} deficiency.[28]

Prokinetic Medications

Prokinetic drugs such as bethanechol chloride, metoclopramide, and cisapride have the potential to be useful in GERD by treating some of the underlying physiological abnormalities. They can increase LES pressure, enhance peristalsis, and improve gastric emptying, thereby reducing duration of esophageal acid exposure.[45] However, their use has been limited by a relatively *high incidence of adverse effects.* Bethanechol has up to 50% efficacy in improving symptoms of GERD, but has adverse cholinergic effects include abdominal cramping, blurred vision, and urinary frequency. Metoclopramide is a dopamine antagonist and smooth muscle stimulant. It may improve symptoms, but does not effectively treat esophagitis. Adverse effects are common and include drowsiness, agitation, tremor, and dystonic reactions. This limits its use in the elderly. Cisapride increases availability of acetylcholine at the myenteric plexus, and is a serotonin agonist on smooth muscle. It relieves nocturnal heartburn and can treat mild to moderate esophagitis.[30] However, the serious adverse reaction of cardiac arrhythmias has caused the manufacturer to stop marketing the drug in the United States. Currently cisapride is only available to patients who meet specific clinical eligibility criteria for a limited-access protocol.

Sucralfate

Another option for medical therapy of elderly patients with GERD is sucralfate. Sucralfate has been shown to be as effective as H2 blockers in relieving symptoms and healing esophagitis in patients with mild disease.[38] Because sucralfate is locally acting and has minimal side effects, it is a safe medication to use for elderly patients.

Role of Surgery

Surgery tends to be reserved for patients with persistent or recurrent symptoms despite medical therapy or with complications of reflux such as strictures, Barrett's metaplasia, or recurrent pulmonary symptoms in association with GERD. The most frequently performed operation is the Nissen fundoplication, which aims at restoring the gastroesophageal junction anatomy and function by repairing underlying hiatal hernia and creating a valve-like effect at the level of the LES. Little data exist comparing the elderly and the general population in terms of procedure safety, tolerability, and long-term outcomes.

Open fundoplication can have up to an 85% success rate in relieving symptoms of GERD and healing esophagitis. Open fundoplication has also previously been shown to be better than medical therapy in complicated GERD.[57] However, this was prior to more effective medical therapy with the development of PPIs. The most common open procedures are the Nissen (complete) and Toupet (partial) fundoplication. Complication rates between young and elderly patients appear to be similar,[1] but likely reflect a selection bias. One potential risk is that an incorrectly performed fundoplication may prevent appropriate relaxation of the LES with swallowing. Laparoscopic techniques of antireflux surgery have also largely replaced open surgery.

Laparoscopic fundoplication is comparable to open fundoplication in terms of safety, short-term efficacy, patient satisfaction, and it also offers shorter hospital stays and recuperative times.[40,46,63] Complication rates between younger and elderly patients appear similar.[24,64] Minimally invasive approaches are more appealing than open surgery to most patients and their physicians. The threshold in terms of perceived surgical risk may also be lower. However, expertise with laparoscopic techniques is of paramount importance.[2]

Endoscopic Therapies

Several endoscopic methods for treating GERD have been recently introduced. The use of radiofrequency energy in the muscle of the lower esophagus (the Stretta procedure) has been shown to eliminate the need of PPI therapy in 60% of cases at 1 year after the procedure.[60,61] Another, similarly effective technique involves transoral endoscopic suturing to strengthen the LES.[12,22] Other endoscopic methods being studied involve the injection of microspheres[10] or injection of a biopolymer into the LES.[7] Although these procedures are promising, experience is limited, and long-term studies on efficacy and safety are not yet available, especially in the elderly.

Conclusion

GERD is common in the elderly. As compared to the general population, older patients frequently present with atypical symptoms, suffer greater complication rates, and have higher mortality. Physicians should have a lower threshold for screening and evaluating the elderly for GERD and its complications. Furthermore, they must aggressively treat elderly patients with either pharmacological or surgical therapy.

Suggested Reading

1. Allen R, Rappaport W, Hixson L, et al: Referral patterns and the results of antireflux operations in patients more than sixty years of age. Surg Gynecol Obstet 173(5): 359–362, 1991.
2. Bais JE, Bartelsman JF, Bonjer HJ, et al: Laparoscopic or conventional Nissen fundoplication for gastrooesophageal reflux disease: Randomised clinical trial. The Netherlands Antireflux Surgery Study Group. Lancet 355(9199):170–174, 2000.
3. Blechman MB, Gelb AM: Aging and gastrointestinal physiology. Clin Geriatr Med 15(3):429–438, 1999.
4. Cameron AJ, Lomboy CT: Barrett's esophagus: Age, prevalence, and extent of columnar epithelium. Gastroenterology 103(4):1241–1245, 1992.
5. Castell DO: Esophageal disorders in the elderly. Gastroenterol Clin North Am 19(2): 235–254, 1990.
6. Collen M, Abdulian J,Chen Y: Gastroesoophageal reflux disease in the elderly: More severe disease that requires aggressive therapy. Am J Gastroenterol 90(7):1053–1057, 1995.
7. Deviere J, Pastorelli A, Louis H, et al: Endoscopic implantation of a biopolymer in the lower esophageal sphincter for gastroesophageal reflux: A pilot study. Gastrointest Endosc 55(3):335–341, 2002.
8. Dodds WJ, Hogan WJ, Helm JF,Dent J: Pathogenesis of reflux esophagitis. Gastroenterology 81(2):376–394, 1981.
9. Fass R, Pulliam G, Johnson C, et al: Symptom severity and oesophageal chemosensitivity to acid in older and young patients with gastro-oesophageal reflux. Age Ageing 29(2):125–130, 2000.
10. Feretis C, Benakis P, Dimopoulos C, et al: Endoscopic implantation of Plexiglas (PMMA) microspheres for the treatment of GERD. Gastrointest Endosc 53(4): 423–426, 2001.
11. Ferriolli E, Oliveira RB, Matsuda NM, et al: Aging, esophageal motility, and gastroesophageal reflux. J Am Geriatr Soc 46(12):1534–1537, 1998.
12. Filipi CJ, Lehman GA, Rothstein RI, et al: Transoral, flexible endoscopic suturing for treatment of GERD: A multicenter trial. Gastrointest Endosc 53(4):416–422, 2001.
13. Flora-Filho R, Zilberstein B: The importance of age as determining factor in hiatus hernia and gastroesophageal reflux. Cross-sectional study. Arq Gastroenterol 36(1): 10–17, 1999.

14. Friedland GW: Progress in radiology: Historical review of the changing concepts of lower esophageal anatomy: 430 B.C.–1977. AJR Am J Roentgenol 131(3):373–378, 1978.

15. Garnett WR: Considerations for long-term use of proton-pump inhibitors. Am J Health Syst Pharm 55(21):2268–2279, 1998.

16. Grande L, Lacima G, Ros E, et al: Deterioration of esophageal motility with age: A manometric study of 79 healthy subjects. Am J Gastroenterol 94(7):1795–1801, 1999.

17. Hatlebakk JG, Berstad A, Carling L, et al: Lansoprazole versus omeprazole in short-term treatment of reflux oesophagitis. Results of a Scandinavian multicentre trial. Scand J Gastroenterol 28(3):224–228, 1993.

18. Holloway R,Dent J: Pathophysiology of gastroesophageal reflux: Lower esophageal sphincter dysfunction is gastroesophageal reflux disease. Gastoenterol Clin North Am 19(3): 517–535, 1990.

19. Howard PJ,Heading RC: Epidemiology of gastro-esophageal reflux disease. World J Surg 16(2):88–293, 1992.

20. James OF,Parry-Billings KS: Comparison of omeprazole and histamine H2-receptor antagonists in the treatment of elderly and young patients with reflux oesophagitis. Age Ageing 23(2):121–126, 1994.

21. Jones MP, Sloan SS, Rabine JC, et al: Hiatal hernia size is the dominant determinant of esophagitis presence and severity in gastroesophageal reflux disease. Am J Gastroenterol 96(6):1711–1717, 2001.

22. Kadirkamanathan SS, Evans DF, Gong F, et al: Antireflux operations at flexible endoscopy using endoluminal stitching techniques: An experimental study. Gastrointest Endosc 44(2):133–143, 1996.

23. Katz P: Gastroesophageal reflux disease. J Am Geriatr Soc 46(12):1558–1565, 1998.

24. Khajanchee YS, Urbach DR, Butler N, et al: Laparoscopic antireflux surgery in the elderly. Surg Endosc 16(1):25–30, 2002.

25. Kinekawa F, Kubo F, Matsuda K, et al: Relationship between esophageal dysfunction and neuropathy in diabetic patients. Am J Gastroenterol 96(7):2026–2032, 2001.

26. Kongara KR,Soffer EE: Saliva and esophageal protection. Am J Gastroenterol 94(6): 1446–1452, 1999.

27. Koop H,Arnold R: Long-term maintenance treatment of reflux esophagitis with omeprazole. Prospective study in patients with H2-blocker-resistant esophagitis. Dig Dis Sci 36(5):552–557, 1991.

28. Laine L, Ahnen D, McClain C, et al: Review article: Potential gastrointestinal effects of long-term acid suppression with proton pump inhibitors. Aliment Pharmacol Ther 14(6):651–668, 2000.

29. Lasch H, Castell DO,Castell JA: Evidence for diminished visceral pain with aging: Studies using graded intraesophageal balloon distension. Am J Physiol 272(1 Pt 1): G1–3, 1997.

30. Lepoutre L, Van der Spek P, Vanderlinden I, et al: Healing of grade-II and III oesophagitis through motility stimulation with cisapride. Digestion 45(2):109–114, 1990.

31. Levine DS, Haggitt RC, Blount PL, et al: An endoscopic biopsy protocol can differentiate high-grade dysplasia from early adenocarcinoma in Barrett's esophagus. Gastroenterology 105(1):40–50, 1993.

32. Lin S, Brasseur JG, Pouderoux P,Kahrilas PJ: The phrenic ampulla: Distal esophagus or potential hiatal hernia? Am J Physiol 268(2 Pt 1):G320–327, 1995.

33. MacIntosh CG, Andrews JM, Jones KL, et al: Effects of age on concentrations of plasma cholecystokinin, glucagon- like peptide 1, and peptide YY and their relation to appetite and pyloric motility. Am J Clin Nutr 69(5):999–1006, 1999.

34. Massey BT, Hogan WJ, Dodds WJ,Dantas RO: Alteration of the upper esophageal sphincter belch reflex in patients with achalasia. Gastroenterology 103(5):574–1579, 1992.
35. Mittal RK,Balaban DH: The esophagogastric junction. N Engl J Med 336(13):924–932, 1997.
36. Mold JW, Reed LE, Davis AB, et al: Prevalence of gastroesophageal reflux in elderly patients in a primary care setting. Am J Gastroenterol 86(8):965–970, 1991.
37. Navarro-Rodriguez T, de Moraes-Filho JP, Arakaki E, et al: The screening sensitivity of endoscopy, acid perfusion test and 24-hour pH-monitoring to evaluate esophagitis in patients with heartburn and histological esophagitis. Arq Gastroenterol 34(3): 148–156, 1997.
38. Orlando RC: Sucralfate therapy and reflux esophagitis: An overview. Am J Med 91 (2A):123S-124S, 1991.
39. Patel RS,Rao SS: Biomechanical and sensory parameters of the human esophagus at four levels. Am J Physiol 275(2 Pt 1):G187-G191, 1998.
40. Peters JH, Heimbucher J, Kauer WK, et al: Clinical and physiologic comparison of laparoscopic and open Nissen fundoplication. J Am Coll Surg 180(4):385–393, 1995.
41. Plant RL: Anatomy and physiology of swallowing in adults and geriatrics. Otolaryngol Clin North Am 31(3):477–488, 1998.
42. Porro GB, Pace F, Peracchia A, et al: Short-term treatment of refractory reflux esophagitis with different doses of omeprazole or ranitidine. J Clin Gastroenterol 15(3):192–198, 1992.
43. Raiha I, Hietanen E, Sourander L: Symptoms of gastro-oesophageal reflux disease in elderly people. Age Ageing 20(5):365–370, 1991.
44. Raiha IJ, Impivaara O, Seppala M, Sourander LB: Prevalence and characteristics of symptomatic gastroesophageal reflux disease in the elderly. J Am Geriatr Soc 40(12): 1209–1211, 1992.
45. Ramirez B, Richter JE: Review article: Promotility drugs in the treatment of gastro-oesophageal reflux disease. Aliment Pharmacol Ther 7(1):5–20, 1993.
46. Rattner DW, Brooks DC: Patient satisfaction following laparoscopic and open antireflux surgery. Arch Surg 130(3):289–293; discussion 293–294, 1995.
47. Ren J, Shaker R, Kusano M, et al: Effect of aging on the secondary esophageal peristalsis: Presbyesophagus revisited. Am J Physiol Gastrointest Liver Physiol 268(5): 772-G779, 1995.
48. Richter JE: Typical and atypical presentations of gastroesophageal reflux disease. The role of esophageal testing in diagnosis and management. Gastoenterol Clin North Am 25(1):75–102, 1996.
49. Richter JE: Gastroesophageal reflux diesase in the older patient: Presentation, treatment, and complications. Am J Gastroenterol 95:(2):368–373, 2000.
50. Schenk BE, Kuipers EJ, Klinkenberg-Knol EC, et al: Omeprazole as a diagnostic tool in gastroesophageal reflux disease. Am J Gastroenterol 92(11):1997–2000.
51. Segal WN,Cello JP: Hemorrhage in the upper gastrointestinal tract in the older patient. Am J Gastroenterol 92(1):42–46, 1997.
52. Smith AB, Dickerman RD, McGuire CS, et al: Pressure-overload-induced sliding hiatal hernia in power athletes. J Clin Gastroenterol 28(4):352–354, 1999.
53. Smith PM, Kerr GD, Cockel R, et al: A comparison of omeprazole and ranitidine in the prevention of recurrence of benign esophageal stricture. Restore Investigator Group. Gastroenterology 107(5):1312–1318, 1994.
54. Sonnenberg A, Massey BT, McCarty DJ,Jacobsen SJ: Epidemiology of hospitalization for achalasia in the United States. Dig Dis Sci 38(2):233–244, 1993.

55. Sonnenberg A, Steinkamp U, Weise A, et al: Salivary secretion in reflux esophagitis. Gastroenterology 83(4):889–895, 1982.

56. Sontag SJ, Schnell TG, Miller TQ, et al: The importance of hiatal hernia in reflux esophagitis compared with lower esophageal sphincter pressure or smoking. J Clin Gastroenterol 13(6):628–643, 1991.

57. Spechler SJ: Comparison of medical and surgical therapy for complicated gastroesophageal reflux disease in veterans. The Department of Veterans Affairs Gastroesophageal Reflux Disease Study Group. N Engl J Med 326(12):786–792, 1992.

58. Spechler SJ: Clinical practice: Barrett's esophagus. N Engl J Med 346(11):836–842, 2002.

59. Stilson WL, Sanders I, Gardiner GA, et al: Hiatal hernia and gastroesophageal reflux. A clinicoradiological analysis of more than 1000 cases. Radiology 93(6):323–1327, 1969.

60. Triadafilopoulos G, Dibaise JK, Nostrant TT, et al: Radiofrequency energy delivery to the gastroesophageal junction for the treatment of GERD. Gastrointest Endosc 53 (4):407–415, 2001.

61. Triadafilopoulos G, DiBaise JK, Nostrant TT, et al: The Stretta procedure for the treatment of GERD: 6- and 12-month follow-up of the U.S. open label trial. Gastrointest Endosc 55(2):149–156, 2002.

62. Triadafilopoulos G, Sharma R: Features of symptomatic gastroesophageal reflux disease in elderly patients. Am J Gastroenterol 92(11):2007–2011, 1997.

63. Trus TL, Laycock WS, Branum G, et al: Intermediate follow-up of laparoscopic antireflux surgery. Am J Surg 171(1):32–35, 1996.

64. Trus TL, Laycock WS, Wo JM, et al: Laparoscopic antireflux surgery in the elderly. Am J Gastroenterol 93(3):351–353, 1998.

65. Zhu H, Pace F, Sangaletti O,Bianchi Porro G: Features of symptomatic gastroesophageal reflux in elderly patients. Scand J Gastroenterol 28(3):235–238, 1993.

66. Zimmerman J, Shohat V, Tsvang E, et al: Esophagitis is a major cause of upper gastrointestinal hemorrhage in the elderly. Scand J Gastroenterol 32(9):906–909, 1997.

HOT TOPICS

Gastroesophageal Reflux Disease and Systemic Disease

chapter
10

Eyal Gal, M.D., and
Yaron Niv, M.D.

Gastroesophageal reflux disease (GERD) is a common, mostly idiopathic medical condition that results from the pathologic reflux of gastric content into the esophagus. Normally, several mechanisms work in combination to prevent reflux. However, systemic disease can affect the defense mechanisms that normally prevent such reflux or can aggravate existing GERD. In this chapter, we describe the systemic diseases affecting gastroesophageal reflux from a pathogenetic point of view.

Four main mechanisms operate in combination to keep the gastric content from refluxing into the esophagus and to clear the esophagus of noxious material. An impairment in any of these can lead to GERD and related conditions (Table 1):

1. Intact lower esophageal sphincter (LES) pressure:
   a. Intrinsic LES pressure (muscular and nervous control)
   b. Extrinsic compression of the LES by the crural diaphragm
   c. Intra-abdominal location of the LES
   d. Integrity of the phrenoesophageal ligament
   e. Preservation of the acute angle of His
2. Transient lower esophageal sphincter relaxations
3. Increased abdominal pressure
4. Clearance of refluxate:
   a. Esophageal peristalsis
   b. Saliva secretion
   c. Intact swallowing mechanism

Scleroderma (Systemic Sclerosis)

Scleroderma is a multisystemic disease characterized by mononuclear cell infiltration, vascular damage, and excessive collagen deposition in the skin and internal organs. Manifestations may include skin involvement, Raynaud's disease, polyarthritis, and lung, kidney, heart, and thyroid disease.[1-3]

TABLE 1.   Gastroesophageal Reflux Disease Mechanisms and Related Conditions

Mechanism	Related Conditions
Decreased LES pressure	Scleroderma, MCTD, rheumatoid arthritis, amyloidosis, pregnancy, smoking
Increased TLESRs	Diabetes mellitus
Reduced saliva secretion	Sjögren's syndrome, smoking, MCTD
Impaired gastric emptying	Diabetes mellitus, polymyositis, amyloidosis
Gastric acid hypersecretion	Zollinger–Ellison syndrome, systemic mastocytosis, short bowel syndrome
Impaired esophageal motility	Scleroderma, polymyositis, variceal sclerotherapy, MCTD, diabetes mellitus, amyloidosis
Increased intra-abdominal pressure	Obesity, pregnancy, smoking

LES = lower esophageal sphincter, MCTD = mixed connective tissue disease, TLESRs = transient lower esophageal relaxations.

The gastrointestinal tract is often involved in scleroderma at all levels, resulting in severe dysmotility. Esophageal involvement, reported in up to 90% of patients, is characterized by decreased or absent peristalsis in the distal two thirds of the esophagus, reduced LES pressure, and, when combined with sicca syndrome, reduced capacity to neutralize acid.[4] Chronic gastroesophageal reflux predisposes affected individuals to the development of esophagitis, Barrett's esophagus, and strictures.

Abu Shakra et al[5] followed 262 patients with scleroderma for 14 years. Heartburn was noted in 71% and dysphagia in 49% to 53%. Esophageal manometry was performed in 121 patients, including 109 with heartburn or dysphagia. The rate of heartburn or dysphagia was significantly higher in patients with reduced LES pressure or motility dysfunction than in patients with normal manometry findings. Of the 122 patients who underwent barium studies or esophagogastroduodenoscopy (EGD), or both, 62% had manifestations of chronic GERD, 39% had esophagitis, 40% had distal esophageal stricture, 3% had esophageal ulceration, 6% had Barrett's metaplasia, and 25% had hiatal hernia.

The primary site of pathologic lesions along the gastrointestinal tract in patients with scleroderma is the muscularis propria.[1] The damage is progressive, with atrophy and fragmentation of the smooth muscle and collagen infiltration followed by fibrosis. In patients with early scleroderma and in healthy individuals, direct cholinergic stimulation by metacholine causes an increase in LES pressure, but edrophonium, a cholinesterase inhibitor, does not. This finding suggests the presence of a primary neural dysfunction with secondary muscle atrophy.[1,6]

Stampfl et al[7] demonstrated a positive correlation between aperistalsis and low LES pressure in 20 patients with scleroderma. The number of reflux episodes was significantly greater in the aperistaltic group. Although another team failed to confirm these results, these authors' aperistaltic patients were characterized by a significantly larger percentage of time of distal esophageal acid exposure than patients with normal peristalsis, supporting the importance of effective esophageal peristalsis.[8] When proximal esophageal acid exposure was measured with a dual pH probe, patients with aperistalsis demonstrated more reflux episodes, a greater percentage of reflux time, and more reflux episodes lasting more than 5 minutes than patients with normal peristalsis.[7,8]

In one series, Barrett's metaplasia was documented in 37% (9 of 27) of patients with scleroderma, compared with 4% to 13% of patients with GERD.[9] Dependent risk factors for the development of Barrett's metaplasia included long duration of dysphagia, low LES pressure, and presence of the CREST syndrome (calcinosis cutis, Raynaud's phenomenon, esophageal dysmotility, sclerodactyly, and telangiectasia). Two patients (7%) had adenocarcinoma of the esophagus. Although higher rates of esophageal adenocarcinoma may be expected in these patients, there are only a few case reports of an association of adenocarcinoma of the esophagus with scleroderma.[10] Screening for esophageal adenocarcinoma in patients with scleroderma may be unjustified because of the low detection rate. Of 680 patients with scleroderma followed for a median of 12 years, only one who did not report GERD symptoms was found to have undifferentiated esophageal carcinoma.[11]

Extraintestinal manifestations of GERD including noncardiac chest pain, hoarseness, sore throat, cough, and recurrent pneumonia also occur in scleroderma.[1] Dynamic lung compliance and lung functions were found to be worse in scleroderma patients with impaired motility and hypotensive LES.[12–14] Aspiration was demonstrated in 85% of affected patients, and arytenoid erythema in 92%.[14] There was no association between pulmonary function tests and esophageal acid exposure (examined by esophageal pH monitoring).[15] Concomitant finding of worsened pulmonary function and esophageal dysmotility might be partially explained by the increased gastroesophageal reflux and aspiration, but it more likely indicates simultaneous involvement of the two systems.

Treatment of GERD is basically similar in patients with and without scleroderma, although there is more emphasis in the former on a high dosage of proton pump inhibitor (PPI) drugs.[1] The combination of omeprazole and cisapride caused better gastric and esophageal emptying, thereby improving control of reflux symptoms and esophagitis.[16] Surgical treatment has a limited role in scleroderma and is considered only in severe, resistant cases. Apart from the increased operative risk due to systemic complications, fundoplication carries an additional risk of worsening dysphagia in an aperistaltic esophagus. Partial wrap of the fundus, as in the Belsey Mark IV and Toupet operations, is preferred over the complete wrap used in Nissen fundoplication. Good results have been reported for combined Collis-Nissen gastroplasty, which creates a continuous esophagus from the gastric fundus and wraps it with the rest of the fundus.[17,18]

Connective Tissue Diseases

In cases of rheumatoid arthritis, findings of low-amplitude peristaltic waves in the middle and lower esophagus and reduced LES pressure are not unusual, although there is no increase in heartburn and dysphagia (Table 2).[19]

In mixed connective tissue disease, upper gastrointestinal symptoms are common and include dysphagia in 38% of patients, heartburn and regurgitation in 48%, dyspepsia in 20%, and vomiting in 3%.[20] In a series of 61 patients followed for a mean of 6.3 years, 3 patients developed esophageal strictures and 1 had recurrent aspirations. Esophageal manometry demonstrated significantly reduced LES and upper esophageal sphincter pressures in addition to lower peristaltic amplitude or aperistalsis in the distal esophagus, as compared with healthy control subjects. Steroid therapy led to a significant improvement in LES pressure and a trend for improvement of peristalsis. Ambulatory pH monitoring, performed in five children and adolescents with mixed connective tissue disease, showed an increased reflux index (pH < 4 for 27.7% of the time) and an increased number of reflux episodes longer than 5 minutes.[21]

Gastrointestinal manifestations are common in patients with Sjögren's syndrome, with 75% of patients reporting dysphagia.[22] This may be related to the lack of saliva and the consequent loss of its buffering effect on acid reflux but also to connective tissue damage to the esophagus and impaired peristalsis, as seen in scleroderma. Esophageal webs are described in 10% of patients.[23] Several studies showed only minor, nonspecific motility abnormalities in one third of patients with Sjögren's syndrome.[22–24] Despite the high rate of dysphagia, there is apparently no correlation between the severity of the dysphagia and motility abnormalities, except in patients with severe dysphagia and increased simultaneous contractions.[24] There are no reports of increased heartburn or esophagitis in this population. It appears that loss of the buffering effect of saliva has only a minor effect on the development of GERD.

The main gastrointestinal tract disturbance in cases of polymyositis is found in the striated muscle of the cricopharyngeus, causing a pharyngeal dysphagia and deglutition disorder.[25] Distal esophageal dysmotility also occurs in about two thirds of patients with impaired peristalsis as an isolated disorder or as part of an overlapping syndrome, causing

TABLE 2. Gastroesophageal Reflux Disease in Connective Tissue Diseases							
Disease	GERD	Dysphagia	LES Pressure	UES Pressure	Proximal Peristalsis	Distal Peristalsis	Saliva Secretion	Gastric Emptying
Scleroderma	+++	++	---	N	N/-	---	N	NA
Mixed connective tissue disease	+	++	---	-	N	---	-	NA
Rheumatoid arthritis	+/-	-	-	N	N	-	N	NA
Polymyositis/dermatomyositis	++	++	N	---	---	N/-	N	-
Systemic lupus erythematosus	+	+/-	N/-	N	N	N/-	N	NA
Sjögren's syndrome	+/-	++	N	N	N	N/-	---	NA
GERD = gastroesophageal reflux disease, LES = lower esophageal sphincter, UES = upper esophageal sphincter, N = normal, NA = not available.							

dysphagia, heartburn, and regurgitation.[25–27] Treatment with antacids improves the esophageal symptoms.[27]

Common gastrointestinal tract symptoms of systemic lupus erythematosus are nausea, vomiting, and anorexia, appearing in about half of patients.[19] Esophageal dysmotility is also common and may cause heartburn and dysphagia. In one study, GERD symptoms were noted in more than half of patients, but esophageal dysmotility was found only in a small percentage and included mostly impaired peristalsis with intact LES pressures.[28,29]

Diabetes Mellitus

Gastrointestinal symptoms are common in diabetic patients, especially those with type I diabetes mellitus, long-standing disease, poor glycemic control, and diabetic autonomic neuropathy.[30] Motility disorders are common, and GERD is found in 44% of unselected patients, most of them asymptomatic.[31–33] Abnormal esophageal body motility was detected in 7 of 20 diabetic patients, all with peripheral neuropathy.[33] In a study of 50 patients with type I diabetes mellitus and no heartburn, 14 patients (28%) had significant reflux on ambulatory 24-hour pH monitoring, mainly patients with cardiovascular autonomic neuropathy.[34] No difference was found in LES length or pressure between patients with diabetes and control subjects.[33] The suggested mechanism of reflux in diabetes patients is increased frequency of transient LES relaxations, mostly in the postprandial period, as shown on analysis of the pH monitor, probably related to impaired vagal autonomic control. An absence of GERD symptoms could be related to desensitization of the esophagus as part of a sensory neuropathy.

Another confounding factor for GERD in patients with diabetes mellitus is gastroparesis, which may affect up to 58% of diabetic patients.[35] It usually develops gradually, with symptoms of early satiety, anorexia, postprandial nausea and vomiting, heartburn, regurgitation, bloating, and epigastric distress, although it may be asymptomatic in a large proportion of patients.[36] Metabolic alterations, such as severe hyperglycemia, hypokalemia, and ketoacidosis, may cause acute gastroparesis and gastric dilatation. EGD is mandatory in these patients to search for other causes of the nausea and vomiting. In a retrospective study of 20 diabetic patients with intractable nausea and vomiting thought to be due to gastroparesis, other sources were found in 11 (55%): candidal esophagitis in 3, erosive esophagitis in 4, gastric ulcer in 2, and duodenal erosions and bile gastritis in 1 each.[37] Management of diabetic gastroparesis is complex and includes correcting metabolic irregularities, stopping medications that can worsen the gastroparesis (anticholinergics, tricyclic antidepressants, benzodiazepines, and ganglionic-blocking agents), gastric decompression, and upper endoscopy with clearing of bezoars. Prokinetic drugs, such as metoclopramide, domperidone, cisapride, and erythromycin, are the mainstay of therapy.[38–40] Dietary modifications include the introduction of small, low-residue meals, liquid formulas, and in severe cases, feeding through a jejunostomy tube or total parenteral nutrition.[41] New experimental motilin receptor agonists are being studied, and gastric pacemakers have been shown to be useful in severe cases.[42]

Treatment of reflux disease in patients with diabetes mellitus consists of reducing gastroparesis with prokinetic drugs and administration of antisecretory drugs. Aluminium- and magnesium-containing antacids may worsen existing diarrhea and should be used cautiously in patients with renal impairment due to aluminium and magnesium toxicity. Histamine-2 blockers have beneficial effects on weight reduction and glycemic control in patients with type II diabetes mellitus and potentiate the hypoglycemic response to glipizide.[43,44] PPIs are the drugs of choice in patients with proven esophagitis or severe GERD. Antireflux surgery should be avoided because of the increased surgical risk and the risk of esophageal and gastric motility dysfunction.

Obesity

Obesity is defined as a body mass index (BMI) above 30. It affects 22.3% of the adult population in the United States.[45,46] The rising incidence of adenocarcinoma of the esophagus and cardia in the Western world may be associated with the obesity epidemic and the consequent increase in the incidence of GERD,[47] although findings are conflicting.[48–54] Lagergren et al[48] interviewed 820 patients for symptoms of GERD and measured their BMI. The authors found no association between GERD and obesity. Accordingly, Lundell et al,[49] did not find significant differences in GERD symptoms and 24 h pH monitoring results, between a group of morbidly obese patients and healthy control subjects.[49] By contrast, Locke et al[50] analyzed a self-report questionnaire completed by 1524 residents of Olmsted County, Minnesota, and found that a BMI above 30 had an odds ratio of 2.8 (95% CI, 1.7–4.5) for GERD symptoms. In another study 12,349 persons were followed for a median of 18.5 years; the hazard ratio for GERD-related hospitalization was 1.22 (95% CI, 1.13–1.32) for persons with a higher BMI.[52] The increased intra-abdominal pressure in obese people may be one of the mechanisms causing increased pressure on the LES[55]; the presence of hiatal hernia causes weakening of the extrinsic pressure on the LES area, thereby promoting reflux. This assumption is supported by findings of a correlation of obesity with the presence of hiatal hernia and GERD.[56,57] A retrospective case-control study of 1382 patients revealed an association of BMI with a finding of hiatal hernia and reflux esophagitis on endoscopy.[57] After controlling for the effect of the hiatal hernia on GERD, obesity was still an independent risk factor for the development of esophagitis.

Manometric studies of obese persons have not yielded a correlation between BMI and LES resting pressure, but 60% of the morbidly obese patients had manometric abnormalities, such as hypotensive LES (25%), nutcracker esophagus (14%), nonspecific esophageal motility disorder (14%), diffuse esophageal spasm (7%), and achalasia (1%).[58] Most of the patients did not have esophageal symptoms. Gastric acid secretion and gastric emptying are similar in obese and nonobese patients,[58] although obese patients may have more bile and pancreatic enzyme secretion. Complications of GERD, such as strictures or ulcers, are not more common in obese patients. However, obesity is a weak risk factor for the development of Barrett's esophagus, especially in young persons.[59] High waist-to-hip ratio, but not BMI, was found to be a risk factor for epithelial cell proliferation, indicating the possibility of progression toward dysplasia and carcinoma in patients with Barrett's esophagus.[60]

Weight loss may reduce heartburn in obese patients, but the results of interventional studies are controversial. A group of 34 obese patients with symptoms of GERD and normal endoscopy findings or mild esophagitis were placed on a weight reduction diet; in 9 patients, the symptoms disappeared completely.[61] However, a randomized, controlled, prospective study of 32 obese patients with GERD failed to demonstrate any benefit of a weight reduction plan for GERD symptoms or 24-hour pH monitoring findings.[62] Surgical bariatric therapy is controversial in the presence of GERD because it may lead to worsening of reflux.[53] Two recently published prospective studies of obese patients evaluated for GERD before and after laparoscopic band gastroplasty showed improvement or complete disappearance of GERD symptoms in more than 90%,[54,63] whereas a Swedish prospective study of 25 morbidly obese patients after vertical banded gastroplasty found no differences in 24-hour pH monitoring.[64] Roux-en-Y gastric bypass with or without an antireflux procedure provides good results for weight reduction and a 90% reduction in GERD symptoms or need for GERD medications.[65] Thus, data are so far insufficient to support the role of weight reduction in improving GERD in obese patients.

The use of pharmacologic agents such as PPIs or H_2 blockers in obese patients should be adjusted according to the lean body mass and not to the actual weight because of the altered pharmacokinetics associated with obesity.[66,67] Cisapride is contraindicated in patients with a prolonged QTc interval, and it should be used with caution in obese patients, who were found to have a 24% prevalence of prolonged QTc.[68] PPIs are probably the best treatment for GERD, but they have not been studied separately in the obese population.

The role of antireflux surgery in obese patients is controversial owing to the risk of increased complications, reduced long-term effectiveness, and need to combine it with bariatric surgery.[69-71] Nissen fundoplication is associated with a high recurrence rate in morbidly obese patients and does not contribute to weight reduction. A combination of vertical banded gastroplasty with anterior fundoplication may be a good option.

Pregnancy

Symptoms of GERD, heartburn, and regurgitation are common in pregnancy and can significantly affect patient comfort and quality of life.[72] There are no large epidemiologic studies of GERD in pregnancy, and no prospective manometric or pH monitoring studies. Thus, the true prevalence in not known. In the Western world, the estimated prevalence of GERD in pregnant women is more than 25%, compared with 10% in nonpregnant adults.[73] In another study of 607 pregnant women, the prevalence of heartburn increased from 22% in the first trimester and 39% in the second to 72% in the third trimester.[74] Regression analysis demonstrated an increased risk of heartburn with gestational age and parity.

The clinical spectrum of GERD during pregnancy does not differ from that in the general population.[75,76] In addition to heartburn, women may experience regurgitation, nausea, dysphagia, and vomiting or extraesophageal symptoms, such as cough, wheezing, or chest pain.[76] Symptoms worsen during the third trimester.

During pregnancy, the displacement of the LES due to increased intra-abdominal pressure together with the placental secretion of estrogen and progesterone cause a decrease in the resting LES pressure in the second trimester, which normalizes after delivery.[75,76] Esophageal clearance also decreases as a result of the increase in the frequency of low-amplitude contractions.

A limited number of studies have examined the role of the LES, esophageal motility, gastric emptying, and increased intra-abdominal pressure in promoting GERD during pregnancy, and the results are controversial. A hypotensive LES and a progressive decrease in LES pressure with the advance of the pregnancy in symptomatic women has been described by several authors [77,78], but was not confirmed by others.[79,80] The combination of estrogen and progesterone is more effective in decreasing LES pressure than each of the hormones alone.[81,82] A similar controversy exists concerning esophageal motility, gastric emptying, and intragastric pressure. A decrease in esophageal clearance during the third trimester, probably secondary to a rapid rise in gestational hormones, was demonstrated in six pregnant women as compared with six control subjects.[83] This change could not be demonstrated between the luteal and follicular phases of the menstrual cycle.[84] Schade et al[85] found no difference in gastric emptying of solids in the first trimester as compared to 6 weeks after therapeutic abortion. Intragastric pressure in pregnant women was twice that of the control groups.[86] Since the increase in intragastric pressure was followed by an increase in LES pressure in the patients with tense ascites, it is unlikely that intra-abdominal pressure is the primary factor in the genesis of GERD.[87]

Diagnosis of GERD in pregnancy is based on clinical grounds, as in the general population; the sensitivity and specificity are 90%. Manometry, pH monitoring, and EGD play a small diagnostic role. Barium swallow study is contraindicated, especially in the first trimester. In the rare cases in which symptoms are intractable and complications of GERD are suspected, EGD is the procedure of choice.[88,89]

In pregnancy, treatment should be directed more toward classic life style modifications, dietary changes, and nonsystemic therapies, such as antacids, alginic acid, and sucralfate, rather than H_2 antagonists, prokinetics, or PPIs.[72,76] In severe cases, category B drugs should be used, such as ranitidine (H_2 antagonist)[90,91] or lansoprazole (PPI)[92]; omeprazole may also be appropriate.[93,94]

Cirrhosis

Gastroesophageal reflux is common in patients with liver cirrhosis; pH monitoring findings are positive in 25% to 64%, and esophagitis is noted in 12%.[95,96] One study found no difference in the presence of GERD between cirrhotic patients with or without ascites, bleeding esophageal varices, encephalopathy, or neuropathy.[97] Others failed to show a decrease in LES pressure in cirrhotic patients, even in the presence of tense ascites and varices.[98,99]

The main mechanism of reflux in cirrhosis is probably reduced esophageal motility, mostly in the distal esophagus, leading to decreased acid clearance from the esophagus, especially in patients with esophageal varices.[100]. The elevated intra-abdominal pressure in patients with tense ascites might play a minor role, since it does not reduce LES pressure.[98] Transjugular intrahepatic portosystemic shunt placement has no effect on LES pressure, but it reverses reduced esophageal motility.[99] According to one theory, bleeding of esophageal varices is caused by abnormalities in LES pressure or by gastroesophageal reflux events. However, this assumption was not supported by studies comparing LES pressure and esophageal acid exposure in cirrhotic patients with or without bleeding varices.[101,102] Indeed, one study suggested a protective role for high-grade esophageal varices against GERD.[103]

Variceal sclerotherapy leads to diminished LES pressure and reduced velocity or amplitude of esophageal peristalsis in the long term, although immediately after sclerotherapy, nonpropagating, simultaneous contractions may be present for up to 1 week, causing chest pain, heartburn, and dysphagia.[95,104,105] An increase in esophageal reflux was demonstrated in one study[103], but was not confirmed in another.[102] Ligation of esophageal varices is not associated with an alteration in esophageal acid exposure unless it is combined with sclerotherapy.[106] Antireflux therapy is recommended at least for 1 week after sclerotherapy or if symptoms occur; in cirrhotic patients, the pharmacokinetic properties of the different drugs should be taken into consideration. The pharmacokinetics of ranitidine and famotidine are not significantly changed in cases of compensated cirrhosis, although ranitidine levels may be elevated in patients with severe cirrhosis.[107–109] PPIs are the treatment of choice in patients with cirrhosis.[110] Serum drug levels of all types of PPIs are higher in cirrhotic patients than in control subjects due to reduced clearance, but they are not associated with additional adverse events.[111]

Amyloidosis

Autopsy studies have yielded a 70% to 100% rate of pathologic involvement of the gastrointestinal tract in systemic amyloidosis; gastrointestinal tract symptoms are present in 30% to 60% of patients.[112] Esophageal disturbances are common, manifested by dysphagia and GERD. In a study of 30 patients with amyloidosis, Rubinow et al[113] found a low resting LES pressure in 14 (46%), of whom 12 had heartburn and 9 had motility abnormalities of the esophageal body.

Manometric studies of patients with familial amyloidosis, which typically manifests with severe polyneuropathy and gastroparesis, have shown severe esophageal motility disorders with reduced LES pressure, decreased amplitude of contractions, or simultaneous contractions.[114] These abnormalities probably represent deposition of amyloid in the esophageal muscles and nervous plexuses.[114,115] Gastroparesis and reduced gastric emptying are common in patients with amyloidosis and may contribute to GERD symptoms. Esophageal erosions were found in 5% of patients with amyloidosis and shallow ulcerations in 3%.[116] Treatment of GERD in this population is similar to that in other patients, although prokinetic drugs should be used when dysmotility and gastroparesis are diagnosed by manometry and scintigraphy.

Smoking

It is a common belief among physicians that cigarette smoking worsens GERD, and patients are often advised to cease smoking as part of GERD treatment. However, the reported data on the effect of smoking on GERD are controversial. Pehl et al[117] performed 24-hour pH monitoring in 280 patients with symptoms of GERD, of whom 78 were smokers and 45 actually smoked during the test. No significant difference was found in reflux parameters among the three groups. Kadakia et al[118] assessed acid reflux by 24-hour pH monitoring in 14 smokers with heartburn and esophagitis after they abstained from smoking for 48 hours and again after they resumed smoking for 48 hours. They found that the duration of pH < 4 increased from 7.4% of the time to 11.1% ($P = 0.007$) in the smoking period due to both an increase in reflux events, especially during the day and in the upright position, and a decrease in esophageal clearance. The patients reported an increase in the number of daytime heartburn episodes, which followed the recorded reflux events. In another study, double-probe, 24-hour pH monitoring was used in 15 patients during smoking and without smoking; again the duration of pH < 4 was significantly longer in both the distal and proximal esophagus during smoking.[119]

The pathogenesis of GERD in association of smoking may be multifactorial and is explained by the following mechanisms[120–123]:

1. A decrease in LES pressure during smoking
2. An increase in reflux events connected with coughing and deep inspiration
3. Reduced salivary secretion-rate and saliva bicarbonate content

The exact ingredients in cigarettes that cause the effects on esophageal motility and salivary glands are unknown; studies in patients wearing nicotine transdermal patches yielded equivocal results as to esophageal acid exposure measured by 24-hour pH monitoring.[124–126] A well-designed manometric study of esophageal motility during nicotine patch use showed a 30% decrease in LES pressure with no relaxation or peristalsis abnormalities.[126] Thus, smoking is a weak risk factor for GERD. Cessation of smoking may be advised as an adjunct to lifestyle changes and as an important general health-care measure.

Hypersecretory States

Zollinger-Ellison Syndrome

General studies of Zollinger-Ellison Syndrome (ZES) reported a 3% incidence of associated GERD.[127–129] When GERD was specifically sought, one third of 32 patients were found to have endoscopically positive signs.[130,131] Miller et al[132] questioned 122 patients with ZES about GERD symptoms and performed upper endoscopy[132]; 61% were found to have either GERD symptoms or endoscopic abnormalities (46% had grade 1 esophagitis, 13% had grade 2 esophagitis, and 41% had grade 3 esophagitis). Barrett's esophagus was found in 17% of the patients with esophagitis, and esophageal peptic strictures in 8%.

The main mechanism of GERD in patients with ZES is the high rate of gastric acid secretion. The relatively low prevalence of GERD found in some series was assumed to be related to the elevation in LES pressure due to high gastrin concentration. However, several later studies failed to find an association between gastrin serum concentration and LES pressure.[130,131,133] Strader et al[133] reported a similar esophageal motility patterns in ZES patients and healthy control subjects. Another possible defense mechanism against esophagitis is the secretion of epidermal growth factor in the saliva and gastric juice. Epidermal growth factor plays a role in maintaining the integrity of the esophageal and gastric mucosa. Salivary and gastric epidermal growth factor output was found to be elevated in ZES patients, thus adding to the protection of esophageal mucosa against reflux.[134]

Systemic Mastocytosis

Gastroesophageal reflux disease may be caused by hypersecretion of acid and has been reported in one case of systemic mastocytosis.[135] Treatment consists mainly of H_1 and H_2 blockers, which inhibit histamine-mediated gastric acid secretion and the systemic effects of histamine. Basophilic leukemia may produce a similar clinical picture.

Short Bowel Syndrome

Resection of a large portion of the small bowel may cause elevated gastrin levels owing to the lack of inhibitory peptides secreted by the small intestine.[136] This hypergastrinemia may cause acid hypersecretion and severe peptic disease resembling ZES.[137] Tang et al[137] described a patient with short bowel syndrome who had recurrent bleeding from severe gastric and esophageal ulcerations. The patient was first treated with intravenous ranitidine, and when this failed, he was given long-term intravenous pantoprazole with good results.

Helicobacter pylori

Eradication of *Helicobacter pylori* is now an established treatment for gastric and a duodenal ulcers and a preventive measure against ulcer recurrence and gastric neoplasia. Its effect on GERD is controversial, however. Case-control studies from Japan have shown a lower prevalence of *H. pylori* infection in patients with GERD, suggesting a protective effect against reflux.[138] Labenz et al[139] were the first to report that patients with duodenal ulcer may develop GERD after successful eradication of *H. pylori*. Other researchers have reached opposing conclusions.[140–143] In a recent multicenter randomized prospective study of 1421 patients with duodenal and gastric ulcers, GERD symptoms improved after *H. pylori* eradication in those with duodenal ulcers but not in those with gastric ulcers. Heartburn at baseline and ulcer relapse were independent factors for post-eradication GERD.

Suggested mechanisms of *H. pylori* augmentation of GERD are:[143]

1. Release of LES-relaxing cytoxins, prostaglandins, and nitric oxide by *H. pylori*.
2. Vagal sensitization causing lower threshold for transient LES relaxations.
3. Increased gastrin release in antrum predominant gastritis.
4. Delayed gastric emptying caused by gastritis.
5. Direct injury to the esophageal mucosa by bacterial cytotoxins.

Suggested mechanisms for *H. pylori* protection against GERD are:

1. Release of gastric acid secretion inhibitors—mostly in corpus gastritis.
2. Secretion of acid-neutralizing ammonia.
3. Progression to atrophic gastritis with low acid output.
4. Hypergastrinemia causing elevated LES pressure—in antral gastritis.

The question of *H. pylori* eradication and GERD is still unresolved, especially its connection with the increasing incidence of adenocarcinoma of the esophagus and gastric cardia in the Western world.

Key Points: Gastroesophageal Reflux Disease and Systemic Disease

∞ Systemic disease can affect the defense mechanisms that normally prevent reflux or can aggravate existing GERD.

∞ Scleroderma often involves the gastrointestinal tract, especially the esophagus. Patients can experience chronic gastroesophageal reflux, which can lead to esophagitis, Barrett's esophagus, and strictures.

∞ Some connective tissue disorders have gastrointestinal and esophageal symptoms, but most do not have an association with GERD.

∞ Gastrointestinal symptoms and motility disorders are common in patients with diabetes mellitus. Gastroparesis, found in more than half of diabetic patients, can confound GERD.

∞ Obesity may be a factor in the increasing incidence of GERD, al-

Key Points (*Continued*)

though findings are conflicting. In some studied patients, weight loss improved GERD symptoms; in others, it did not.

☞ Pregnant women often experience GERD symptoms, which are worst in the third trimester.

☞ Gastroesophageal reflux is common in patients with liver cirrhosis, probably because of reduced esophageal motility.

☞ Esophageal disturbances, manifested by dysphagia and GERD, are common in patients with amyloidosis.

☞ It is a common belief among physicians that cigarette smoking worsens GERD, although reported data are controversial.

☞ One third of patients with ZES are found to have GERD. Elevated salivary and gastric epidermal growth factor output may protect these patients against reflux.

☞ The effect of *Helicobacter pylori* infection and eradication on GERD is controversial. *H. pylori* may have a protective effect against reflux.

Suggested Reading

1. Rose S, Young MA, Reynolds JC: Gastrointestinal manifestations of scleroderma. Gastroenterol Clin North Am 27:563–594, 1998.

2. Kim DD, Ryan JC: Gastrointestinal manifestations of systemic diseases. In Sleisenger & Fordtran's, Gastrointestinal and Liver Disease: Pathophysiology/Diagnosis/Management, 7th ed. Philadelphia, WB Saunders, 2002, pp 507–537.

3. Clouse RE, Diamant NE: Esophageal motor and sensory function and motor disorders of the esophagus. In Sleisenger & Fordtran's, Gastrointestinal and Liver Disease: Pathophysiology/Diagnosis/Management, 7th ed. Philadelphia, WB Saunders, 2002, pp 561–598.

4. Weston S, Thumshirn M, Wiste J, et al: Clinical and gastrointestinal motility features in systemic sclerosis and related disorders. Am J Gastroenterol 93:1085–1089, 1998.

5. Abu-Shakra M, Guillemin F, Lee P: Gastrointestinal manifestations of systemic sclerosis. Semin Arthritis Rheum 24:29–39, 1994.

6. Cohen S, Fisher R, Lipshutz W, et al: The pathogenesis of esophageal dysfunction in scleroderma and Raynaud's disease. J Clin Invest 51:2663, 1972.

7. Stampfl D, Denuna S, Varga J, et al: Relations between dysmotility and acid exposure in scleroderma (SSc). Am J Gastroenterol 85:1226, 1990.

8. Yarze JC, Varga J, Stampfl D, et al: Esophageal function in systemic sclerosis: A prospective evaluation of motility and acid reflux in 36 patients. Am J Gastroenterol 88:870–876, 1993.

9. Katzka DA, Reynolds JC, Saul SH, et al: Barrett's metaplasia and adenocarcinoma of the esophagus in scleroderma. Am J Med 87:46–52, 1987.

10. Niv Y, Abu-Avid S, Yelin A, et al: Barrett's epithelium and esophageal adenocarcinoma in scleroderma. Am J Gastroenterol 83:792–793, 1988.

11. Segel MC, Campbell WL, Medsger TA Jr, Roumm AD: Systemic sclerosis (sclero-

derma) and esophageal adenocarcinoma: Is increased patient screening necessary? Gastroenterology 89:485–488, 1985.

12. Johnson DA, Drane WE, Curran J, et al: Pulmonary disease in progressive systemic sclerosis: A complication of gastroesophageal reflux and occult aspiration? Arch Intern Med 149:589–593, 1989.

13. Marie I, Dominique S, Levesque H, et al: Esophageal involvement and pulmonary manifestations in systemic sclerosis. Arthritis Rheum 45:346–354, 2001.

14. Lock G, Pfeifer M, Straub RH, et al: Association of esophageal dysfunction and pulmonary function impairment in systemic sclerosis. Am J Gastroenterol 93:341–345, 1998.

15. Troshinski MB, Kane GC, Varga J, et al: Pulmonary function and gastroesophageal reflux in systemic sclerosis. Ann Intern Med 121:6–10, 1994.

16. Horowitz M, Maddern GJ, Maddox A, et al: Effects of cisapride on gastric and esophageal emptying in systemic sclerosis. Gastroenterology 93:311–315, 1987.

17. Poirier NC, Taillefer R, Topart P, et al: Antireflux operations in patients with scleroderma. Ann Thorac Surg 58:66–73, 1994.

18. Orringer MB, Orringer JS, Dabich L, et al: Combined Collis gastroplasty-fundoplication operations for scleroderma reflux esophagitis. Surgery 90:624–630, 1981.

19. Levine JS: Gastrointestinal manifestation of systemic diseases. In Tadanaka Yamada Textbook of Gastroenterology, 3rd ed. Philadelphia, Lippincott Williams & Wilkins, 1999, pp. 2504–2546.

20. Marshall JB, Kretchmar JM, Gerhardt DC, et al: Gastrointestinal manifestations of mixed connective tissue disease. Gastroenterology 98:1232–1238, 1990.

21. Weber P, Ganser G, Frosch M, et al: Twenty-four hour intraesophageal pH monitoring in children and adolescents with scleroderma and mixed connective tissue disease. J Rheumatol 27:2692–2695, 2000.

22. Kjellen G, Fransson SG, Lindstrom F, et al: Esophageal function, radiography, and dysphagia in Sjögren's syndrome. Dig Dis Sci 31:225–229, 1986.

23. Grande L, Lacima G, Ros E, et al: Esophageal motor function in primary Sjogren's syndrome. Am J Gastroenterol 88:378–381, 1993.

24. Anselmino M, Zaninotto G, Costantini M, et al: Esophageal motor function in primary Sjogren's syndrome: Correlation with dysphagia and xerostomia. Dig Dis Sci 42:113–118, 1997.

25. de Merieux P, Verity MA, Clemens PJ, et al: Esophageal abnormalities and dysphagia in polymyositis and dermatomyositis. Arthritis Rheum 26:961–968, 1983.

26. Jacob H, Berkowitz D, McDonald E, et al: The esophageal motility disorder of polymyositis: A prospective study. Arch Intern Med 143:2262–2264, 1983.

27. Horowitz M, McNeil JD, Maddern GJ, et al: Abnormalities of gastric and esophageal emptying in polymyositis and dermatomyositis. Gastroenterology 90:434–439, 1986.

28. Gutierrez F, Valenzuela JE, Ehresmann GR, et al: Esophageal dysfunction in patients with mixed connective tissue disease and systemic lupus erythematosus. Dig Dis Sci 27:592–597, 1982.

29. Lapadula G, Muolo P, Semeraro F, et al: Esophageal motility disorders in rheumatic diseases: A review of 150 patients. Clin Exp Rheumatol 12:515–521, 1994.

30. Verne NG, Sninski CA: Diabetes and the gastrointestinal tract. Gastroenterol Clin North Am 27:861–874, 1998.

31. Holloway RH, Tippett MD, Horowitz M, et al: Relationship between esophageal motility and transit in patients with type I diabetes mellitus. Am J Gastroenterol 94:3150–3157, 1999.

32. Jackson AL, Rashed H, Cardoso S, et al: Assessment of gastric electrical activity and autonomic function among diabetic and nondiabetic patients with symptoms of gas-

troesophageal reflux. Dig Dis Sci 45:1727–1730, 2000.

33. Murray FE, Lombard MG, Ash J, et al: Esophageal function in diabetes mellitus with special reference to acid studies and relationship to peripheral neuropathy. Am J Gastroenterol 82:840–843, 1987.

34. Lluch I, Ascaso JF, Mora F, et al: Gastroesophageal reflux in diabetes mellitus. Am J Gastroenterol 94:919–924, 1999.

35. Jackson AL, Rashed H, Cardoso S, et al: Assessment of gastric electrical activity and autonomic function among diabetic and non diabetic patients with symptoms of gastroesophageal reflux. Dig Dis Sci 45:1727–1730, 2000.

36. Horowitz M, Edelbrock M, Fraser R, et al: Disordered gastric motor function in diabetes mellitus: Recent insights into prevalence, pathophysiology, clinical relevance, and treatment. Scand J Gastroenterol 26:673–684, 1991.

37. Parkman HP, Schwartz SS: Esophagitis and gastroduodenal disorders associated with diabetic gastroparesis. Arch Intern Med 147:1477–1480, 1987.

38. Brown CK, Khanderia U: Use of metoclopramide, domperidone, and cisapride in the management of diabetic gastroparesis. Clin Pharmacol 9:357–365, 1990.

39. Kendal BJ, Kendal ET, Soykan I, et al: Cisapride in the long-term treatment of chronic gastroparesis: A 2-year open-label study. J Int Med Res 25:182–189, 1997.

40. Janssens J, Peeters TL, Vantrappen G, et al: Improvement of gastric emptying in diabetic gastroparesis by erythromycin: Preliminary studies. N Engl J Med 322:1028–1031, 1990.

41. Fontana RJ, Barnett JL: Jejunostomy tube placement in refractory diabetic gastroparesis: A retrospective review. Am J Gastroenterol 91:2174–2178, 1996.

42. McCallum RW, Chen JD, Lin Z, et al: Gastric pacing improves emptying and symptoms in patients with gastroparesis: Gastroenterology 114:456–461, 1998.

43. Stoa-Birketvedt G, Paus PN, Ganss R, et al: Cimetidine reduces weight and improves metabolic control in overweight patients with type 2 diabetes. Int J Obes Relat Metab Disord 23:550–551, 1998.

44. Feely J, Collins WC, Cullen M, et al: Potentiation of the hypoglycemic response to glipizide in diabetic patients by histamine H2-receptor antagonists. Br J Clin Pharmacol 35:321–323, 1993.

45. Barak N, Ehrenpreis ED, Harrison JR, et al: Gastro-esophageal reflux disease in obesity: Pathophysiological and therapeutic considerations. Obes Rev 3:9–15, 2002.

46. Denke MA: Anorexia nervosa, bulimia nervosa and obesity. In Sleisenger & Fordtran's Gastrointestinal and Liver Disease: Pathophysiology /Diagnosis/ Management, 7th ed. Philadelphia, W.B. Saunders, 2002, pp 310–338.

47. Devesa SS, Blot WJ, Fraumeni JF Jr: Changing patterns in the incidence of esophageal and gastric carcinoma in the United States. Cancer 83:2049–2053, 1998.

48. Lagergren J, Bergstrom R, Nyren O: No relation between body mass and gastro-oesophageal reflux symptoms in a Swedish population based study. Gut 47: 26–29, 2000.

49. Lundell L, Ruth M, Sandberg N, Bove-Nielsen M: Does massive obesity promote abnormal gastroesophageal reflux? Dig Dis Sci 40:1632–1635, 1995.

50. Locke GR 3rd, Talley NJ, Fett SL, et al: Risk factors associated with symptoms of gastroesophageal reflux. Am J Med 106:642–649, 1999.

51. Romero Y, Cameron AJ, Locke GR III, et al: Familial aggregation of gastroesophageal reflux in patients with Barrett's esophagus and esophageal adenocarcinoma. Gastroenterology 113:1449–1456, 1997.

52. Ruhl CE, Everhart JE: Overweight, but not high dietary fat intake, increases risk of gastroesophageal reflux disease hospitalization: The NHANES I Epidemiologic Followup Study. Ann Epidemiol 9:424–435, 1999.

53. Forsell P, Hallerback B, Glise H, et al: Complications following Swedish adjustable gastric banding: A long-term followup. Obes Surg 9:11–16, 1999.

54. Iovino P, Angrisani L, Tremolaterra F, et al: Abnormal esophageal acid exposure is common in morbidly obese patients and improves after a successful lap-band system implantation. Surg Endoscopy 20 (e-published), 2002.

55. Sugerman HJ: Increased intra-abdominal pressure in obesity. Int J Obes Relat Metab Disord 22:1138, 1998.

56. Stene-Larsen G, Weberg R, Froyshov Larsen I, et al: Relationship of overweight to hiatus hernia and reflux esophagitis. Scand J Gastroenterol 23:427–432, 1988.

57. Wilson LJ, Ma W, Hirschowitz BI: Association of obesity with hiatal hernia and esophagitis. Am J Gastroenterol 94:2840–2844, 1999.

58. Wisen O, Johansson C: Gastrointestinal function in obesity: Motility, secretion, and absorption following a liquid test meal. Metabolism 41:390–395, 1992.

59. Caygill CP, Johnston DA, Lopez M, et al: Lifestyle factors and Barrett's esophagus. Am J Gastroenterol 97:1328–1331, 2002.

60. Vaughan TL, Kristal AR, Blount PL, et al: Nonsteroidal anti-inflammatory drug use, body mass index, and anthropometry in relation to genetic and flow cytometric abnormalities in Barrett's esophagus. Cancer Epidemiol Biomarkers Prev 11:745–752, 2002.

61. Fraser-Moodie CA, Norton B, Gornall C, et al: Weight loss has an independent beneficial effect on symptoms of gastro-oesophagel reflux in patients who are overweight. Scand J Gastroenterol 34:337–340, 1999.

62. Kjellin A, Ramel S, Rossner S, et al: Gastroesophageal reflux in obese patients is not reduced by weight reduction. Scand J Gastroenterol 31:1047–1051, 1996.

63. Dixon JB, O'Brien PE: Gastroesophageal reflux in obesity: The effect of lap-band placement. Obes Surg 9:527–531, 1999.

64. Frederiksen SG, Johansson J, Johnsson F, et al: Neither low-calorie diet nor vertical banded gastroplasty influence gastro-oesophageal reflux in morbidly obese patients. Eur J Surg 166:296–300, 2000.

65. Smith SC, Edwards CB, Goodman GN: Symptomatic and clinical improvement in morbidly obese patients with gastroesophageal reflux disease following Roux-en-Y gastric bypass. Obes Surg 7:479–484, 1997.

66. Davis RL, Quenzer RW, Bozigian HP, et al: Pharmacokinetics of ranitidine in morbidly obese women. DICP Ann Pharmacother 24:1040–1043, 1990.

67. Abernethy DR, Greenblat DJ, Matlis R: Cimetidine disposition in obesity. Am J Gastroenterol 79:91–94, 1984.

68. Frank S, Colliver JA, Frank A: The electrocardiogram in obesity: Statistical analysis in 1,029 patients. J Am Coll Cardiol 7:295–299, 1986.

69. Schauer P, Hamad G, Ikramuddin S: Surgical management of gastroesophageal reflux disease in obese patients. Semin Laparosc Surg 8:256–264, 2001.

70. Perez AR, Moncure AC, Rattner DW: Obesity adversely affects the outcome of antireflux operations. Surg Endosc 15:986–989, 2001.

71. Chiasson PM, Perey BJ, Valdhuyzen Van Zanten SJ: Initial experience with the surgical management of morbid obesity associated with symptomatic gastro-esophageal reflux: A comparison between gastroplasty alone and and gastroplasty with anterior fundoplication. Obes Surg 4:340–343, 1994.

72. Katz PO, Castell DO: Gastroesophageal reflux disease during pregnancy. Gastroenterol Clini North Am 27:153–167,1998.

73. Nebel OT, Fornes MF, Castell DO: Symptomatic gastroesophageal reflux: Incidence and precipitating factors. Am J Dig Dis (Dig Dis Sci) 21:953–956, 1976.

74. Ho K, Kang JY, Viegas OA: Symptomatic gastroesophageal reflux in pregnancy: A

prospective study among Singaporean women. J Gastroenterol Hepatol 13: 1020–1026,1998.

75. Baron TH, Richter JE: Gastroesophageal reflux disease in pregnancy. Gastroenterol Clin North Am 21:777–791, 1992.

76. Riely CA, Davila R: Pregnancy–related hepatic and gastrointestinal disorders. In Shleisenger & Fordtran's Gastrointestinal and Liver Disease, 7th ed. Philadelphia, W.B. Saunders, 2002, pp 1448–1461.

77. Nagler R, Spiro HM: Heartburn in late pregnancy: Manometric studies of esophageal motor function. J Clin Invest 40:954–970, 1961.

78. Van Thiel DH, Gavaler JS, Joshi SN, et al: Heartburn of pregnancy. Gastroenterology 72:666–668, 1977.

79. Lind JF, Smith AM, McIver DK, et al: Heartburn in pregnancy: A manometric study. Can Med Assoc J 98:571–574, 1968.

80. Fisher RS, Roberts GS, Grabowski CJ, et al: Altered lower esophageal sphincter function during early pregnancy. Gastroenterology 74:1233–1237, 1978.

81. Schulze K, Christensen J: Lower sphincter of the opossum esophagus in pseudo-pregnancy. Gastroenterology 73:1082–1085, 1977.

82. Van Thiel DH, Gavaler JS, Stremple JL, et al: Lower esophageal sphincter pressure in women using sequential oral contraceptives. Gastroenterology 71:232–234, 1976.

83. Ulmsten U, Sundstrom G: Esophageal manometry in pregnant and nonpregnant women. Am J Obstet Gynecol 132:260–264, 1978.

84. Mohuiddin A, Pursnaki K, Katzka DA, et al: Does circadian hormonal changes during normal menstruation cycle affect esophageal motility? Gastroenterology 111: A1126, 1996.

85. Schade RR, Pelekanos MJ, Tauxe WN, et al: Gastric emptying during pregnancy. Gastroenterology 86:1234–1237, 1984.

86. Spence AA, Moir DD, Finlay WEI: Observations on intragastric pressure. Anesthesia 22:249–256, 1967.

87. Van Thiel DH, Wald A: Evidence refuting a role for increased abdominal pressure in the pathogenesis of the heartburn associated with pregnancy. Am J Obstet Gynecol 140:420–422, 1981.

88. Cappel MS, Sidhom OA: A multicenter, multiyear study of the safety and clinical utility of esophagogastroduodenoscopy in 20 concecutive pregnant femaleswith follow-up of fetal outcome. Am J Gastroenterol 88:1990–1995, 1993.

89. Cappel MS, Colon VJ, Sidhom OA: A study of eight medical centers of the safety and clinical efficacy of esophagogastroduodenoscopy in 83 pregnant females with follow up of fetal outcome and with comparison to control groups. Am J Gastroenterol 91:348–344, 1996.

90. Briggs GG, Freeman RK, Yaffe SJ: Ranitidine. In Drugs in Pregnancy and Lactation: A Reference Guide to Fetal and Neonatal Risk, 4th ed. Baltimore, Williams & Wilkins, 1994, pp 763–764.

91. Sifton DW, Westlet GI, Pfohl B (eds): Physician's Desk Reference. Montvale, NJ, Medical Economics Data Production Company, 1997.

92. Broussard CN, Richter JE: Treating gastroesophageal reflux disease during pregnancy and lactation: what are the safest therapy options? Drug Saf 19:325–337, 1998.

93. Marshall JK, Thompson AB, Armstrong D: Omeprazole for refractory gastroesophageal reflux disease during pregnancy and lactation. Can J Gastroenterol 12: 225–227, 1998.

94. Ramakrishnan A, Katz PO: Pharmacologic management of gastroesophageal reflux disease. Curr Treat Options Gastroenterol 5:301–310, 2002.

95. Fass R, Landau O, Kovacs TO, et al: Esophageal motility abnormalities in cirrhotic

patients before and after endoscopic variceal treatment. Am J Gastroenterol 92:941–946, 1997.

96. Ahmed AM, al Karawi MA, Shariq S, et al: Frequency of gastroesophageal reflux in patients with liver cirrhosis. Hepatogastroenterology 40: 478–480, 1993.

97. Arsene D, Bruley des Varannes S, et al: Gastro-oesophageal reflux and alcoholic cirrhosis: A reappraisal. J Hepatol 4:250–258, 1987.

98. Van Thiel DH, Stremple JF: Lower esophageal sphincter pressure in cirrhotic men with ascites: before and after diuresis. Gastroenterology 72:842–844, 1977.

99. Iwakiri K, Kanazawa H, Matsuzaka S, et al: Effects of transjugular intrahepatic portosystemic shunt (TIPS) on esophageal motor function and gastroesophageal reflux. J Gastroenterol 33:305–309, 1998.

100. Passaretti S, Mazzotti G, deFranchis R, et al: Esophageal motility in cirrhotics with and without esophageal varices. Scand J Gastroenterol 24:334–338, 1989.

101. Eckardt VF, Grace ND: Gastroesophageal reflux and bleeding esophageal varices. Gastroenterology 76:39–42, 1979.

102. Eckardt VF, Grace ND, Kantrowitz PA: Does lower esophageal sphincter incompetency contribute to esophageal bleeding? Gastroenterology 71:185–189, 1976.

103. Iwakiry K, Kobayashi M, Sesoko M, et al: Gastroesophageal reflux and esophageal motility in patients with esophageal varices. Gastroenterol Jpn 28:477–482, 1993.

104. Ghoshal UC, Saraswat VA, Aggarwal R, et al: Oesophageal motility and gastro-oesophageal reflux: Effect of variceal eradication by endoscopic sclerotherapy. Gastroenterol Hepatol 13:1033–1038, 1998.

105. Kinoshita Y, Kitajima N, Itoh T, et al: Gastroesophageal reflux after endoscopic injection sclerotherapy. Am J Gastroenterol 87:282–286, 1992.

106. de la Pena J, de las Heras G, Sanchez Antolin G, et al: [Prospective study of gastroesophageal reflux after esophageal variceal band ligation] [in Spanish]. Gastroenterol Hepatol 22:386–390, 1999.

107. Morichau-Beauchant M, Houin G, Mavier P, et al: Pharmacokinetics and bioavailability of ranitidine in normal subjects and cirrhotic patients. Dig Dis Sci 31:113–118, 1986.

108. Gonzalez-Martin G, Paulos C, Veloso B, et al: Ranitidine disposition in severe hepatic cirrhosis. Int J Clin Pharmacol Ther Toxicol 25:139–142, 1987.

109. Walker S, Krishna DR, Klotz U, et al: Frequent non-response to histamine H2-receptor antagonists in cirrhotics. Gut 30:1105–1109, 1989.

110. Walker S, Klotz U, Sarem-Aslani A, et al: Effect of omeprazole on nocturnal intragastric pH in cirrhotics with inadequate antisecretory response to ranitidine. Digestion 48:179–184, 1991.

111. Pique JM, Feu F, De Prada G, et al: Pharmacokinetics of omeprazole given by continuous intravenous infusion to patients with varying degrees of hepatic dysfunction. Clin Pharmacokinet 41:999–1004, 2002.

112. Friedman S, Janowitz HD: Systemic amyloidosis and the gastrointestinal tract. Gastroenterol Clin North Am 27:595–614, 1998.

113. Rubinow A, Burakoff R, Cohen AS: Esophageal manometry in systemic amyloidosis: A study of 30 patients. Am J Med 75:951–956, 1983.

114. Burakoff R, Rubinow A, Cohen AS: Esophageal manometry in familial amyloid polyneuropathy. Am J Med 79:85–89, 1985.

115. Bjerle P, Ek B, Linderholm H: Oesophageal dysfunction in familial amyloidosis with polyneuropathy. Clin Physiol 13:57–69, 1993.

116. Tada S, Iida M, Iwashita A, et al: Endoscopic and biopsy findings of the upper digestive tract in patients with amyloidosis. Gastrointest Endosc 36:10–14, 1990.

117. Pehl C, Pfeiffer A, Wendl B, et al: Effect of smoking on the results of esophageal pH measurement in clinical routine. J Clin Gastroenterol 25:503–506, 1997.

118. Kadakia SC, Kikendall JW, Maydonovitch C, et al: Effect of cigarette smoking on gastroesophageal reflux measured by 24-h ambulatory esophageal pH monitoring. Am J Gastroenterol 90:1785–1790, 1995.

119. Smit CF, Copper MP, van Leeuwen JA, et al: Effect of cigarette smoking on gastropharyngeal and gastroesophageal reflux. Ann Otol Rhinol Laryngol 110:190–193, 2001.

120. Pandolfino JE, Kahrilas PJ: Smoking and gastro-oesophageal reflux disease. Eur J Gastroenterol Hepatol 12:837–842, 2000.

121. Kahrilas PJ, Gupta RR: Mechanisms of acid reflux associated with cigarette smoking. Gut 31:4–10, 1990.

122. Chattopadhyay DK, Greaney MG, Irvin TT: Effect of cigarette smoking on the lower oesophageal sphincter. Gut 18:833–835, 1977.

123. Trudgill NJ, Smith LF, Kershaw J, et al: Impact of smoking cessation on salivary function in healthy volunteers. Scand J Gastroenterol 33:568–571, 1998.

124. Wright RA, Goldsmith LJ, Ameen V, et al: Transdermal nicotine patches do not cause clinically significant gastroesophageal reflux or esophageal motor disorders. Nicotine Tob Res 1:371–374, 1999.

125. Rahal PS, Wright RA: Transdermal nicotine and gastroesophageal reflux. Am J Gastroenterol 90:919–921, 1995.

126. Kadakia SC, De La Baume HR, Shaffer RT: Effects of transdermal nicotine on lower esophageal sphincter and esophageal motility. Dig Dis Sci 41:2130–2134, 1996.

127. Pisegna JR: Zollinger Ellison syndrome and other hypersecretory states. In Sleisenger & Fordtran's Gastrointestinal and Liver Disease: Pathophysiology/Diagnosis/Management. Philadelphia, W.B. Saunders, 2002, pp 782–796.

128. Ellison EH, Wilson SD: The Zollinger-Ellison syndrome: Reappraisal and evaluation of 260 registered cases. Ann Surg 160:512–530, 1964.

129. Regan PT, Malagelada JR: A reappraisal of clinical, roentgenographic, and endoscopic features of the Zollinger-Ellison syndrome. Mayo Clin Proc 49:44–51, 1978.

130. McCallum RW, Walsh JH: Relationship between lower esophageal sphincter pressure and serum gastrin concentration in Zollinger-Ellison syndrome and other clinical settings. Gastroenterology 76:76–81, 1979.

131. Richter JE, Pandol SJ, Castell DO, et al: Gastroesophageal reflux disease in the Zollinger-Ellison syndrome. Ann Intern Med 95:37–43, 1981.

132. Miller LS, Vinayek R, Frucht H, et al: Reflux esophagitis in patients with Zollinger-Ellison syndrome. Gastroenterology 98:341–346, 1990.

133. Strader DB, Benjamin SB, Orbuch M, et al: Esophageal function and occurrence of Barrett's esophagus in Zollinger-Ellison syndrome. Digestion 56:347–356, 1995.

134. Sarosiek J, Jensen RT, Maton PM, et al: Salivary and gastric epidermal growth factor in patients with Zollinger-Ellison syndrome: Its protective potential. Am J Gastroenterol 95:1158, 2000.

135. Rozmanic V, Ahel V, Rozmanic J: Asthma and gastroesophageal reflux in a girl with urticaria pigmentosa. Pediatr Int 42:568–569, 2000.

136. Straus E, Gerson CD, Yalow RS: Hypersecretion of gastrin associated with the short bowel syndrome. Gastroenterology 64:175–180, 1974.

137. Tang SJ, Nieto JM, Jensen D, et al: The novel use of an intravenous proton pump inhibitor in a patient with short bowel syndrome: Case report and literature review. J Clin Gastroenterol 34:62–63, 2002.

138. Mihara M, Haruma K, Kamada T, et al: Low prevalence of Helicobacter pylori infection in patients with reflux esophagitis [abstract]. Gut 39(suppl 2):A94, 1996.

139. Labenz J, Blum AL, Bayerdörffer E, et al: Curing *Helicobacter pylori* infection inpa-

tients with duodenal ulcer may provoke reflux esophagitis. Gastroenterology 112: 1442–1447, 1997.

140. Schweizer W, Thumshirn M, Dent J, et al: Helicobacter pylori and symptomatic relapse of gastro-oesophageal reflux disease: A randomized controlled trial. Lancet 357:1738–1742, 2001.

141. O'Connor HJ, McGee C, Ghabash NM, et al: Prevalence of esophagitis in *H. pylori*-positive peptic ulcer disease and the impact of eradication therapy. Hepatogastroenterology 48:1064–1068, 2001.

142. Malfertheiner P, Dent J, Zeijlon I, et al: Impact of *Helicobacter pylori* eradication on heartburn in patients with gastric or duodenal ulcer disease-results from a randomized trial program. Aliment Pharmacol Ther 16:1431–1442, 2002.

143. Labenz J, Malfertheiner P: *Helicobacter pylori* in gastro-oesophageal reflux disease: causal agent, independent or protective factor? Gut 41:277–280, 1997.

Noncardiac Chest Pain

Ronnie Fass, M.D.

chapter
11

Chest pain of esophageal origin, or noncardiac chest pain (NCCP), defined as recurring angina-like substernal chest pain of noncardiac origin, is very common. The overall prevalence of NCCP was 23.1% in one population-based study.[1] In this study, NCCP was inversely associated with increasing age, and 40% of the subjects reported having symptoms for more than 5 years. Despite the high prevalence of NCCP, it is still unclear what percentage of patients seek medical attention for their chest pain and thus become avid, and sometime relentless, consulters of the medical system. Although chest pain may signify a cardiac event, only 15% to 34% of ambulatory patients who present with chest pain are diagnosed ultimately with coronary artery disease.[2]

Because of the nature of the symptoms in patients with NCCP that are described as squeezing or burning substernal chest pain, which may radiate to the back, neck, arms, and jaws, most of these patients are evaluated initially by a cardiologist.[3] The extent of work-up that is required to exclude a cardiac cause is individually determined. History of retrosternal chest discomfort, pressure, or heaviness that lasts several minutes; pain that is induced by exertion, emotion, exposure to cold, or a large meal; and pain that is relieved by rest or nitroglycerin usually signifies typical cardiac angina. Any two of these clinical characteristics are suggestive of atypical cardiac angina, and only one or none of these characteristics is indicative of NCCP.

Although the impact of chest pain on the quality of life of patients with NCCP has not been fully evaluated, it is likely to match other functional gastrointestinal disorders, such as irritable bowel syndrome.[4] Lack of reassurance is a strong motivating factor for these patients to continue to seek medical attention. The seeking of such reassurance leads to frequent visits to the same physician or multiple physicians.[5] Additionally, repeated emergency department visits, hospitalizations, and testing are not uncommon.

Causes

Figure 1 summarizes the different underlying mechanisms of NCCP. Our current understanding of esophageal symptom perception remains relatively poor. An association with gastroesophageal reflux disease (GERD) has been demonstrated by abnormal 24-hour esophageal pH monitoring and upper endoscopy findings in up to 60% of patients with NCCP.[6] Marked improvement in symptoms with the use of antireflux medications in the vast majority of these patients suggests causality. However, it is still unclear why a similar stimulus (acid) leads to different types of symptoms (chest pain and heartburn) in different patients or in the same patient. Furthermore, as in patients with GERD, most acid reflux events in patients with GERD-related NCCP are not perceived, emphasizing the importance of peripheral and central factors in enhancing the perception of intraesophageal stimuli.[7]

The role of esophageal dysmotility in patients with NCCP remains to be elucidated. Additionally, esophageal manometry appears to have a

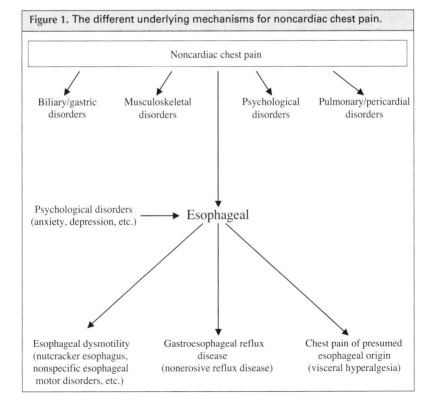

Figure 1. The different underlying mechanisms for noncardiac chest pain.

relatively poor sensitivity. More than 70% of patients with non-GERD-related NCCP are found to have normal esophageal motility.[8] Furthermore, patients rarely experience chest pain during esophageal manometry, regardless of whether esophageal dysmotility was documented.[9] Unfortunately, unlike GERD, clinicians still lack highly effective pharmacologic compounds that can eliminate esophageal dysmotility and thus can be used to demonstrate a causal relationship.[9]

Studies that focused primarily on patients with non-GERD-related NCCP have consistently documented alteration in pain perception regardless of whether esophageal dysmotility was present. The underlying mechanisms for esophageal hypersensitivity in patients with NCCP remain an area of intense research.

Rao et al.[10] performed graded balloon distensions of the esophagus using impedance planimetry in 16 consecutive patients with NCCP (normal esophageal evaluation) and 13 healthy control subjects. Patients who experienced chest pain during the balloon distension were subsequently restudied after receiving intravenous atropine. Balloon distensions reproduced chest pain at lower sensory thresholds in most NCCP subjects than in control subjects. Similar findings were documented after atropine administration despite relaxed and more deformable esophageal wall. Thus, the investigators concluded that hyperalgesia, rather than motor dysfunction, is the predominant mechanism for functional chest pain.

Several studies have documented altered autonomic function in patients with NCCP. In a recent study, Tougas et al.[11] assessed autonomic activity using power spectral analysis of heart rate variability before and during esophageal acidification in patients with NCCP and matched healthy control subjects. Of the patients with NCCP, 68% were considered acid sensitive (developed angina-like symptoms during esophageal acidification). The acid-sensitive patients had a higher baseline heart rate and lower baseline vagal activity than the acid-insensitive patients. During acid infusion, vagal cardiac outflow increased in acid-sensitive but not in acid-insensitive patients. The same investigators have already documented an increase in vagal activity in patients with NCCP during other intraesophageal stimuli (mechanical and electrical). The role that altered autonomic function plays in the pathogenesis of NCCP remains speculative. As has been stated by Tougas,[12] in most cases in which both central and autonomic factors are involved, it is the effect of the former that most likely leads to the occurrence of the latter.

As with other functional bowel disorders, psychological comorbidity is common in patients with NCCP. Studies have reported a prevalence of psychiatric disorders as high as 70%, the most common being anxiety and affective disorders.[10–14] In some patients, chest pain is part of a host of symptoms that characterize panic attack.[16] In a large study that encompassed 441 consecutive ambulatory patients presenting with chest pain to the emergency department of a heart center, 25% were diagnosed as suffering from a panic attack.[17] In another study, it was estimated that 17% to 43% of patients with NCCP suffer from a psychological abnormality, primarily anxiety/panic disorder and hypochondriasis.[23] Song et al.[18] evaluated the psychological profiles of 113 patients with chest pain and a variety of esophageal motility abnormalities, 23 symptomatic control subjects (similar symptoms but without esophageal motility abnormalities), and 27 asymptomatic control subjects. All participants were assessed by the Beck Depression Inventory, Spielberger State-Trait Anxiety Inventory, and the psychosomatic symptom checklist. Patients with esophageal symptoms and either hypertensive lower esophageal sphincter, nutcracker esophagus, or hypotensive contractions exhibited increased somatization, anxiety, and depression. Among esophageal symptoms, chest pain was closely correlated with psychometric abnormalities. Psychological comorbidity may be a driving force for nonconsulters with NCCP to seek medical attention rather than the direct *cause* of their chest pain symptoms, as has been observed with other functional gastrointestinal disorders.

Lastly, in two letters to the editor, physicians have pointed out that biliary pain is frequently felt most severely in the sternal area.[19,20] Anecdotal cases are described in these letters concerning patients with biliary diseases who first presented with acute retrosternal chest pain to the emergency room. Although evaluation of the biliary tree is not considered to be part of a routine work-up for NCCP, these cases demonstrate the diversity of underlying mechanisms that can lead to chest pain and the importance of keeping an open mind when evaluating this challenging group of patients.

Noncardiac Chest Pain Related to Gastroesophageal Reflux Disease

Gastroesophageal reflux disease has been reported to be the most common esophageal cause of NCCP. Several studies[21] have demonstrated that GERD may be present in 25% to 60% of patients with NCCP, depending on the patient population evaluated. The mechanism by which acid reflux causes heartburn in some patients and chest pain in others remains poorly understood. This is compounded by the fact that a subset of patients with NCCP report heartburn in addition to their chest pain symptom. The prevalence of erosive esophagitis in patients with GERD-related NCCP has been reported to be as low as 10% and as high as 70%.[6,22–24] The reason for such a wide range in percentage is likely to be related to the different patient populations that were evaluated in these studies. The true prevalence is yet to be determined by large, population-based studies carried out in the community. Abnormal acid exposure has been demonstrated in up to 60% of patients presenting with NCCP.[6,25] The role of symptom index (percentage of symptoms that correlate with acid reflux events) in improving the sensitivity of the pH test has been overemphasized.

The presence of abnormal acid exposure in patients with NCCP suggests an *association* with GERD but not necessarily causality. In contrast, the improvement of symptoms in patients with NCCP after antireflux treatment strongly suggests causality. In several studies, up to 80% of the NCCP patients with either abnormal upper endoscopy or pH testing findings responded to potent antireflux treatment.[6,8] These data suggest that in most NCCP patients with evidence of GERD, a pH abnormality is the cause of their symptoms.

The introduction of the proton pump inhibitor (PPI) test provided an attractive alternative to the assortment of invasive tests that patients with NCCP had to endure as part of their diagnostic evaluation. The PPI test (high-dose PPI during a short period of time) is highly sensitive and specific for diagnosing GERD-related NCCP.[26] The test is readily available, is at the disposal of primary care physicians, is noninvasive, and offers significant cost savings (Table 1).[27] In general, the need for the test increases as the true prevalence of GERD decreases in the different GERD-related disorders.[27]

In using the PPI test in patients with NCCP, there was a significant correlation between the extent of esophageal acid exposure, as determined by ambulatory 24-hour esophageal pH monitoring before the test, and the improvement in symptom intensity score at the end of the test.[26] This suggests that the higher the esophageal acid exposure is, the greater the response to the PPI test is in patients with GERD-related NCCP.

Ofman et al.[28] compared the costs and clinical outcomes of the PPI test with those of the traditional diagnostic strategies that have been recommended for patients with NCCP. Decision analysis was developed to

TABLE 1. The Proton Pump Inhibitor Test—Why?
• Readily available and at the disposal of primary care physicians
• Increases the role of primary care physicians in evaluating and treating patients with spectrum of gastroesophageal reflux disease
• Decreases patients' discomfort—less invasive tests
• Offers significant cost savings
From Fass R: Empirical trials in treatment of gastroesophageal reflux disease. Dig Dis 18(1):20–26, 2000; with permission.

evaluate the clinical and economic outcomes of two diagnostic strategies that begin with the PPI test, followed sequentially by invasive testing (endoscopy, pH testing, and esophageal manometry) as compared with two traditional strategies involving sequential invasive diagnostic tests. The strategy of the PPI test, followed, if necessary, by pH testing, manometry, and finally endoscopy, was both the most effective and the least expensive. This strategy led to an 11% improvement in diagnostic accuracy and a 43% reduction in the use of invasive diagnostic tests, yielding an average cost savings of US$454 per patient, as compared with the strategy of beginning with endoscopy, then pH monitoring, and then esophageal manometry. Richter[29] commented that the cost of the PPI test would become increasingly less expensive with the competitive pricing of the different PPIs that are currently available on the market and the imminent introduction of omeprazole in a generic form. Table 2 provides a list of studies assessing the value of the PPI test in NCCP patients.

As is true with extraesophageal manifestations of GERD, a potent antireflux medication that provides a long-term and consistent antisecretory effect is needed for GERD-related NCCP. When omeprazole 20 mg twice daily was administered over a period of 8 weeks to NCCP patients in a double-blind, placebo-controlled trial, 81% reported symptomatic improvement (compared with only 6% on placebo).[8] Patients with GERD-related NCCP may require more than 2 months of therapy for optimal symptom response. In rare cases, up to 6 months of treatment may be required. Step-down therapy to histamine-2 receptor antagonists is rarely successful and should be avoided. Furthermore, many patients with GERD-related NCCP demonstrate a long-term need for high-dose PPI (at least twice daily) for symptom control. Although attempts to reduce the dose are justified, such a reduction may result in symptom relapse.

TABLE 2. The Proton Pump Inhibitor Test in Patients with Noncardiac Chest Pain

Group (First Author)	Patients, n	Proton Pump Inhibitor	Dose	Cutoff symptom improvement, %	Duration, days	Sensitivity, %
Young	30	Omeprazole	80 mg/day	75	1	80
Squillace	17	Omeprazole	80 mg/day	50	1	69
Fass	37	Omeprazole	40 mg AM/ 20 mg PM	50	7	78
Fass	36	Rabeprazole	20 mg AM/ 20 mg PM	50	7	78
Fass	40	Lansoprazole	60 mg AM/ 30 mg PM	50	7	78

Adapted from Fass R: Empirical trials in treatment of gastroesophageal reflux disease. Dig Dis 18(1):20–26, 2000.

If the patient fails to respond to proper antireflux treatment, then evaluation by 24-hour esophageal pH monitoring while the patient is on therapy should be considered.

Esophageal Dysmotility and Noncardiac Chest Pain

In patients with lack of any evidence of GERD, esophageal dysmotility is commonly entertained. Various esophageal motility abnormalities may manifest with chest pain only or, more commonly, with other esophageal-related symptoms (such as dysphagia). The motility abnormalities include diffuse esophageal spasm, nutcracker esophagus, achalasia, long-duration contractions, multipeaked waves, and hypertensive lower esophageal sphincter.[30] However, esophageal manometry appears to have a relatively poor sensitivity in evaluating patients with NCCP. When evaluated by esophageal manometry, most patients with NCCP demonstrate normal esophageal motor function. In a tertiary referral center with a major interest in esophageal motility, only 28% of the patients evaluated by esophageal manometry for NCCP were found to have some type of esophageal dysmotility.[31] Furthermore, patients rarely experienced chest pain during esophageal manometry, regardless of whether esophageal dysmotility was documented.[32]

Obviously, this raises the question about the relationship between documented esophageal dysmotility and patients' chest pain. Unlike for GERD, clinicians still lack highly effective drugs that can easily correct a patient's motility abnormalities and consequently be used to demonstrate causal relationship. Some authorities suggest that motility abnormalities in patients with NCCP should be used as a marker of an underlying esophageal motor disorder that may be responsible for the patient's symptoms.[32] The use of ambulatory 24-hour esophageal manometry has been suggested as a means to improve the sensitivity of the test in NCCP; however, the results varied considerably.[33,34] In fact, in these studies, a significant number of patients (between 27% and 43%) reported no symptoms at all during the 24-hour recordings. Moreover, in only 13% to 24% of the patients were the investigators able to relate the pain episodes to a recorded esophageal dysmotility. These results question the routine use in clinical practice of ambulatory 24-hour esophageal manometry for the evaluation of patients with NCCP.

The distribution of esophageal motility disorders in patients presenting with non-GERD-related NCCP has been scarcely investigated. In a commonly cited study, 910 NCCP patients were evaluated by esophageal manometry, and of those 255 (28%) were found to have an esophageal motility disorder.[31] By far the most common motor disorder was nutcracker esophagus, followed by nonspecific esophageal motility disorders, diffuse esophageal spasm, hypertensive lower esophageal sphincter, and achalasia. Although this is an experience of one tertiary referral center with a major interest in esophageal motor disorders, the finding of high prevalence of nutcracker esophagus in NCCP patients is common and highly intriguing. Manometrically defined as high-amplitude contractions in the distal esophagus (>180 mm Hg), nutcracker esophagus remains an area of intense controversy. Investigators have long argued about the clinical relevance of this manometric phenomenon.[35] However, Achem et al[36] reported that most patients with chest pain associated with nutcracker esophagus responded symptomatically to antireflux treatment. Normalization of the nutcracker motility phenomenon was documented only in a minority of the patients, suggesting that GERD was the likely cause of their symptoms rather than the high-amplitude contractions in the distal esophagus.

The edrophonium test (Tensilon test) has been used to pharmacologically induce esophageal dysmotility and chest pain in patients with NCCP. Intravenous administration of edrophonium has been shown to induce esophageal manometric changes and chest pain in up to 30% of the patients.[37,38] Response to this provocative test may not necessarily indicate that a motility abnormality is responsible for the patient's symptoms; rather, a hypersensitivity to augmented esophageal motor events may be responsible.[32]

Noncardiac Chest Pain and Visceral Hyperalgesia

In most patients with non-GERD-related NCCP, there is no evidence of a motility disorder with a recognized pathologic basis. These patients are defined, by the Rome II committee for functional esophageal disorders, as having functional chest pain of presumed esophageal origin.[39]

The mechanisms of pain in patients with non-GERD-related NCCP are not fully understood. Numerous studies that focused primarily on this group of patients have consistently documented alteration in pain perception regardless of whether esophageal dysmotility was present. The underlying mechanisms for esophageal hypersensitivity in patients with NCCP remain an area of intense research. Peripheral and central sensitization of esophageal sensory afferents and spinal cord neurons has been suggested to result in heightened responses to innocuous and noxious intraesophageal stimuli.[6,40] It has been postulated that inflammation or other injuries to the esophageal mucosa sets off a cascade of events that leads to upregulation of receptors, which, in turn, induces the development of visceral hypersensitivity through peripheral and central sensitization.[6] The presence of esophageal hypersensitivity can be demonstrated long after the original stimulus has disappeared and the mucosa has healed. It is still unclear what factors determine the long-term persistence of esophageal hypersensitivity.

The use of balloon distension studies in patients with chest pain of presumed esophageal origin should be reserved only for experimental protocols. The therapeutic approach is unlikely to be altered by the results of such provocative tests.

Treatment

Treating esophageal motility abnormalities in patients with NCCP is generally less than rewarding, primarily because of the paucity of clinically effective, motility-related drugs. A treatment algorithm is given in Figure 2. In patients with nutcracker esophagus, antireflux treatment should be tried before smooth-muscle relaxants are considered.[36] Diltiazem (at doses of 60–90 mg four times daily) has been shown to improve chest pain score significantly more than placebo in small trials of patients with NCCP and documented nutcracker esophagus on esophageal manometry.[41,42] Nifedipine at doses of 10 to 30 mg three times daily demonstrated a limited symptomatic response in these patients.[43] Symptom improvement lasted only 2 weeks and was noted only after a lag time of 3 weeks. By the end of the sixth week of therapy, nifedipine appears to completely lose its efficacy. A limited effect of calcium channel blockers has also been documented in the other spastic motility disorders described in association with NCCP. Evidence supporting the use of nitrates in patients with NCCP and esophageal motility abnormalities is scarce and primarily anecdotal.[44] Overall, it appears that the smooth-muscle relaxants have a very limited role, if any at all, in patients with NCCP and documented esophageal motor disorder.

Pain modulators such as tricyclic antidepressants and trazodone have been shown to improve symptoms in NCCP patients regardless of whether esophageal motility was present. Antidepressants have a neuromodulatory effect and visceral analgesic properties, which appear to benefit patients independent of the psychotropic effects of the drugs.[45] Furthermore, tricyclics are commonly administered in non-mood-altering doses.[46] It is preferable to initiate therapy with a low dose and to then slowly increase administration as tolerated by the patient, until the target dose of 50 to 100 mg is reached. For example, if amitriptyline is used, then starting with a 10 mg dose at bedtime and increasing by 10 mg increments weekly to a target dose of 50 mg daily represents a cautious approach that allows careful monitoring for the development of side effects. Because receptor (acetylcholine, histamine and α-adrenergic)

Figure 2. Diagnosis and treatment flow chart for noncardiac chest pain. (PPI = proton pump inhibitor; GERD = gastroesophageal reflux disease.)

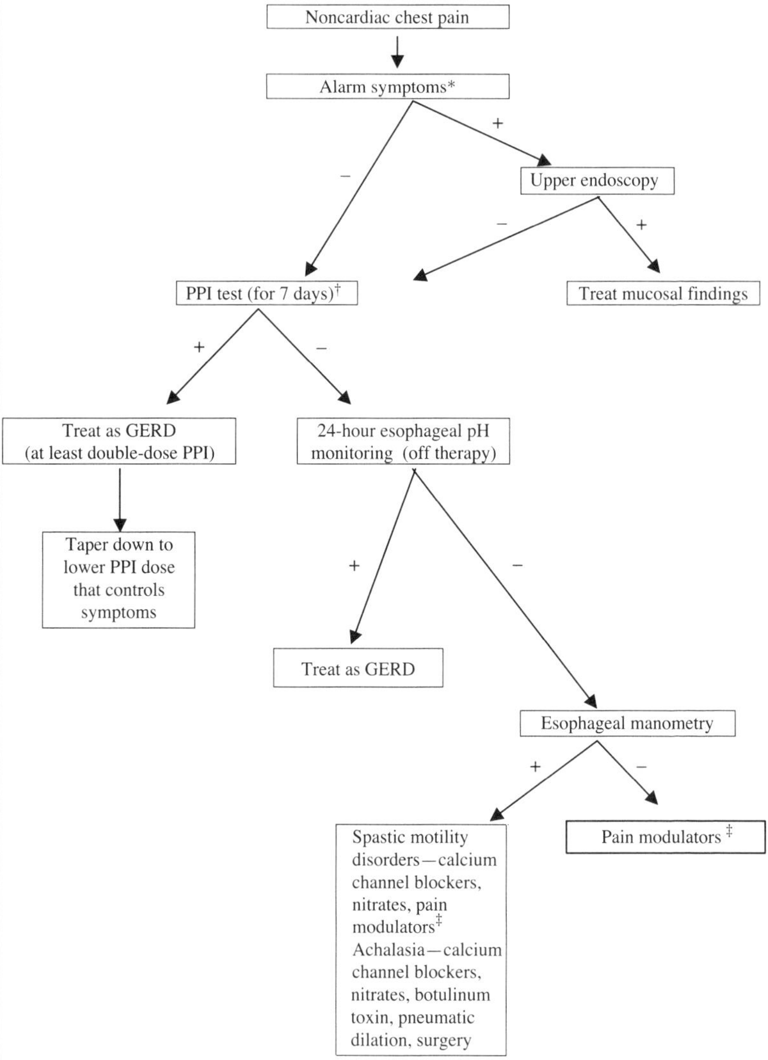

*Dysphagia, odynophagia, weight loss, anorexia, anemia, etc.
†Data are available for omeprazole, lansoprazole, and rabeprazole.
‡Tricyclic antidepressants, trazodone, and selective serotonin reuptake inhibitors.

affinity varies with the tricyclic agent used, switching to another compound if one has failed may prove helpful.[47]

Trazodone given in doses of 100 to 150 mg daily has been used in a placebo-controlled trial of patients with chest pain and esophageal contraction abnormalities.[48] The drug appeared to be significantly more effective than placebo in controlling symptoms, despite the observation that the esophageal manometric changes were not influenced by treatment or clinical response.

The use of selective serotonin reuptake inhibitors (SSRIs) has been scarcely studied. Recently, Varia et al.[49] performed a randomized trial that assessed the efficacy, tolerability, and safety of sertraline in patients with NCCP. This was a double-blind, placebo-controlled trial that included 30 subjects. Patients were randomly selected to receive sertraline or placebo in doses starting at 50 mg and adjusted to a maximum of 200 mg. By using intention-to-treat analysis, investigators demonstrated that patients receiving sertraline reported a significant reduction in their pain scores as compared with those who received placebo, regardless of concomitant improvement in psychological scores.[50] This study further confirms the potential role of SSRIs in treating patients with NCCP. As with tricyclic antidepressants, the SSRIs' effect on visceral pain perception appears to be independent of their effect on mood.

The role of other potential pain modulators in NCCP has yet to be determined. Alosetron, a 5-hydroxytryptamine type 3 antagonist that was recently removed from the market, appears to have a visceral analgesic effect, probably by altering the initiation, transmission, or processing of extrinsic sensory information from the gastrointestinal tract. A recent case report suggested that alosetron at a dose of 1 mg twice daily can markedly improve chest pain in patients with NCCP.[51] Further studies are needed to explore the clinical role and safety profile of the 5-hydroxytryptamine type 3 antagonists in patients with NCCP.

Investigators from Temple University recently proposed a provocative approach to NCCP in patients with documented spastic motility abnormalities: 100 units of botulinum toxin were injected in five circumferential injections of 20 units each at the gastroesophageal junction.[52] The investigators reported a 79% reduction in the mean chest pain score (post- vs. pre-injection). Approximately half of the patients had complete relief of chest pain. The mean duration of the response for chest pain was 7.3 months.

Because psychological comorbidity is common in patients with NCCP, identifying and treating these psychiatric disorders is an important part of any therapeutic scheme that is tailored for patients with NCCP.

Key Points: Noncardiac Chest Pain

∞ GERD is the most common cause for NCCP. Proper treatment with at least double-dose PPI should be initiated for a period of up to 6 months to ensure symptom control.

∞ In patients with negative evaluation for GERD or lack of response to proper antireflux treatment, the esophageal manometry may reveal a variety of motility abnormalities in about 30% of the patients.

∞ Currently, the role of esophageal manometry in patients with NCCP is probably limited to excluding achalasia due to similar efficacy to pain modulators in patients who are with and those who without spastic esophageal motility disorders.

∞ Smooth muscle relaxants have a limited role in treating patients with NCCP and esophageal motor disorders.

∞ Tricyclic agents, trazodone, and SSRIs are currently the most effective therapeutic modalities in treating patients with non-GERD-related NCCP.

Suggested Reading

1. Locke III GR, Talley NJ, Fett SL, et al. Prevalence and clinical spectrum of gastroesophageal reflux: a population-based study in Olmstead Count, Minnesota. Gastroenterology 112:1448–1456, 1997.

2. Katerndahl DA, Trammell C. Prevalence and recognition of panic state in STARNET patients presenting with chest pain. J Fam Pract 45:54–63, 1997.

3. Richter JE. Chest pain and gastroesophageal reflux disease. J Clin Gastroenterol. 30(suppl)39–41, 2000.

4. Gralnek IM, Hays RD, Kilbourne A, Naliboff B, Mayer EA. The impact of irritable bowel syndrome on health-related quality of life. Gastroenterology. 119:654–660, 2000.

5. Richter JE, Bradley LA, Castell DO. Esophageal chest pain: current controversies in pathogenesis, diagnosis and therapy. Ann Intern Med. 100:68–78, 1989.

6. Fass R, Fennerty MB, Ofman JJ, et al. The clinical and economic value of a short course of omeprazole in patients with noncardiac chest pain. Gastroenterology 115:42–49, 1998.

7. Fass R, Fennerty MD, Vakil N. Nonerosive reflux disease—current concepts and dilemmas. Am J Gastroenterol 96(2):303–314, 2001.

8. Achem SR, Kolts BE, MacMath T, et al. Effects of omeprazole versus placebo in treatment of noncardiac chest pain and gastroesophageal reflux. Dig Dis Sci. 42:2138–2145, 1997.

9. Fass R, Winters GF. Evaluation of the patient with noncardiac chest pain: is gastroesophageal reflux disease or an esophageal motility disorder the cause? Medscape Gastroenterol 3:1–10, 2001.

10. Rao SS, Hayek B, Summers RW. Functional chest pain of esophageal origin: hyperalgesia or motor dysfunction. Am J Gastroenterol 96(9):2584–2589, 2001.

11. Tougas G, Spaziani R, Hollerbach S, et al. Cardiac autonomic function and oe-

sophageal acid sensitivity in patients with non-cardiac chest pain. Gut 49(5): 706–712, 2001.

12. Tougas G. The autonomic nervous system in functional bowel disorders. Gut 47(Suppl 4):iv78-iv80, 2000.

13. Clouse RE, Carney RM. The psychological profile of non-cardiac chest pain patients. Eur J Gastroenterol Hepatol. 7:1160–1165, 1987.

14. Clouse RE. Spastic disorders of the esophagus. The Gastroenterologist. 5(2):112–127, 1997.

15. Cormier LE, Karon W. Russo J, et al. Chest pain with negative cardiac diagnostic studies. Relationship to psychiatric illness. J Nerv Men Dis. 176:351–358, 1988.

16. Potokar JP, Nutt DJ. Chest pain: panic attack or heart attack? Int J Clin Pract 54(2):110–114, 2000.

17. Fleet RP, Dupuis G, Marchand A, et al. Panic disorder in emergency department chest pain patients: prevalence, comorbidity, suicidal ideation, and physician recognition. Am J Med 101(4):371–380, 1996.

18. Song CW, Lee SJ, Jeen YT, et al. Inconsistent association of esophageal symptoms, psychometric abnormalities and dysmotility. Am J Gastroenterol. 96(8):2312–2316, 2001.

19. Hugh TB. Letter: Non-cardiac chest pain. Med J Aust. 174(9):482–483, 2001.

20. Jones KS. Letter: Non-cardiac chest pain: a variant on Murphy's sign. Med J Aust 175(7):391, 2001.

21. Azpiroz F, Dapoigny M, Pace F, et al. Nongastrointestinal disorders in the irritable bowel syndrome. Digestion 62:66–72, 2000.

22. Cherian P, Smith LF, Bardhan KD, et al. Esophageal tests in the evaluation of non-cardiac chest pain. Dis Esophagus. 8:129–133, 1995.

23. Frobert O, Funch-Jensen P, Jacobsen NO, et al. Upper endoscopy in patients with angina and normal coronary angiograms. Endoscopy. 27:365–370, 1996.

24. Hsia P, Maher K, Lewis J, et al. Utility of upper endoscopy in the evaluation of non-cardiac chest pain. Gastrointest Endosc. 37:22–26, 1991.

25. Hewson EG, Sinclair JW, Dalton CB, Richter JE. Twenty-four hour esophageal pH monitoring. The most useful test for evaluating noncardiac chest pain. Am J Med. 90:576–583, 1991.

26. Fass R, Fennerty MC, Johnson, C, et al. Correlation of ambulatory 24-hour esophageal pH monitoring results with symptom improvement in patients with noncardiac chest pain due to gastroesophageal reflux disease. J Clin Gastroenterol 28(1):36–39, 1999.

27. Fass R: Empirical trials in treatment of gastroesophageal reflux disease. Dig Dis 18(1):20–26, 2000.

28. Ofman JJ, Gralnek IM, Udani, J, et al. The cost-effectiveness of the omeprazole test in patients with noncardiac chest pain. 107(3):219–227, 1999.

29. Richter JE. Cost-effectiveness of testing for gastroesophageal reflux disease: what do patients, physicians, and health insurers want? Am J Med. 107(3):288–289, 1999.

30. Kahrilas PJ, Clouse RE, Hogan WJ. An American Gastroenterological Association medical position statement on the clinical use of esophageal manometry. Gastroenterology. 107:1865–1884, 1994.

31. Katz PO, Dalton CB, Richter JE, Wu WC, Castell DO. Esophageal testing in patients with noncardiac chest pain or dysphagia: results of three years' experience with 1161 patients. Ann Intern Med. 106:593–597, 1987.

32. DiMarino Jr. AJ, Allen ML, Lynn RB, Zamani S. Clinical value of esophageal motility testing. Dig Dis. 16:198–204, 1998.

33. Breumelhof R, Nadorp JHSM, Akkemans LMA, Smout AJPM. Analysis of 24-hour

esophageal pressure and pH data in unselected patients with noncardiac chest pain. Gastroenterology. 99:1257–1264, 1990.

34. Lam HGT, Dekker W, Kan G, Breedjijk M, Smout AJPM. Acute noncardiac chest pain in a coronary care unit: evaluation by 24-hour pressure and pH recording of the esophagus. Gastroenterology 102:453–460, 1992.

35. Kahrilas PJ. Nutcracker esophagus: Editorial: An idea whose time has gone? Am J Gastroenterol. 88:167–169, 1993.

36. Achem SR, Kolts BE, Wears R, Burton L, Richter JE. Chest pain associated with nutcracker esophagus: A preliminary study of the role of gastroesophageal reflux. Am J Gastroenterol. 88:187–192, 1993.

37. Dalton CB, Hewson EG, Castell DO, Richter JE. Edrophonium provocation test in noncardiac chest pain. Dig Dis Sci. 35:1445–1451, 1990.

38. Fass R, Offman JJ, Sampliner RE, Camargo L, Wendel C, Fennerty MB. The omeprazole test is as sensitive as 24-h oesophageal pH monitoring in diagnosing gastrooesophageal reflux disease in symptomatic patients with erosive esophagitis. Aliment Pharmacol Ther. 14:389–396, 2000.

39. Drossman DA, Corazziari R, Talley NJ, et al, and the Rome II Multinational Working Teams: Rome II. In The Functional Esophageal Disorders, edn 2. Edited by Drossman DA. Lawrence: Allen Press, Inc.; 2000.

40. Mayer EA. The neurobiology of stress and gastrointestinal disease. Gut 46:861–869, 2000.

41. Cattau Jr. EL, Castell DO, Johnson DA, et al. Diltiazem therapy for symptoms associated with nutcracker esophagus. Am J Gastroenterol. 86:272–276, 1991.

42. Richter JE, Spurling TJ, Cordova CM, Castell DO. Effects of calcium blocker, diltiazem, on esophageal contractions. Studies in volunteers and patients with nutcracker esophagus. Dig Dis Sci. 29:649–656, 1987.

43. Richter JE, Dalton CB, Bradley LA, Castell DO. Oral nifedipine in the treatment of noncardiac chest pain in patients with the nutcracker esophagus. Gastroenterology. 93:21–28, 1987.

44. Mellow MH. Effect of isosorbide and hydralazine in painful primary esophageal motility disorders. Gastroenterology. 83:264–370, 1982.

45. Camilleri M. Management of the irritable bowel syndrome. Gastroenterology. 120:652–668, 2001.

46. Cannon R, Epstein S. "Microvascular angina" as a cause of chest pain and angiographically normal coronary arteries. Am J Cardiol. 61:1338–1343, 1988.

47. Clouse RE. Psychotropic medications for the treatment of functional gastrointestinal disorders. Clin Perspect Gastroenterol. 2:348–356, 1999.

48. Clouse RE, Lustman PJ, Eckert TC, et al. Low-dose trazodone for symptomatic patients with esophageal contraction abnormalities. A double-blind, placebo-controlled trial. Gastroenterology. 92(4):1027–1036, 1987.

49. Varia I, Logue E, O'Connor C, et al. Randomized trial of sertraline in patients with unexplained chest pain of noncardiac origin. Am Heart J 140:367–372, 2000.

50. Krishman KR. Selected summary: Chest pain and serotonin: a possible link. Gastroenterology 121:495–496, 2001.

51. Burbige EJ. Use of a 5-HT_3 antagonist in a patient with noncardiac chest pain. Am J Gastroenterol 96:S183, 2001.

52. Sujata V, Pullela SV, Parkman HP, et al. Treatment of chest pain in patients with nonachalasia spastic esophageal motor disorders using botulinum toxin injection. Am J Gastroenterol 96:S23, 2001.

53. Van Peski-Oosterbaan AS, Spinhoven P, Van der Does AJ, et al. Cognitive change following cognitive behavioural therapy for non-cardiac chest pain. Psychother Psychosom. 68(4):214–220, 1999.

Quality of Life and Cost Analysis for Gastroesophageal Reflux Disease

chapter

12

Lauren B. Gerson M.D., M.Sc.

Patients with chronic gastroesophageal reflux disease (GERD) suffer from diminished health-related quality of life,[1] and must confront potentially high costs of lifetime drug therapy to achieve satisfactory symptom control. While state-of-the-art proton pump inhibitor (PPI) therapy can effectively heal erosive esophagitis and reduce symptoms in 85% to 90% of patients with chronic GERD,[2–4] the cost per pill is several times greater than the price of histamine-2 receptor antagonist (H_2RAs), which heal esophagitis in approximately 50% of patients. When costs of therapy increase in conjunction with improved efficiency, cost-effectiveness analyses provide useful insight regarding the role for newer and more expensive therapies in disease management. The costs associated with medical therapy for GERD include both direct costs (cost of drugs, other diagnostic tests such as endoscopy, and physician visits) and indirect costs (time lost from work and decreased productivity). Therefore, although the price per pill for H_2-blockers is considerably lower than for PPIs, the decreased efficacy of H_2-blockers in healing erosive esophagitis may lead to increased endoscopy rates for refractory symptoms, more physician visits, and therefore higher overall costs compared to use of PPIs for GERD patients. This chapter focuses on cost-effectiveness assessments in the area of GERD, and the impact on health-related quality-of-life from this chronic disease.

Cost-Effectiveness Analyses

The purpose of a cost-effectiveness analysis is to illustrate the trade-offs involved in choosing among different interventions with varying clinical outcomes and costs.[6] A cost-effectiveness ratio comparing two alternatives is calculated by the difference in costs between the two alternatives divided by the difference in effectiveness. This ratio can be

197

expressed as dollars per life-year gained or dollars per quality-adjusted life-year gained. When comparing alternative treatments, interventions associated with the lowest cost and highest efficiency or quality of life are always the preferred strategy. However, when one treatment (such as PPI therapy for GERD) is more expensive yet more effective than another therapy (such as H_2RA for GERD), the calculation of a cost-effectiveness ratio may demonstrate that the cost per quality-adjusted life-year is lower for the PPI despite the increased cost.

To perform cost-effectiveness analyses in the area of GERD, information regarding costs and effectiveness associated with treatment is needed. The cost of a medication is usually based on the average whole-sale price from the Drug Topics Book,[7] and the effect of variations in cost is tested by means of a sensitivity analysis. The costs associated with diagnostic testing are usually obtained from the perspective of a third-party payer. The effectiveness of therapy can be derived from the medical literature. Estimation of life-years gained can be based on current US life expectancy tables, or quality-adjusted life years can be based on patient preferences (also known as utilities, discussed in the next section). The decision model can be created using Excel (Microsoft Excel 2000, Microsoft Corporation, Redmond, WA) or programs designed for decision analysis such as DATA 4.0 (Treeage Software, Williamstown, MA) or SMLTREE software (version 2.9, J. Hollenberg, New York, NY). The analysis can occur as a decision tree, in which patients are followed over time until particular outcomes occur, or a Markov model, in which patients can cycle through states over time until all patients reach the terminal state, or death. An example of a decision tree showing "step-up" therapy from a cost-effectiveness analysis comparing intermittent PPI therapy to other treatment options is shown in Figure 1. Circles represent chance nodes (where the outcome depends upon chance), squares decision nodes (where the physician would decide upon the next step), and triangles end nodes (after which point no more outcomes would occur).

Costs used for a decision analysis should reflect as broad as a perspective as possible and should reflect a consistent focus throughout the analysis. For example, the cost for the PPI omeprazole is approximately $3.87 per pill, according to the average wholesale price listing in the Drug Topics Book,[7] but can be as low as $1.66 through the Department of Veterans Affairs Health Care System[8] and other managed care plans. If one were to use drug costs from the VA Health Care System for a model, it would be preferable to obtain costs for upper endoscopy and other services from the perspective of the Department of Veterans Affairs as well. Current procedural terminology codes and Medicare costs are often used for procedures such as upper endoscopy with biopsy (code 42329, 1999), including conscious sedation (code 99141) and patho-

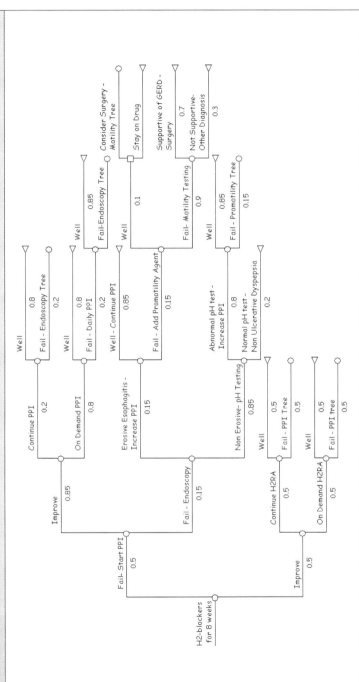

pump inhibitor therapy; circles = chance nodes; squares = decision nodes; triangles = end nodes, where patients remain for the duration of the study. The percentage of patients responding to each intervention is listed below each arm of the tree. Patients who fail a PPI at any point are referred for an upper endoscopy. Prokinetic therapy is given if a patient remains symptomatic on twice-daily PPI therapy. Motility studies and/or surgery is performed if patients elect to undergo surgery or fail medical management. (From Gerson LB, Robbins AS, Garber A, et al: A cost-effectiveness analysis of prescribing strategies in the management of gastroesophageal reflux disease. Am J Gastroenterol 95:395–407, 2000; with permission.)

logic interpretation of endoscopic biopsies (code 88305). In addition to the procedure costs, many decision analyses often include the additional facility fee of the hospital for the procedure. The following section presents the results from cost-effectiveness analyses that have been published to determine the optimal treatment strategy for patients with chronic GERD.

What is the Most Cost-Effective Medical Therapy for Gastroesophageal Reflux Disease?

Management options for patients with chronic GERD include lifestyle modifications; H_2RA therapy, PPIs, promotility agents, "step-up" therapy, "step-down" therapy, intermittent therapy, or "on demand" therapy. Cost-effectiveness analyses in the literature (Table 1) have attempted to determine whether initial treatment for GERD should consist of PPI or H_2RA, and whether maintenance therapy should be intermittent (4–8 weeks of medication for symptoms followed by cessation of medication), on demand (medication taken as need for several days or weeks for symptoms), or continuous. Other maintenance strategies include the "step-down" option, in which patients responding to PPI are then prescribed H_2RAs for maintenance therapy, or "step-up" option, in which patients are started on H_2RAs and then prescribed PPIs for symptom failure. An additional option includes the PPI test, which includes 7 days of omeprazole 40 mg daily and 20 mg at night, followed by the step-down approach for responders.

In general, PPI therapy followed by on-demand therapy or step-down treatment is more cost-effective than the traditional step-up approach (see Fig. 1) due to decreased rates of endoscopy for lack of symptom control on H_2RAs. Since 50% of patients do not respond to H_2RAs, more patients undergo diagnostic testing, as compared to a scenario in which all patients receive PPIs from the outset.

Although initial cost-effectiveness analyses based response rates on endoscopic healing rates in patients with erosive esophagitis, it is now well documented that patients with nonerosive gastroesophageal reflux disease do not differ from patients with erosive esophagitis in terms of symptom severity or response to medical therapy.[9] Therefore, most analyses use symptom control in lieu of endoscopic healing as an end point for medical therapy. In addition, although most studies use a time horizon of 1 to 5 years for evaluation of cost-effectiveness, the ideal time span for the study should be a lifetime perspective, since initial cost savings, for example, those associated with surgical therapy, may be offset by medical therapy costs later in life because of symptomatic recurrence. In addition, costs during the first year of a model are increased

TABLE 1. Cost-Effectiveness Studies in Management of Gastroesophageal Reflux Disease

Study	End Point	Time Horizon	Treatment Arms	Result	Sensitivity Analysis	Incremental Cost-Effectiveness Ratio
Ofman et al[40] (2002, USA)	Symptom relief	1 year	a. Step-up approach b. PPI test* and step-down approach	PPI test followed by step-down cost-effective	Step-up preferred if PPI test cost > $4521 or cost of PPI per week > $242 or < 47% of patients with positive PPI test stepped down	PPI Test: $510/cure or $2822–$10160/QALY
Wahlqvist et al[41] (2002, UK)	Symptom relief (nonerosive only)	6 months	a. On demand†esomeprazole b. Intermittent omeprazole c. Continuous omeprazole	On demand most cost-effective	Intermittent cost-effective if cost of esomeprazole increases by 30%, cost of omeprazole decreases by 50%, or cost of relapse doubles	On-demand dominant
Gerson et al[42] (2000, USA)	Symptom relief	Lifetime	a. Intermittent PPI‡ b. Continuous PPI c. Step-up approach d. Step-down approach e. Lifestyle modifications	Intermittent most cost-effective	Step-up if efficacy of intermittent < 59%	Mild GERD: $37,923/QALY Moderate GERD: $20,934/QALY
Ofman et al[43] (2000, USA)	Symptom relief	1 year	a. Rabeprazole b. Ranitidine	Rabeprazole more cost-effective	Did not change results	Rabeprazole: $2748/ recurrence prevented
Goeree et al[44] (1999, Canada)	Healing of EE	1 year	a) Intermittent PPI‡ b. Continuous PPI c. Step Down approach d. Step-Up approach	Intermittent PPI most cost-effective	Step-up if generic: H₂RA	Intermittent PPI Can$8/GERD week

(continued)

TABLE 1. Cost-Effectiveness Studies in Management of Gastroesophageal Reflux Disease (*Continued*)

Study	End Point	Time Horizon	Treatment Arms	Result	Sensitivity Analysis	Incremental Cost-Effectiveness Ratio
Stal JM et al[45] (1998, UK)	Esophageal stricture maintenance	1 year	a. Omeprazole b. Ranitidine	Omeprazole cost-effective	Results sensitive to drug costs, disutility of dysphagia and dilation	Omeprazole: Can$49,630/QALY
Harris et al[46] (1997, USA)	Healing of EE	1 year	a. Continuous PPI b. Intermittent PPI‡ (with continuous PPI for 1 or 2 recurrences)	Intermittent PPI most cost-effective	Continuous PPI if esophagitis causes >22% decrement in quality of life	Intermittent PPI $73/recurrence prevented
Harris et al[47] (1997, USA)	Maintenance for EE	1 year	a. PPI b. H₂RAs, high dose c. H₂RAs, standard	PPI most cost-effective	H₂RAs preferred if utility of EE less than 0.91	PPI $59 (average whole-sale pric ng) to $677/recurrence (govern-ment costs) prevented

*PPI test includes 7 days of omeprazole 40 mg PO AM ± 20 mg PM followed by step-down approach
†"On-demand" defined as single doses of medications to relieve symptoms
‡Intermittent defined as 4 to 8 week course of therapy for symptoms
EE = erosive esophagitis; GERD = gastroesophageal reflux disease; H₂RA = histamine-2 receptor antagonist; QALY = quality-adjusted life-year; PPI = proton pump i nhibitor.

due to costs of diagnostic procedures typically performed within the first year of presentation of symptoms.

Ofman et al[40] (see Table 1) compared the traditional step-up approach to a PPI testing followed by a step-down arm. They found that the traditional management strategy resulted in a greater than fivefold increase in the utilization of upper endoscopy, which was partially offset by a 47% reduction in the use of ambulatory 24-hour esophageal pH monitoring. The PPI test and step-down approach was preferred unless the cost of the PPI exceeded $242/week or less than 47% of patients with a positive PPI test are stepped down to H_2RA therapy.

Recently, the on-demand strategy for GERD symptoms has been shown to be effective for most GERD patients.[10,11] In work by Talley et al,[10] most patients achieved adequate symptom control on esomeprazole 20 mg or 40 mg every third day for a 6-month study duration. In the only cost-effectiveness analysis to date to examine an on-demand strategy, Wahlqvist et al[41] compared (a) esomeprazole 20 mg on-demand therapy to (b) intermittent therapy with omeprazole 20 mg for 4 weeks for symptomatic relapses or (c) continuous therapy with omeprazole 20 mg after the first relapse. An on-demand approach (defined as medication taken on a daily basis as needed for symptoms) was less costly and more effective than intermittent or continuous therapy. In sensitivity analysis, intermittent therapy was preferred if the price of esomeprazole increased by 30% or the cost of omeprazole decreased by 50%.

A decision analysis published by Gerson et al[42] in 2000 compared a strategy using intermittent therapy (defined as 8 weeks of omeprazole 20 mg daily for symptomatic recurrences) to other strategies, which included step-up therapy, a step-down approach, continuous PPI, and lifestyle modifications, which included use of antacids (the reference treatment). Endoscopy was reserved in all arms for patients who failed to respond to PPI therapy. Using data from US life tables, patients were followed until death, providing the perspective of lifetime costs. Since published utility values were not available based on severity of GERD symptoms, it was assumed that patients with severe GERD would have a utility of 0.95 (see utility section following; utilities range from a scale of 0 to 1, where 0 is a state equivalent to death and 1 is perfect health) and that patients with mild GERD would have a utility of 0.98. The intermittent therapy was the most cost-effective approach, with a discounted incremental cost-effectiveness ratio of $20,934 for severe GERD, and $37,923 for mild GERD. Sensitivity analysis showed that the step-up arm would be preferred if the efficacy of the on-demand approach was less than 59%. The results did not change when other parameters were varied such as the costs of medications, success rate of

Nissen fundoplication, length of on-demand therapy, costs of office visits, or success rate of the lifestyle arm.

The study by Goeree et al[44] examined healing of erosive esophagitis from the perspective of the Canandian Health System. The strategies included (a) intermittent omprazole 20 mg daily for 8 weeks, which was repeated for symptom recurrence; (b) omeprazole 20 mg daily; (c) standard H$_2$RAs (150 mg ranitidine twice daily) for acute and maintenance therapy; (d) step-down therapy with prokinetic therapy (cisapride 10 mg four times daily for 12 weeks, then 10 mg twice daily for maintenance therapy); (e) step-down PPI to H$_2$RA therapy with omeprazole for 8 weeks followed by ranitidine 150 mg twice daily for maintenance; and (f) step-down PPI with omeprazole 20 mg for 8 weeks followed by 10 mg daily for maintenance therapy. Patients who did not experience endoscopic healing on H$_2$RAs or prokinetic therapy received omeprazole 20 mg daily; if healing still did not occur, the dose of PPI was then doubled for 8 weeks. Surgery was reserved for patients who failed to heal on double-dose PPI therapy. Using the H$_2$RA arm as the baseline strategy (since it was associated with the lowest costs), the intermittent omeprazole arm was the most cost-effective and required an additional Can$8 per week that GERD was averted as compared with the step-down strategy from PPI to H$_2$RAs, which required an additional Can$44 per week that GERD was averted. Costs used in this study were based on professional and facility fees from the Ontario Case Costing Program. Sensitivity analysis demonstrated that the step-up arm dominated the PPI intermittent therapy if costs for generic H$_2$RAs were used.

The issue of esophageal stricture maintenance therapy was examined in a 1998 decision analysis by Stal et al[45] comparing the incremental cost-utility of omeprazole 20 mg once daily with that of ranitidine 150 mg twice daily for 1 year. Input variables were estimated from the literature and local hospital data. Utility data were collected using the time-tradeoff technique (see Quality of Life Assessments section) involving patients with peptic stricture and health professionals. The incremental cost of omeprazole compared with that of ranitidine was $556 per patient treated, and the incremental utility gain of omeprazole was 0.0112 quality-adjusted life-years. Overall, the incremental cost-utility ratio of omeprazole in maintenance therapy for patients with peptic stricture was $49,600 per quality-adjusted life-year gained. Sensitivity analysis revealed that the estimates with the greatest impact on the cost-effectiveness analysis were disutility associated with dysphagia and dilation, the probability of requiring redilation, and the cost of medications.

Harris and colleagues published two studies in 1997 that examined healing and maintenance therapy for erosive esophagitis. In the first study,[46] patients with healed erosive esophagitis received maintenance therapy with (1) lansoprazole 15 mg daily with dose escalation to 30 mg or 45 mg in the setting of symptom recurrence; (2) maintenance PPI after one symptom recurrence; or (3) maintenance PPI after two symptom recurrences. Drug costs were based on average wholesale prices and procedural costs on government procurement prices. Expert opinion was used to estimate the decrement in symptom-free days with recurrence. As expected, waiting until the second recurrence was the least costly strategy but also was associated with the most symptomatic recurrences. Intermittent PPI with continuous PPI for one recurrence was the most cost-effective strategy.

In the second study,[47] maintenance therapy with PPI was compared to maintenance with standard or high-dose H2RAs. Average wholesale costs were used for drugs. The PPI strategy was cost-effective if the utility for erosive esophagitis was 0.91 and average wholesale costs were used (annual cost of omeprazole $1360 and ranitidine $1337). However, if government procurement costs were used (annual omeprazole cost $867 compared to $598 for ranitidine), the utility associated with erosive esophagitis would need to be 0.75 for the PPI strategy to be cost-effective. The authors concluded that using PPI therapy from the outset would cost $1360 and lead to 0.15 recurrences per year as compared to standard H2RAs, which cost $1337 and lead to 0.549 recurrences per year.

Is Surgery More Cost-Effective Than Medical Therapy?

Three published studies have compared surgical therapy (laparoscopic Nissen fundoplication [LNF]) to medical therapy as a maintenance treatment for chronic GERD. Romagnuolo et al[48] compared LNF to maintenance therapy with omeprazole 20 mg daily. The authors' base case was a 45-year-old man with erosive esophagitis refractory to H2RAs. Direct costs were estimated from the perspective of a provincial health ministry in Canada. Utilities were derived from an abstract[12] in which standard gamble and time trade-off techniques (see Quality of Life Assessments section) were employed in patients with severe GERD. Reflux symptoms were associated with a utility between 0.90 and 0.97, depending on the technique used; the mean utility value (0.935) was used for this model.

In the medical arm of the study, patients were initially healed with omeprazole, followed by maintenance therapy that could be increased to a maximum of 60 mg/day. The authors assumed that 20% of patients requiring 60 mg of omeprazole daily would opt for LNF annually. In the surgical arm of the study, the healing phase was considered to be the surgery itself. Patients with recurrent symptoms after LNF could have a repeat surgery via the open approach (30%) or continue on omeprazole

40 mg/day. Over the 5-year time horizon of the model, LNF was less costly (Can$3520) than omeprazole (Can$5465), and the quality-adjusted life-years between the two arms did not differ significantly (4.35 years for omeprazole and 4.34 for LNF). Therefore, the incremental cost-effectiveness ratio for medical therapy was $129,667 per quality-adjusted life-year gained, and LNF was a cost-effective approach.

Sensitivity analysis showed that the medical arm was preferred if the cost of omeprazole was less than Can$38.60 per month, if the cost of LNF exceeded $5296, or if the length of hospital stay exceeded 4.2 days. A potential limitation of this study is the 5-year time horizon, which might favor surgical therapy. Recent reports have suggested that a majority of patients will experience recurrent GERD symptoms more than 10 years after Nissen fundoplication, requiring ongoing medical therapy.[13]

A 1997 study by Heudebert et al[49] compared LNF to omeprazole 20 mg daily for patients with erosive esophagitis over a 5-year time horizon. After healing of erosive esophagitis, patients received escalating doses of omeprazole for symptom relief, up to 60 mg/day. Patients failing on 60 mg/day received LNF. Costs for the model were calculated using Blue Cross/Blue Shield reimbursement figures, and average wholesale prices were used for medications. The cost for a LNF was $7500. The decrement in quality of life due to reflux symptoms was 0.82, based on expert opinion. The authors also assumed that patients who had undergone LNF or were on chronic omeprazole usage would have a utility of 1.0, a state equivalent to perfect health.

Similar to the study published by Romagnuolo et al,[48] this study found that the two treatments were equally effective (4.33 quality-adjusted life-years per patient) but that omeprazole was less expensive than LNF ($6053 compared with $9452 per patient). Sensitivity analysis revealed that costs of LNF and omeprazole were equivalent if the cost of LNF was reduced to $4100, if the cost of omeprazole increased to $120 per month, or at 10 years of follow-up. In addition, the two strategies were equivalent in terms of effectiveness when the utility for GERD symptoms was less than 0.7.

Limitations of this model were the short time horizon, the low utility value used for GERD symptoms (see Quality of Life Assessments section), and the assumption that all patients were symptom-free after surgery. Recent studies have demonstrated that many patients suffer from dysphagia, inability to belch, and gas-bloat syndrome, despite the fact that they are free of GERD symptoms.[14] The effect of these symptoms on utility assessments after LNF has not been formally studied.

In a 1996 study by Van Den Boom et al[50] maintenance therapy with omeprazole was compared to LNF after an initial healing phase. Costs for

TABLE 2. Cost-Effectiveness Analysis Comparing Medical and Surgical Therapy

Study	End Point	Time Horizon	Treatment Arms	Result	Sensitivity Analysis	Incremental Cost-Effectiveness Ratio
Romagnuolo et al[48] (2001, Canada)	Healing of EE	5 years	a. LNF b. Omeprazole	LNF more cost-effective at 3.3 yrs	Omeprazole preferred if cost < Can$38.60/month or cost LNF > Can$5274 or stay > 4.2 days	Omeprazole Can$129,665/QALY
Heudebert et al[49] (1997, USA)	Healing of EE	5 years	a. LNF b. Omeprazole	Omeprazole more cost-effective	LNF = omeprazole if U of GERD < 0.7, cost LNF $4100 or cost of omeprazole $120/month.	Omeprazole $1398/QALY
Van Den Boom et al[50] (1996, Netherlands)	Symptom relief	4 years	a. LNF b. Omeprazole	LNF more cost-effective	Omeprazole preferred if duration of treatment < 1.4 yrs	LNF Dutch guilders 4748/year

EE = erosive esophagitis; GERD = gastroesophageal reflux disease; LNF = laparoscopic Nissen fundoplication; QALY = quality-adjusted life-year; U = utility.

omeprazole were based on wholesale prices in the Netherlands, and the cost of endoscopy was based on the mean of reimbursements by the National Health Insurance and private insurers. The study assumed an 88% effectiveness of omeprazole for symptom control, compared with a 98% effectiveness for LNF (the latter based on a 3-month follow-up study of LNF in which 98.5% of patients had normal esophageal mucosa, but symptom relief was not assessed[15]). The study concluded that LNF would become cost-effective at 1.4 years of follow-up and would be the preferred strategy at 10 years of follow-up. The study did not consider the possibility of failure of the wrap over time. Results were not sensitive to variations in hospital stay or cost, cost of endoscopy, or price of omeprazole.

Willingness to Pay Analysis

Willingness to pay is defined as an indication of the monetary value of a commodity or service. In a population with chronic GERD symptoms, patients can be asked about the amount of money they would be willing to pay for symptom relief as well as medical therapy, such as the use of a PPI as compared with H_2RAs. In a study by Kleinman et al,[16] a computer-administered questionnaire was given to patients with chronic GERD to assess willingness to pay for complete relief of GERD symptoms. Four attributes of treatment relevant to the analysis included time to relief (2–14 days for symptom resolution), amount of relief (complete or not), side effects from medication, and out-of-pocket costs per month of medication (ranging from $5–60). Of the 205 patients completing the study, more than half had moderate GERD symptoms as defined by the Gastrointestinal Severity Rating Scale. Respondents were willing to pay $2.50 per month for a 1-day reduction in time to onset of relief, $35 per month for an increase in amount of symptom relief from little to some, $110 per month for an increase in amount of symptom relief from little to complete, and $41.66 per month for a change in side effects from presence of side effects to no side effects. Therefore, the marginal willingness to pay for a drug that has no side effects and improves the amount of relief from little to complete and reduces the time to relief of symptoms from 2 weeks to 2 days is $181.66 ([$2.50 × 12] + $110 + $41.66). Patients with GERD were willing to pay nearly $200 additionally per month for complete symptom relief. This information can be useful when making decisions about newer but more costly therapies for GERD.

Is Screening for Barrett's Esophagus Cost-Effective?

Patients with GERD are at risk of developing Barrett's esophagus and subsequent esophageal cancer. Male patients with longstanding GERD are at the greatest risk for the development of Barrett's esophagus.[17] Once Barrett's esophagus is present, the risk of developing cancer is approximately 0.4% per year.[18] Whether screening for Barrett's esophagus in all patients with GERD is cost-effective has not yet been established. Soni et al[19] published a decision analysis examining whether screening for high-grade dysplasia is cost-effective. In the model, the base case patient, a 60-year-old undergoing one-time endoscopy to screen for Barrett's esophagus, would undergo esophagectomy if high-grade dysplasia or esophageal adenocarcinoma was detected. Costs were analyzed from the perspective of a third-party payer. Compared with no endoscopic screening, endoscopy cost $24,700 per life-year screened. Screening was no longer effective if the sensitivity of endoscopy for high-grade dysplasia in Barrett's esophagus was less than 70%, or if the prevalence of Barrett's esophagus or high-grade dysplasia was less than 4%. In addition, it was assumed that esophagectomy would not markedly affect patient's health-related quality of life. A 16% drop in health-related quality of life after esophagectomy would render screening ineffective. Other cost-effectiveness analyses, published to date in abstract form, have supported the concept of once in a lifetime screening for Barrett's esophagus as a cost-effective approach.[20,21]

Quality-of-Life Assessments

Although GERD is a chronic disease with a very small risk of associated malignancy, multiple studies have demonstrated that chronic heartburn adversely impacts patients' health-related quality of life (Table 3).[22] Quality of life has been defined by the World Health Organization as "not only the absence of disease and infirmity but also the presence of physical, mental, and social well-being."[23] Health-related quality of life can further be defined as the impact of an individual's health status on physicial functioning as well as social and psychological function. In the case of a chronic disease such as GERD, therefore, it is important to measure the impact of the disease on the patient's overall health status.

A variety of health-related quality of life instruments are available to the clinical investigator studying GERD. Instruments are tested for the following properties: validity (ability to measure what it is intended to measure), reliability (reproducibility of the measure), responsiveness (ability of the score to correspond to the clinical condition and its change), and coverage (ability to address the disease in question).[24] The types of such instruments include generic instruments, disease-specific questionnaires, and utility assessments, which are obtained using standard gamble and time-tradeoff methods.

	TABLE 3. Health-Related Quality-of-Life Studies in Gastroesophageal Reflux Disease			
Author	**Patients**	**Instrument**	**Intervals**	**Final Results**
Fisher et al[51] (2002, USA)	BE undergoing surveillance (n = 15)	QOLRAD Utilities program	Baseline on medications	QOLRAD scores higher than age-matched cohort without GERD or BE
Johanson JF et al[52] (2002, USA)	Patients with EE in open-label study of rabeprazole	SF-36	Baseline and at 8 weeks	Improvement on rabeprazole in all SF-36 subscales
Damiano et al[53] (2002, USA)	187 patients with non-erosive GERD	SF-36 GSAS	Baseline and after 4 weeks of therapy	GSAS more useful than SF-36 for detecting change in symptom severity over time
Wahlquist[54] (2001, Sweden)	136 patients with GERD	WPAI-GERD QOLRAD SF-36	One-time assessment of Swedish working population	GERD patients lost a mean of 2.5 hours from work per week with 23% decreased productivity. Productivity during daily activities decreased by 30%.
Farup et al[55] (2001, USA)	a. Controls (n = 268) b. Daytime GERD (n = 339) c. Nocturnal GERD (n = 945)	SF-36	Random-sample telephone survey	Non-nocturnal GERD patients had lower scores on SF-36 physical and mental component summary scores than controls; nocturnal GERD patients had even more impairment on all subscales of SF-36
Eluobeidi et al[56] (2001, USA)	a. GERD (n = 104) b. BE (n = 107)	SF-36 GERQ	One-time assessment	No difference between BE and GERD; both scored below US norms on all subscales
Kaplan-Machlis et al[57] (2000, USA)	Clinical trial of omeprazole vs ranitidine in GERD	GSRS PGWB SF-36	2, 4, 12, and 24 wks	Omeprazole with improved HRCL at 2 and 4 weeks
Revicki et al[58] (1999, USA)	Three clinical trials comparing omeprazole to ranitidine (n = 1351)	PGWB SF-36	Baseline and follow-up data (varied from 4–24 weeks)	Resolution of GERD symptoms associated with higher HRQL
Havelund et al[59] (1999, Denmark)	a. Omeprazole 20 mg (n = 163) b. Omeprazole 10 mg (n = 163)	PGWB GSRS	Baseline After omeprazole or placebo for 4 weeks	GSRS reflux scale significantly improved on omeprazole 20 mg compared to omeprazole 10 mg and placebo, and omeprazole 10 mg compared to placebo. Total PGWB score

Study	Groups	Instruments	Assessment times	Results
	c. Placebo (n = 82)			improved on omeprazole compared to placebo.
Kaplan-Machlis et al[60] (1999, USA)	a. GERD with comorbidity (n = 164) b. GERD alone (n = 104)	GSRS PGWB	Patients off medications for at least 1 month	Statistically lower scores for severe compared to mild GERD symptoms on PGWB, GSRS, and physical function, bodily pain, social function, and mental health scale of SF-36. Group without comorbidity had lower SF-36 compared with normal population
Revicki et al[61] (1998, USA)	a. Omeprazole 20 mg (n = 156) b. Ranitidine 150 bid (n = 161)	GSRS PGWB	a. Baseline b. After 8 weeks of omeprazole or ranitidine	After 8 weeks, omeprazole group had statistically higher scores on GSRS and total PGWB scores
Revicki et al[62] (1998, USA)	a. Controls b. Ranitidine 150 bid	SF-36	Baseline and 6 weeks of treatment	SF-36 scores for GERD patients worse than diabetes or hypertension patients
McDougall et al[63] (1998, UK)	EE patients treated with omeprazole 20 mg (n = 77)	SF-36	a. Baseline b. After 14 weeks	Baseline SF-36 bodily pain, vitality, social function scores lower than normal; 7/8 subscales improved significantly after omeprazole. SF-36 improved regardless of endoscopic healing.
Wilklund et al[64] (1998, Sweden)	a. Omeprazole 20 mg b. Omeprazole 10 mg c. Ranitidine150 bid d. (n = 704)	PGWB GSRS	2 weeks, 4 weeks, and 1 year follow-up	PGWB and GSRS scores improved more on omeprazole compared to ranitidine
McDougall et al[65] (1996, Ireland)	EE (n = 152)	SF-36	Telephone survey 10 years after diagnosis	SF-36 physical and social function scores lower than normal Northern Ireland population

BE = Barrett's esophagus; EE = erosive esophagitis; GERD = gastroesophageal reflux disease; GSAS = GERD Symptom Assessment Scale; GSRS = Gastroesophageal Symptom Rating Scale; HRQL = health-related quality of life; PGWB = Psychological General Well-Being Index; QOLRAD = Quality of Life in Reflux and Dyspepsia questionnaire; SF-36 = Medical Outcomes Short Form-36; WPAI-GERD = Work Productivity and Activity Impairment in GERD questionnaire.

Generic Instruments

Generic instruments include the Medical Outcomes Study Short Form-36 (SF-36)[25] and the Sickness Impact Profile.[26] The SF-36 has been widely used in the assessment of GERD and contains eight domains (36 questions), including physical functioning, role limitations-physical, bodily pain, general health, vitality, social functioning, role limitations-emotional, and mental health. Scores range from 0 to 100, with the higher scores reflecting better health-related quality of life. Two overall summary scores (physical and mental component summary scores) can also be obtained. In patients with chronic GERD, scores on all dimensions of the SF-36 have been lower than scores for normal US population controls (Fig. 2).

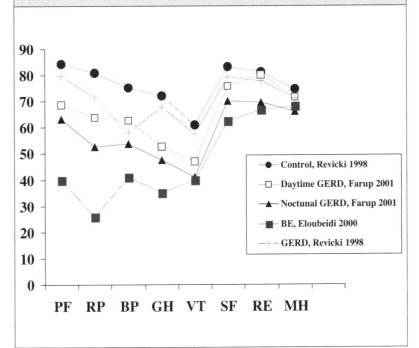

Figure 2. Mean SF-36 scores for patients with gastroesophageal reflux disease (GERD) compared to normal control subjects. In all studies, the scores for GERD patients were lower than the score for the normal US population and improved after therapy. In the study by Eloubeidi and colleagues[56] there was no significant difference between patients with GERD and patients with Barrett's esophagus (BE). (PF = physical function, RP = role limitation-physical, BP = bodily pain, GH = general health perceptions, VT = vitality, SF = social function, RE = role limitations-emotional, MH = mental health)

In the study by Revicki et al,[62] patients with GERD experienced worse pain, social functioning, and emotional well-being than patients with diabetes or hypertension. After treatment with ranitidine for 6 weeks, the health-related quality of life in patients responsive to therapy improved to the level of the control population. In the study by Farup et al,[55] subjects with nonnocturnal GERD had significant decrements on the SF-36 physical and mental component summary scores as compared with the US general population surveyed without GERD. Scores for patients reporting nocturnal GERD were significantly more impaired than scores for subjects with only daytime GERD on the physical and mental component summary.

In another study by Johanson et al,[52] baseline SF-36 scores in a cohort of patients with erosive esophagitis were significantly poorer than general US population scores, and follow-up scores after 8 weeks of rabeprazole therapy for four of the subscales (role limitations due to physical problems, social functioning, role limitations due to emotional problems, and mental health) were comparable to general population scores.

Another generic instrument, the Psychological General Well-Being Index (PGWB),[27] consists of 22 items measuring anxiety, depression, self-control, positive well-being, general health, and vitality. A 6-point scale is used to grade each question. The mean value of the total score in a normal population was 102.9 (95% CI, 102.1–103.8).[59] The higher the value, the better the patient's well-being. In the study by Havelund et al,[58] the mean PGWB score in a cohort of 499 patients with nonerosive GERD was 97. This score improved from 96.8 to 103.9 for patients on omeprazole 20 mg ($P = 0.02$ compared to placebo), from 98.4 to 106 on omeprazole 10 mg ($P = 0.007$ compared to placebo), and from 98 to 100.6 on placebo. All dimensions of the PGWB index improved in patients on omeprazole. Studies have shown differences in overall PGWB scores between patients with mild, moderate, and severe GERD symptoms, with the last group having the lowest score.[57]

Disease-Specific Instruments

An example of disease-specific instruments is the Gastroesophageal Symptom Rating Scale (GSRS). The GSRS is a self-administered questionnaire in which patients are asked to what extent they are bothered by their gastrointestinal symptoms.[28] The GSRS is a symptom survey and not a health-related quality of life instrument, however. It consists of 15 items that evaluate common gastrointestinal symptoms, including abdominal pain, heartburn, nausea, bloating, belching, constipation, diarrhea, and urgency. Each question is rated using a 7-point Likert scale ranging from no discomfort (score of 1) to very severe discomfort (score of 7). Subscores are available for reflux by summing the scores from the reflux-related questions. The lower the score is on the GSRS, the less the gastrointestinal disturbance is. In a normal population, the mean score was 1.53 (95% CI, 1.50–1.55).[59] The mean score in the study by Havelund et al.[58] was 2.35 at baseline. After 4 weeks of omeprazole, the reflux score improved significantly in patients on omeprazole 20 mg or 10 mg as compared with those taking placebo, while the scores on the other subscales did not change.

The Quality of Life in Reflux and Dyspepsia (QOLRAD) is a disease-specific questionnaire designed to measure quality of life for patients with GERD and dyspepsia.[29] Five domains are assessed, including emotions, vitality, sleep, eating/drinking, and physical/social functioning. Questions are graded using a 7-point Likert scale from 1 (symptom present all of the time, lowest health-related quality of life) to 7 (symptom absent, highest health-related quality of life). The minimally relevant change is 0.5 units, and an important change 1.5 units.[30] In a study of 1143 patients with nonerosive GERD treated with esomeprazole 20 mg daily, esomeprazole 40 mg daily, or omeprazole 20 mg daily for 4 weeks, QOLRAD scores were shown to be reliable with retesting and sensitive to change in symptomatic status (talley). Clinical trials using the QOLRAD have recently been published. For example, in a study of 41 GERD patients undergoing the Stretta procedure (radiofrequency application to the lower esophageal sphincter), the mean QOLRAD score was 3.7 + 0.2, and it increased to 5.1 + 0.2 6 months after therapy.[31]

The Gastroesophageal Reflux Questionnaire (GERQ) used in the study by Eluobeidi et al[32] is a self-reported instrument consisting of 80 questions and a psychosomatic symptom checklist, a measure of somatization. The first 32 questions assess symptoms of heartburn, regurgitation, dysphagia, and chest pain. The remaining questions inquire about family history, medication usage, extraesophageal manifestations, clinic visits and other disorders. Symptom frequency is graded from 1, indicating none in the past year, to 6, indicating daily. Symptom severity is graded from 1, indicating mild (can be ignored) to 4, indicating very severe (markedly affects lifestyle).

The GERD Symptom Assessment Scale (GSAS) is a self-adminstered questionnaire designed to measure symptom distress in GERD patients.[33] Patients are asked to report the frequency, severity, and degree of bother during the previous week for 15 symptoms, including heartburn, chest pressure, regurgitation, gurgling in the stomach, nausea, bloating, belching, flatulence, early satiety, bad breath, cough, and hoarseness. Scores are rated from 0, indicating not at all to 3, indicating very much. In the study by Damiano and colleagues,[53] changes in the GSAS distress scale and SF-36 scale scores improved significantly when patients improved on medical therapy.

A questionnaire designed to measure the impact of GERD symptoms on work productivity and activity, called the Work Productivity and Activity Impairment in GERD (WPAI-GERD), was developed and tested in a study by Wahlqvist et al.[34] In the Swedish working population with GERD symptoms who completed the WPAI-GERD, workers lost an average of 2.5 hours per week due to GERD symptoms and suffered 23% decreased productivity.

Utility Assessments

Utility measurements are designed to provide a numerical indication of health-related quality of life on a scale of 0 to 1, where 0 represents death or a state equivalent to death, and 1 represents ideal health, or a state without a particular disease such as GERD. Utility measurements are useful in cost-effectiveness analyses when a measurement of quality-adjusted life-years is desired. Two techniques are available for the measurement of utilities: the standard gamble and time-tradeoff methods. In the standard gamble technique, patients are asked to compare life in a particular health state, say life with chronic GERD, to a gamble with a probability, P, that perfect health (life without any more GERD) is the outcome and $1 - P$ that immediate death is the outcome. The probability P is varied until the preference for the perfect health is equal to the preference for the gamble.[35] For example, a 50-year-old man with GERD who prefers to take a 5% chance of death and a 95% chance of perfect health would have a utility of 0.95.

In the time-tradeoff technique, patients are asked to trade off life-years in a state of less-than-perfect health for a shorter life span in a state of perfect health. The ratio of the number of years of perfect health that is equivalent to a longer life span in less-than-perfect health provides a measure of the preference for that health state. If we interviewed a 40-year-old man with GERD who is expected to live another 31 years and prefers to trade 10 years to eliminate his GERD symptoms, the associated utility would be $1 - (10/31)$ or 0.677. On the other hand, if the patient wanted to trade 1 year of his life to eliminate his GERD, the utility would be $1 - (1/31)$, or 0.968.

To date, utility data in GERD patients have been published only in abstract form. In a 1998 study involving 40 patients with GERD on medications, the mean standard gamble and time-tradeoff scores were 0.90 and 0.97, respectively.[36] In a study by Gerson et al[37] using a custom-designed computer program, 90 patients with GERD were interviewed while on and off PPI therapy. The mean values for GERD patients (mean ± SEM time-tradeoff score of 0.91 ± 0.2 and standard gamble score of 0.93 ± 0.2) did not differ significantly from patients with Barrett's esophagus ($n = 18$, mean time-tradeoff 0.91 ± 0.3, mean standard gamble

0.96 ± 0.1). In addition, standard gamble and time-tradeoff scores did not differ significantly for patients on or off therapy for GERD (mean time-tradeoff score off medication was 0.93 and on medication was 0.94; mean standard gamble off medication was 0.95 and on medication was 0.96), whereas significant differences were seen in the reflux scale of the GSRS and food and drink subscale of the QOLRAD. No difference were seen when comparing GERD patients with and without comorbid conditions.

Recently, Fisher et al[51] administered 16 scenarios describing possible Barrett's esophagus surveillance outcomes (including dysplasia, esophageal cancer, perforation, and complications from esophagectomy) to 15 patients with Barrett's esophagus in a surveillance program. The median utility was 4.0, with a range from 0 to 8 depending on the scenario. The authors found that the utility measurement did not correlate with the disease-specific instrument (the QOLRAD), suggesting that the concerns of patients undergoing surveillance are different from their reflux symptoms.[51]

Health-Related Quality of Life after Surgical Therapy

Most studies examining health-related quality of life after fundoplication for reflux use the Gastrointestinal Quality of Life Index (GIQLI,[38] Fig. 3 & Table 4). The instrument consists of 36 items and uses a 5-grade Likert scale (from 0 to 4), giving a maximum score of 144. This score includes five dimensions: symptoms, emotions, vitality, social relations, and medical treatment. The questions inquire about how frequently a symptom has interfered with the person's life over the past 2 weeks. In a population of 150 GERD patients before LNF, the mean (±SD) GIQLI score was 90 ± 8.9, and it improved to 123.7 ± 9.8 3 years after surgery.[67] In the most recent study by Granderath et al[66] in 27 patients 3 to 5 years after repeat fundoplication for GERD, the mean GIQLI score was 113.4, and most (93%) of the patients were satisfied and off of medical therapy.

The GIQLI scores are lower in patients with comorbid conditions such as major depression; in a study by Kamoltz et al[69] comparing the outcome of 38 patients with LNF and depression to 38 patients undergoing LNF without depression, the mean GIQLI scrore was 71.8 in the depressed group and 91.1 in the nondepressed group.[69] After 1-year of follow-up post-LNF, the scores were 99.3 in the group with depression, compared with 121.9 in the cohort without depression.

Most studies have shown improvement after LNF to the level of the normal population (see Table 4), but Lochnegies et al[75] found that the score on the GIQLI did not improve after LNF to the level of the control

TABLE 4. Health-Related Quality-of-Life Studies after Fundoplication

Study	Patients, n	Setting	Instrument	Result
Granderath et al[66] (2002, Austria)	27	Failed fundoplication with redo 3–5 yrs later	GIQLI	Mean GIQLI 113.4 3–5 years postoperatively. Most (93%) satisfied.
Granderath et al[67] (2002, Austria)	150	LNF follow-up 3 months, 1 year, 3 yrs	GIQLI	GIQLI improved to level of healthy controls 3 yrs postoperatively
Kamoltz et al[68] (2002, Austria)	84	a. Healthy controls b. Primary or repeat fundoplication with 5-year follow-up	GIQLI SF-36	Baseline GIQLI 122.6 for controls, 90.4 for GERD prior to LNF; 5 years after surgery score 120.8
Kamoltz et al[69] (2002, Austria)	76	a. 38 LNF & depression b. 38 with LNF	GIQLI	Preoperative GIQLI 71.8 in depressed group and 91.1 in nondepressed group; 1 year postoperative GIQLI 99.3 in depressed and 121.9 in nondepressed.
Luketich et al[70] (2002, USA)	80	Reoperation with mean 18 mo follow-up	SF-36 GERD-HRQL	Mean SF-36 physical and mental scores of 42 and 47 (normal = 50). HRQL scores excellent in 65%. 18% of patients dissatisfied.
Contini et al[71] (2002, Italy)	32	Assessment 1 week pre-LNF and 2 yrs post-LNF	SF-36	Mean SF-36 scores lower than healthy Italian population and improved to the level of controls 2 years after surgery
Fernando et al[72] (2002, USA)	120 LNF	1 year post-LNF compare to 50 GERD patients on medications	SF-36 GERD-HRQL	Mean HRQL scores better for surgical group (mean score 4) than medical group (score 21). SF-36 improved in 6 of 8 domains for surgical patients
Streets et al[73] (2002, USA)	105	LNF in 72; open LNF in 33 with 2 yrs post-LNF data	SF-36	SF-36 scores equal between two groups; transthoracic patients used less medication and had better satisfaction

(continued)

TABLE 4. Health-Related Quality-of-Life Studies after Fundoplication (*Continued*)

Study	Patients, *n*	Setting	Instrument	Result
Barrat et al (2001, France)	50 LNF 50 Controls	HRQL assessed pre-LNF, 1 mo, 3 mo, 6 mo, 1 yr, and 2 yrs post-LNF	GIQLI	Preoperative LNF group scores 86.7 and controls 123.8. At 3-month to 2-yr follow-up, score 119.3 and equal to control population
Capelluto et al[74] (2001, France)	30 LNF 30 Controls	HRQL assessment pre-LNF, 1 mo, 3 mo, 6 mo, and 1 yr post-LNF	GIQLI	Preoperative GIQLI score: LNF group 87 and 123.4 in controls; post-LNF score 115.3 (equal to controls)
Lochegnies et al[75] (Belgium 2001)	31 LNF 110 Controls	Assessment pre-LNF and 3 years post-LNF	GIQLI	Pre-LNF score 71 for GERD pat ents and 123 for controls; post-LNF score 109 (significantly less than control)
Kamoltz et al[76] (2001, Austria)	72 Patients mean age 71 years	Assessment pre-LNF, 1 mo, 3 mo, and 1 year post-LNF	GIQLI	Preoperative score 86, 3 mo score 120.1, 1 year score 119.3.
Lundell et al[77] (2001, Sweden)	310	155 randomized to omeprazole 155 randomized to open Nissen Follow-up 2 mo, 6 mo, annually for 5 years	PGWB GSRS	No difference between omeprazole or Nissen patients for 60 mont's between scores. PGWB scores normal within 2 months of therapy.
Slim et al[78] (2000, France)	50	Assessment pre-LNF, 3 mo and 1 year post-LNF	GIQLI	Preoperative score 95.6, 3 mo '03.6, 1 year 111.4 (significantly lower than normal control score of 126)
Trus et al[79] (1999, USA)	345	Assessment pre-LNF, 6 weeks and 1 year post-LNF	SF-36	Low pre-LNF scores that imprcved 6 weeks and 1 year after surgery

GERD = gastroesophageal reflux disease; GIQLI = Gastrointestinal Quality of Life Index; HRQL = health-related quality of life; LNF = laparoscopic Nissen fundoplication; SF-36 = Medical Outcomes Short Form-36.

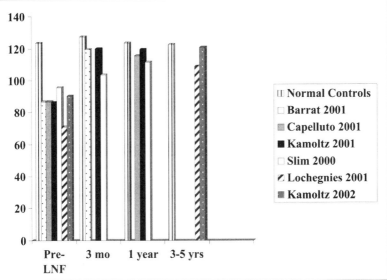

Figure 3. Mean Gastrointestinal Quality of Life Index scores pre- and post-laparoscopic Nissen fundoplication (LNF). Scores improved to baseline 3 months after LNF and remained normal at 1 year and 5 years of follow-up.

subjects (mean score post-LNF cohort of 109 ± 21). In this study, the postoperative symptom score remained significantly lower in the LNF group, a finding that the authors attributed to postoperative symptoms of bloating and dysphagia.

The GERD-HRQL scale, developed by Velanovich,[39] measures GERD-related quality of life using 10 questions. The survey inquires about the severity of symptoms related to various activities such as eating, lying down, standing up, and sleeping and the impact of medication on daily activities. Responses are scored from 0 (no symptoms) to 5 (symptoms are incapacitating, preventing daily activities), with a total score ranging from 0 to 50. Scores on the GERD-HRQL have been shown to improve after LNF.[70,72]

Key Points: Cost Analysis and Quality of Life

- ☞ GERD is a chronic disease that affects physical, mental, and social functioning as assessed by generic instruments, such as the SF-36.
- ☞ Disease-specific instruments, such as the QOLRAD (see page 214), have shown that GERD symptoms adversely affect patients' health-related quality of life.

Key Points (*Continued*)

☞ Scores on generic and disease-specific instruments have been shown to improve after medical or surgical therapy for GERD.

☞ Cost-effectiveness analyses suggest that proton pump inhibitor therapy is cost-saving, particularly if it can be used as on-demand or intermittent therapy.

☞ Laparoscopic Nissen fundoplication has been shown to be another cost-effective approach, but further analyses are needed to assess whether LNF would remain cost-effective over the course of an individual's lifetime.

Suggested Reading

1. Revicki DA, Wood M, Maton PN, et al: The impact of gastroesophageal reflux disease on health-related quality of life. Am J Med 104:252–258, 1998.

2. Robinson M, Sahba B, Avner D, et al: A comparison of lansoprazole and ranitidine in the treatment of erosive oesophagitis. Aliment Pharmacol Ther 9:25–31, 1995.

3. Vantrappen G, Rutgeerts L, Schurmans P, et al: Omeprazole (40mg) is superior to ranitidine in short-term treatment of ulcerative reflux esophagitis. Dig Dis Sci 33:523–529, 1998.

4. Zeitoun P, Desjars De Keranroue N, Isal JP: Omeprazole versus ranitidine in erosive oesophagitis. Lancet 2:621–622, 1987.

5. http://www.ncbi.nlm.nih.gov/PubMed/

6. Russell LB, Siegel JE, Daniels N, et al: Cost-effectiveness analysis as a guide to resource allocation in health: Roles and limitations. In Gold MR, Siegel JE, Russell LB, Weinstein MC (eds): Cost-Effectiveness in Health and Medicine. New York, Oxford University Press, 1996, pp 3–24.

7. Drug Topics Red Book. New Jersey, Medical Economics, 1997.

8. Gerson LB, Hatton BN, Ryono R, et al: Clinical and fiscal impact of lansoprazole intolerance in veterans with gastro-oesophageal reflux disease. Aliment Pharmacol Ther 14:397–406, 2000.

9. Johansson KE, Ask P, Boeryd B, et al: Oesophagitis, signs of reflux, and gastric acid secretion in patients with symptoms of gastro-oesophageal reflux disease. Scand J Gastroenterol 21:837–847, 1986.

10. Talley NJ, Venables TL, Green JR, et al: Esomeprazole 40 mg and 20 mg is efficacious in the long-term management of patients with endoscopy-negative gastro-oesophageal reflux disease: A placebo-controlled trial of on-demand therapy for 6 months. Eur J Gastroenterol Hepatol 14:857–863, 2002.

11. Lind T, Havelund T, Lundell L, et al: On demand therapy with omeprazole for the long-term management of patients with heartburn without oesophagitis: A placebo-controlled randomized trial. Aliment Pharmacol Ther 13:907–914, 1999.

12. Ethiopia A, Gregor JC, Preiksaitis HG, et al: An evaluation of utility measurement in gastroesophagogeal reflux disase (GERD) [abstract]. Gatroenterology 114:A116, 1998.

13. Spechler SJ, Lee E, Ahnen D, et al: Long-term outcome of medical and surgical ther-

apies for gastroesophageal reflux disease: Follow-up of a randomized controlled trial. JAMA 285:2331–2338, 2001.

14. Beldi G, Glattli A: Long-term gastrointestinal symptoms after laparoscopic nissen fundoplication. Surg Laparosc Endosc Percutan Tech 12:316–319, 2002.

15. Dallemagne B, Weerts JM, Jehaes C, et al: Techniques and results of endoscopic fundoplication. Endosc Surg Allied Technol 1:72–75, 1993.

16. Kleinman L, McIntosh E, Ryan M, et al: Willingness to pay for complete symptom relief of gastroesophageal reflux disease. Arch Intern Med 162:1361–1366, 2002.

17. Gerson LB, Edson R, Lavori PW, et al: Use of a simple symptom questionnaire to predict Barrett's esophagus in patients with symptoms of gastroesophageal reflux. Am J Gastroenterol 96:2005–2012, 2001.

18. Drewitz DJ, Sampliner RE, Grewal HS: The incidence of adenocarcinoma in Barrett's esophagus: A prospective study of 170 patients followed 4.8 years. Am J Gastroenterol 92:212–215, 1997.

19. Soni A, Sampliner RE, Sonnenberg A: Screening for high-grade dysplasia in gastroesophageal reflux disease: Is it cost-effective? Am J Gastroenterol 95:2086–2093, 2000.

20. Inadomi J, Lieberman D, Lagergren J, et al: Cost-effectiveness of once in a lifetime screening unsedated endoscopy in 50 year old white males with uncomplicated GERD [abstract]. Gastroenterology 118:AB2116, 2001.

21. Gerson LB, Triadafilopous G: A cost-effectiveness analysis of screening for Barrett's esophagus in patients with chronic gastroesophageal reflux disease [abstract]. Gastrointest Endosc 55:AB158, 2002.

22. Revicki DA, Wood M, Maton PN, et al: The impact of gastroesophageal reflux disease on health-related quality of life. Am J Med 104:252–258, 1998.

23. Constitution of the World Health Oranization: World Health Organization Handbook of Basic Documents, 5th ed. Geneva, Palais des Nations, 1952.

24. Eisen GM, Locke GR 3rd, Provenzale D: Health-related quality of life: A primer for gastroenterologists. Am J Gastroenterol 94:2017–2021, 1999.

25. Stewart AL, Greenfield S, Hays RD, et al: Functional status and well-being of patients with chronic conditions: Results from the Medical Outcomes Study. JAMA 262:907–913, 1989.

26. Bergner M, Bobbitt RA, Carter WB, et al: The Sickness Impact Profile: Development and final revision of a health status measure. Med Care 19:787–805, 1981.

27. Dupuy HJ: The psychological general well-being (PGWB) index. In Wender NK, Mattson ME, Furber CD, Elinson J (eds): Assessment of Quality of Life in Clinical Trials of Cardiovascular Therapies. New York, Le Jacq, 1984, pp 170–183.

28. Svedlund J, Sjodin I, Dotevall G: GSRS—a clinical rating scale for gastrointestinal symptoms in patients with irritable bowel syndrome and peptic ulcer disease. Dig Dis Sci 33:129–134, 1998.

29. Wiklund IK, Junghard O, Grace E, et al: Quality of life in reflux and dyspepsia patients: Psychometric documentation of a new disease-specific questionnaire (QOL-RAD). Eur J Surg Suppl 583:41–49, 1998.

30. Talley NJ, Fullerton S, Junghard O, et al: Quality of life in patients with endoscopy-negative heartburn: Reliability and sensitivity of disease-specific instruments. Am J Gastroenterol 96:1998–2004, 2001.

31. Houston H, Khaitan L, Holzman M, et al: First year experience of patients undergoing the Stretta procedure Surg Endosc 17:401–404, 2003.

32. Locke GR, Talley NJ, Weaver AL, et al: A new questionnaire for gastroesophageal reflux disease. Mayo Clin Proc 69:539–547, 1994.

33. Rothman M, Farup C, Stewart W, et al: Symptoms associated with gastroesophageal

reflux disease: development of a questionnaire for use in clinical trials. Dig Dis Sci 46:1540–1549, 2001.

34. Wahlqvist P, Carlsson J, Stalhammar NO, et al: Validity of a Work Productivity and Activity Impairment questionnaire for patients with symptoms of gastro-esophageal reflux disease (WPAI-GERD): results from a cross-sectional study. Value Health 5:106–113, 2002.

35. Gold MR, Patrick DL, Torrance GW, et al: Identifying and valuing outcomes. In Gold MR, Siegel JE, Russell LB, Weinstein MC, (eds). Cost-Effectiveness in Health and Medicine. New York, Oxford University Press, 1996, pp 82–134.

36. Ethiopia A, Gregor JC, Preiksaitis HG, et al: An evaluation of utility measurement in gastroesophageal reflux disease [abstract]. Gastroenterology 114:G0477, 1998.

37. Gerson LB, Ullah N, Chandal A, et al: Patient-derived health state utilities for GERD and Barrett's esophagus: Impact of medical therapy and comorbid conditions [abstract]. Gastrointest Endosc 2003:

38. Eypasch E, Williams JI, Wood-Dauphinee S, et al: Gastrointestinal quality of life index: Development, validation and application of a new instrument. Br J Surg 82:216–222, 1995.

39. Velanovich V: Comparison of generic (SF-36) vs. disease-specific (GERD-HRQL) quality-of-life scales for gastroesophageal reflux disease. J Gastrointest Surg 2:141–145, 1998.

40. Ofmann JJ, Dorn GH, Fennerty MB, et al: The clinical and economic impact of competing management strategies for gastro-oesophageal reflux disease. Aliment Pharmacol Ther 16:261–273, 2002.

41. Wahlqvist P, Junghard O, Higgins A, et al: Cost effectiveness of proton pump inhibitors in gastro-oesophageal reflux disease without oesophagitis: Comparison of on-demand esomeprazole with conventional omeprazole strategies. Pharmacoeconomics 20:267–277, 2002.

42. Gerson LB, Robbins AS, Garber A, et al: A cost-effectiveness analysis of prescribing strategies in the management of gastroesophageal reflux disease. Am J Gastroenterol 95:395–407, 2000.

43. Ofman JJ, Yamashita BD, Siddique RM, et al: Cost effectiveness of rabeprazole versus generic ranitidine for symptom resolution in patients with erosive esophagitis. Am J Manag Care 6:905–916, 2000.

44. Goeree R, O'Brien B, Hunt R, et al: Economic evaluation of long-term management strategies for erosive oesophagitis. Pharmacoeconomics 16:679–697, 1999.

45. Stal JM, Gregor JC, Preiksaitis HG, et al: A cost-utility analysis comparing omeprazole with ranitidine in the maintenance therapy of peptic esophageal stricture. Can J Gastroenterol 12:43–49, 1998.

46. Harris RA, Kuppermann M, Richter JE: Prevention of recurrences of erosive reflux esophagitis: A cost-effectiveness analysis of maintenance proton pump inhibition. Am J Med 102:78–88, 1997.

47. Harris RA, Kuppermann M, Richter JE: Proton pump inhibitors or histamine-2 receptor antagonists for the prevention of recurrences of erosive reflux esophagitis: A cost-effectiveness analysis. Am J Gastroenterol 92:2179–2187, 1997.

48. Romagnuolo J, Meier MA, Sadowski DC: Medical or surgical therapy for erosive reflux esophagitis: Cost-utility analysis using a Markov model. Ann Surg 236:191–202, 2002.

49. Heudebert GR, Marks R, Wilcox CM, et al: Choice of long-term strategy for the management of patients with severe esophagitis: A cost-utility analysis. Gastroenterology 112:1078–1086, 1997.

50. Van Den Boom G, Go PM, Hameeteman W, et al: Cost effectiveness of medical versus surgical treatment in patients with severe or refractory gastroesophageal reflux

disease in the Netherlands. Scand J Gastroenterol 31:1–9, 1996.

51. Fisher D, Jeffreys A, Bosworth H, et al. Quality of life in patients with Barrett's esophagus undergoing surveillance. Am J Gastroenterol 97:2193–2200, 2002.

52. Johanson JF, Siddique R, Damiano AM, et al: Rabeprazole improves health-related quality of life in patients with erosive gastroesophageal reflux disease. Dig Dis Sci 47:2574–2578, 2002.

53. Damiano A, Handley K, Adler E, et al: Measuring symptom distress and health-related quality of life in clinical trials of gastroesophageal reflux disease treatment: Further validation of the Gastroesophageal Reflux Disease Symptom Assessment Scale (GSAS). Dig Dis Sci 47:1530–1537, 2002.

54. Wahlqvist P: Symptoms of gastroesophageal reflux disease, perceived productivity, and health-related quality of life. Am J Gastroenterol 96:S57–61, 1996.

55. Farup C, Kleinman L, Sloan S, et al: The impact of nocturnal symptoms associated with gastroesophageal reflux disease on health-related quality of life. Arch Intern Med 161:45–52, 2001.

56. Eloubeidi MA, Provenzale D: Health-related quality of life and severity of symptoms in patients with Barrett's esophagus and gastroesophageal reflux disease patients without Barrett's esophagus. Am J Gastroenterol 95:1881–1887, 2000.

57. Kaplan-Machlis B, Spiegler GE, Zodet MW, et al: Effectiveness and costs of omeprazole vs ranitidine for treatment of symptomatic gastroesophageal reflux disease in primary care clinics in West Virginia. Arch Fam Med 9:624–630, 2000.

58. Revicki DA, Crawley JA, Zodet MW, et al: Complete resolution of heartburn symptoms and health-related quality of life in patients with gastro-oesophageal reflux disease. Aliment Pharmacol Ther 13:1621–1630, 1999.

59. Havelund T, Lind T, Wiklund I, et al: Quality of life in patients with heartburn but without esophagitis: Effects of treatment with omeprazole. Am J Gastroenterol 94:1782–1789, 1999.

60. Kaplan-Machlis B, Spiegler GE, Revicki DA: Health-related quality of life in primary care patients with gastroesophageal reflux disease. Ann Pharmacother 33:1032–1036, 1999.

61. Revicki DA, Sorensen S, Maton PN, et al: Health-related quality of life outcomes of omeprazole versus ranitidine in poorly responsive symptomatic gastroesophageal reflux disease. Dig Dis Sci 16:284–291, 1998.

62. Revicki DA, Wood M, Maton PN, et al: The impact of gastroesophageal reflux disease on health-related quality of life. Am J Med 104:252–258, 1998.

63. McDougall NI, Collins JS, McFarland RJ, et al: The effect of treating reflux oesophagitis with omeprazole on quality of life. Eur J Gastroenterol Hepatol 10:459–464, 1998.

64. Wiklund I, Bardhan KD, Muller-Lissner S, et al: Quality of life during acute and intermittent treatment of gastro-oesophageal reflux disease with omeprazole compared with ranitidine: Results from a multicentre clinical trial. The European Study Group. Ital J Gastroenterol Hepatol 30:19–27, 1998.

65. McDougall NI, Johnston BT, Kee F, et al: Natural history of reflux oesophagitis: A 10 year follow up of its effect on patient symptomatology and quality of life. Gut 38:481–486, 1996.

66. Granderath FA, Kamolz T, Schweiger UM, et al: Long-term follow-up after laparoscopic refundoplication for failed antireflux surgery: Quality of life, symptomatic outcome, and patient satisfaction. J Gastrointest Surg 6:812–818, 2002.

67. Granderath FA, Kamolz T, Schweiger UM, et al: Quality of life, surgical outcome, and patient satisfaction three years after laparoscopic Nissen fundoplication. World J Surg 26:1234–1238, 2002.

68. Kamolz T, Granderath PA, Bammer T, et al: Mid- and long-term quality of life as-

sessments after laparoscopic fundoplication and refundoplication: A single unit review of more than 500 antireflux procedures. Dig Liver Dis 34:470–476, 2002.

69. Kamolz T, Granderath FA, Pointner R: Does major depression in patients with gastroesophageal reflux disease affect the outcome of laparoscopic antireflux surgery? Surg Endosc 17:55–60, 2003.

70. Luketich JD, Fernando HC, Christie NA, et al: Outcomes after minimally invasive reoperation for gastroesophageal reflux disease Ann Thorac Surg 74:328–331, 2002.

71. Contini S, Bertele A, Nervi G, et al: Quality of life for patients with gastroesophageal reflux disease 2 years after laparoscopic fundoplication. Evaluation of the results obtained during the initial experience. Surg Endosc 16:1555–1560, 2002.

72. Fernando HC, Schauer PR, Rosenblatt M, et al: Quality of life after antireflux surgery compared with nonoperative management for severe gastroesophageal reflux disease. J Am Coll Surg 194:23–27, 2002.

73. Streets CG, DeMeester SR, DeMeester TR, et al: Excellent quality of life after Nissen fundoplication depends on successful elimination of reflux symptoms and not the invasiveness of the surgical approach. Ann Thorac Surg 74:1019–1024, 2002.

74. Capelluto E, Barrat C, Catheline JM, et al: Quality of life one year after laparoscopic fundoplication is close to that of a control group: Prospective study. Ann Chir 126:440–444, 2001.

75. Lochegnies A, Hauters P, Janssen P, et al: Quality of life assessment after Nissen fundoplication. Acta Chir Belg 101:20–24, 2001.

76. Kamolz T, Bammer T, Granderath FA, et al: Quality of life and surgical outcome after laparoscopic antireflux surgery in the elderly gastroesophageal reflux disease patient. Scand J Gastroenterol 36:116–120, 2001.

77. Lundell L, Miettinen P, Myrvold HE, et al: Continued (5-year) followup of a randomized clinical study comparing antireflux surgery and omeprazole in gastroesophageal reflux disease. J Am Coll Surg 192:172–179, 2001.

78. Slim K, Bousquet J, Kwiatkowski F, et al: Quality of life before and after laparoscopic fundoplication. Am J Surg 180:41–45, 2000.

79. Trus TL, Laycock WS, Waring JP, et al: Improvement in quality of life measures after laparoscopic antireflux surgery. Ann Surg 229:331–336, 1999.

Novel Treatment Approaches for Gastroesophageal Reflux Disease

chapter
13

Nimish Vakil, M.D.

Gastroesophageal reflux disease (GERD) is a chronic disorder in the vast majority of cases, and, as a cure of this disease has proved elusive, treatment strategies have focused on chronic maintenance therapies that would prevent reflux into the esophagus. The traditional approaches to therapy consist of drugs to reduce acid production, which is effective by reducing the volume of gastric content and raising its pH. Other approaches that have had limited success, include the use of prokinetic drugs that stimulate gastric emptying. In this chapter, novel methods of treatment are discussed. These methods include new ways of using traditional drugs (on-demand and intermittent therapy), combinations of treatment (proton pump inhibitors combined with histamine-2 receptor antagonists), new drugs (acid pump inhibitors such as soraprazam, and drugs that decrease transient lower esophageal sphincter (LES) relaxations (baclofen).

New Ways of Using Traditional Drugs

Proton pump inhibitors are the most commonly used drugs in the treatment of GERD. Although the disease is chronic in the majority of patients, relapses are infrequent in some patients. Observational studies in primary care suggest that many patients do not take their medications on a daily basis either because they do not need daily therapy to control their symptoms or because they cannot afford the cost of daily proton pump inhibitor therapy.[1] New approaches to managing patients with proton pump inhibitors are designed to reduce the cost of maintenance therapy by decreasing the frequency of administration. These strategies are "on-demand" and "intermittent" therapy.

Intermittent therapy can be defined as the administration of short predetermined courses of therapy when symptoms recur. The course may

225

be 1 or 2 weeks in duration. *On-demand therapy* is patient driven, and there are no fixed periods of administration. Instead, patients are told to take medications when they have symptoms for as long as they choose. These strategies are interesting because they reduce the cost of therapy and may also decrease the rebound in acid secretion that is seen after prolonged continuous therapy. In a recent study of intermittent therapy, 677 patients with nonerosive reflux disease or Los Angeles grade A or B erosive esophagitis in a primary care setting were randomized to ranitidine 150 mg twice daily, low-dose omeprazole (10 mg) or standard dose omeprazole (20 mg) for 2 weeks.[2] If they had symptom relief, they continued with the maintenance phase of the study, in which they received 2-week courses of intermittent therapy with the regimen that had worked in the first instance. Of the 677 patients entering the study, 318 reached the 1-year time-point with intermittent therapy, without a need for daily maintenance therapy. Omeprazole 20 mg was significantly superior to ranitidine at week 2. However, the long-term response was similar in the responders in the three groups. Twenty-two percent to 27% of patients required daily maintenance therapy, and 46% to 48% of patients were managed with intermittent therapy over the ensuing 12 months. Most patients relapsed infrequently on intermittent treatment, 271 (40%) had no relapses, 203 (30%) had one, 102 (15%) had two, and 54 (8%) had three. The median number of days without treatment for the entire cohort was 142 days. Therefore, approximately half the population did not need therapy for at least 6 months of the year of maintenance therapy. A cost analysis based on this study found no difference between the cost of the omeprazole arm and the cost of the ranitidine arm. These results did not change when costs from each of the countries that participated in the trial were used. These data suggest that on a cost basis, there is little to be gained from stepping down to intermittent H_2 receptor antagonist therapy after initial treatment with a proton pump inhibitor.[3]

In a short-term study of on-demand therapy with low-dose H_2 receptor antagonist therapy, Galmiche et al[4] showed that ranitidine administered in a dose of 75 mg up to three times a day on demand was effective in the short-term relief of heartburn (defined as a 75% improvement of symptoms). Forty-one percent of patients reported improvement in heartburn in this short-term trial of 15 days.[4]

Two studies have evaluated the efficacy of on-demand proton pump inhibitor therapy over longer periods. In one study, 424 patients with nonerosive reflux disease were randomized to placebo or proton pump inhibitor (omeprazole 20 mg or omeprazole 10 mg) on demand.[5] Over the 6-month follow-up period, a total of 29% of patients failed on-demand therapy and required daily maintenance therapy. However,

83% of patients randomized to on-demand therapy with omeprazole 20 mg a day were satisfactorily maintained over the 6-month time-frame. The mean number of omeprazole capsules used per day was 0.43, and the total amount of medication used was reduced by approximately 50%. In another recent study of esomeprazole therapy, 320 patients with nonerosive reflux disease who had complete symptom resolution after 4 weeks of therapy with either esomeprazole 20 mg or omeprazole 20 mg were randomized to receive esomeprazole 20 mg or placebo on-demand for 6 months.[6] Patients were permitted to use antacids as rescue medications. Patients were instructed to take no more than one dose of the medication a day for the relief of heartburn and to stop when the symptoms were adequately controlled. Medication intake was measured using electronic data recorders mounted into the caps of the medication containers. A total of 110 patients discontinued therapy due to insufficient control of heartburn (14% in the esomeprazole group and 51% in the placebo group). In the esomeprazole group, 52% of patients took medications for a maximum of 3 days at a time, as measured by the electronic sensors in the cap of the medication bottle. Twenty-two percent of patients took esomeprazole for 4 to 6 consecutive days and 11% required medication for 7 to 13 days. Mean antacid use was significantly lower in the esomeprazole group (0.59 tablets/day) compared to the placebo group (1.04 tablets/day). On average, esomeprazole was taken once every 3 days. In an economic analysis of on-demand therapy, Wahlquist et al[7] evaluated the cost-effectiveness of on-demand therapy in the United Kingdom using clinical data from this and other trials and suggested that on-demand therapy was cost-effective as compared with conventional maintenance therapy.

In another recent study, patients with nonerosive reflux disease who achieved complete resolution of heartburn after short-term esomeprazole or omeprazole treatment (n = 721) were randomized to esomeprazole 20 mg (n = 282) or 40 mg (n = 293) or placebo (n = 146) on demand (maximum one dose/day) for 6 months.[8] The primary and secondary efficacy end points were time to study discontinuation due to (1) unwillingness to continue and (2) inadequate control of heartburn, respectively. Both doses of esomeprazole were more effective than placebo. During the 6-month period, 42% of placebo recipients discontinued treatment due to unwillingness to continue, compared with 8% and 11% of esomeprazole 20 mg and 40 mg recipients, respectively. Overall, more patients treated with esomeprazole were free from gastrointestinal symptoms after 6 months of on-demand therapy. More than 90% of patients were willing to continue on-demand treatment with esomeprazole 20 mg over a 6-month period.

Combinations of Proton Pump Inhibitors and Histamine-2 Receptor Antagonists

Nocturnal reflux has been shown to play an important role in the development of complications of reflux disease because natural defense mechanisms such as swallowing are affected. Acid contact time in the distal esophagus can be prolonged. Conventional wisdom argues against the simultaneous administration of proton pump inhibitors and H_2 receptor antagonists. This is because proton pump inhibitors act at the final point of acid secretion, and blocking the histamine receptor is unlikely to add benefit if the drugs are given simultaneously. Recent studies have shown, however, that intragastric pH in healthy volunteers and patients with GERD on proton pump inhibitor therapy can fall below 4 in the nocturnal period (Fig. 1).[9] Although intragastric pH may drop below 4, nocturnal symptoms are uncommon in patients on proton pump inhibitors.[10] Studies in human volunteers have shown that the addition of small doses of H_2 receptor antagonists at bedtime can prevent the nocturnal drop in pH in patients taking proton pump inhibitors.[11] Preliminary data from another recent study, however, suggest

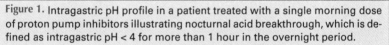

Figure 1. Intragastric pH profile in a patient treated with a single morning dose of proton pump inhibitors illustrating nocturnal acid breakthrough, which is defined as intragastric pH < 4 for more than 1 hour in the overnight period.

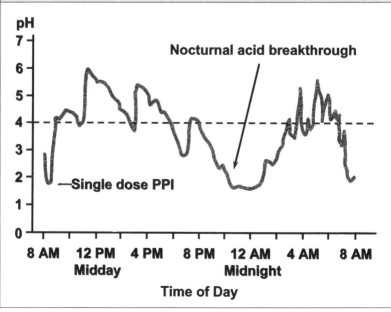

that the effect may be short-lived and that tachyphylaxis may occur within 2 weeks of commencing H_2 receptor antagonist therapy.[12] There are few data on nocturnal symptoms at the present time and little information on the long-term efficacy of a combination of proton pump inhibitor therapy with H_2 receptor antagonists. One study suggested that in patients with symptoms despite proton pump inhibitor use, nocturnal acid breakthrough occurred in 71% of patients, but only one third of symptomatic episodes were associated with reflux.[13]

Further data are awaited on the use of H_2 receptor antagonists in combination with proton pump inhibitors.

Drugs that Affect Transient Lower Esophageal Sphincter Relaxation: Baclofen

Transient lower esophageal sphincter relaxation is defined as spontaneous, abrupt, prolonged and complete relaxation of the lower esophageal sphincter associated with inhibition of the crural diaphragm and not preceded by a swallow.[14] This is an important cause for reflux-related symptoms. The selective $GABA_B$ agonist baclofen, currently used for the treatment of spasticity in patients with neurologic disorders, reduces the incidence of gastroesophageal reflux episodes by inhibiting transient lower esophageal sphincter relaxations. The reduction in transient esophageal sphincter relaxations in ferrets and dogs is close to 100% and in healthy human subjects may be up to 60%.[15-17] Although acid inhibitory agents are effective in symptom relief and healing of esophagitis, they do not change the frequency of nonacid reflux episodes. Recent studies have shown that baclofen reduces reflux episodes.[18] In a small study of nine patients with GERD, baclofen reduced postprandial acid and nonacid reflux and their associated symptoms, as measured by pH testing and impedance.[19] In a double-blind, placebo-controlled, two-way crossover study that was performed to study the effect of baclofen on heartburn and acid regurgitation after a provocative test meal in 37 patients with GERD, the authors found that baclofen decreased postprandial acid reflux by reducing the incidence of transient lower esophageal sphincter relaxations.[20] No effect of a single dose of baclofen on reflux symptoms could be demonstrated in this 3-hour postprandial study. The 40 mg dose of baclofen used in GERD studies is higher than the single dose of the drug used in spastic disorders (usually 10–25 mg) and was associated with a significant fatigue in 40% of the patients in one study.[21] Adverse effects related to the central nervous system are predictable because the spinal fluid concentration of baclofen is approximately 10% of the plasma concentration. Other common central nervous system effects that may be encountered are confusion and insomnia. These side-effects limit the use of baclofen in patients with GERD, but active research is being pursued for the development of new $GABA_\beta$ agonists that have fewer side-effects.

Acid Pump Inhibitors

A new class of proton pump inhibitors is being developed that may offer significant advantages over conventional agents. The acid pump inhibitors do not require activation by acid and bind to actively secreting and nonsecreting pumps. These agents are highly potent and raise intragastric pH in a very short period of time (20–30 minutes) in preliminary studies. The first of these agents (soraprazan) is currently in phase II testing and the results are awaited.

Suggested Reading

1. Hungin AP, Rubin G, O'Flanagan H: Factors influencing compliance in long-term proton pump inhibitor therapy in general practice. Br J Gen Pract 49:463–464, 1999.
2. Bardhan KD, Muller-Lissner S, Bigard M, et al: Symptomatic gastro-esophageal reflux disease: Double blind controlled study of intermittent treatment with omeprazole or ranitidine. BMJ 318:502–507, 1999.
3. Stalhammer NO, Carlsson J, Peacock R, et al: Cost-effectiveness of omeprazole and ranitidine in intermittent treatment of symptomatic GERD. Pharmacoeconomics 16:485–497, 1999.
4. Galmiche J, Shi G, Simon B, et al: On-demand treatment of gastro-esophageal reflux symptoms: A comparison of ranitidine 75 mg with cimetidine 200 mg or placebo. Alment Pharmacol Ther 12:909–917, 1998.
5. Lind T, Havelund T, Lundell L, et al: On demand therapy with omeprazole for the long-term management of patients with heartburn without esophagitis: A placebo-controlled randomized trial. Ailment Pharmacol Ther 13:907–914, 1999.
6. Talley N, Lauritsen K, Tunturi-Hihnala H, et al: Esomeprazole 20 mg maintains symptom control in endoscopy-negative GERD: A controlled trial of on-demand therapy for 6 months. Aliment Pharmacol Ther 15:347–358, 2001.
7. Wahlqvist P, Higgins A, Green J: Esomeprazole is cost-effective compared with omeprazole for the acute treatment of patients with non-endoscoped GORD in the UK. Value Health 3:360–364, 2000.
8. Talley NJ, Venables TL, Green JR, et al: Esomeprazole 40 mg and 20 mg is efficacious in the long-term management of patients with endoscopy-negative gastro-oesophageal reflux disease: A placebo-controlled trial of on-demand therapy for 6 months. Eur J Gastroenterol Hepatol 14:857–863, 2002.
9. Peghini P, Katz P, Bracy N, Castell D: Nocturnal recovery of gastric acid secretion with twice daily dosing of proton pump inhibitors. Am J Gastroenterol 93:763–767, 1998.
10. Vakil N, Katz P, Hwang C, Levine J: Nocturnal heartburn is rare in patients with erosive esophagitis treated with esomeprazole [abstract]. Gastroenterology 120:A-441, 2001.
11. Katz PO, Andersen C, Khoury R, Castell D: Gastroesophageal reflux associated with

nocturnal acid breakthrough on omeprazole: A controlled study in normal subjects. Gastroenterology 115:1335–1333, 1998.

12. Fackler W, Ours T, Vaezi M, Richter J: H2 Ras do not provide sustained suppression of nocturnal acid breakthrough [abstract]. Gastroenterology 120:A33, 2001.

13. Nzeako U, Murray J: An evaluation of the clinical implications of acid breakthrough in patients on proton pump inhibitor therapy. Aliment Pharmacol Ther 16:1309–1318, 2002.

14. Holloway RH, Penagini R, Ireland AC: Criteria for objective definition of transient lower oesophageal sphincter relaxation. Am J Physiol 286:G128–133, 1995.

15. Lidums I, Lehman A, Checklin H, et al: Control of transient lower oesophageal sphincter relaxations and reflux by the GABA$_B$ agonist baclofen in normal subjects. Gastroenterology 118:7–13, 2000.

16. Lehman A, Antonsson M, Bremner-Danielsen M, et al: Activation of the GABA$_B$ receptor inhibits transient lower esophageal sphincter relaxations in dogs. Gastroenterology 117:1147–1154, 1999.

17. Blackshaw LA, Staunton E, Lehman A, et al: Inhibition of transient LES relaxations and reflux in ferrets by GABA receptor agonists. Am J Phys 277:G867–874, 1999.

18. Zhang Q, Lehman A, Rigda R, et al: Control of transient lower oesophageal sphincter relaxations and reflux by the GABA$_B$ agonist baclofen in patients with gastro-oesophageal reflux disease. Gut 50:19–24, 2002.

19. Vela MF, Tutuian R, Katz PO, Castell DO: Baclofen decreases acid and non-acid post-prandial gastro-oesophageal reflux measured by combined multichannel intraluminal impedance and pH. Aliment Pharmacol Ther 17:243–251, 2003.

20. Van Herwaarden MA, Samsom M, Rydholm H, Smout AJPM: The effect of baclofen on gastro-oesophageal reflux, lower oesophageal sphincter function and reflux symptoms in patients with reflux disease. Aliment Pharmacol Ther 16:1655–1662, 2002.

21. Cange L, Johnsson E, Rydholm H, et al: Baclofen-mediated gastro-oesophageal acid reflux control in patients with established reflux disease. Aliment Pharmacol Ther 16:869–873, 2002.

Surgical and Endoscopic Treatment of Gastroesophageal Reflux Disease

chapter
14

J. Patrick Waring, M.D.

Since its introduction about 10 years ago, laparoscopic surgery for gastroesophageal reflux disease (GERD) has become one of the more common operations performed in the United States. It is interesting that there is still not a consensus among physicians as to the proper role of this procedure in the management of GERD. In the 1970s and 1980s, open antireflux surgery was associated with long postoperative recovery times and poor long-term results. Consequently, there were few surgical referrals, amounting to about one operation per general surgeon per year. The surgery was reserved for patients with refractory or complicated GERD. In the early 1990s, laparoscopic antireflux surgery became available. The short recovery time greatly increased the interest of patients and their physicians regarding this form of therapy. This has led to widespread use of laparoscopic antireflux surgery by physicians with a variety of different skill levels. Consequently, a wide variety of results have been seen.

In most published series, the average patient undergoing antireflux surgery has nearly complete relief of their symptoms and a markedly improved quality of life.[1–14] In fact, most comparative studies demonstrate the superiority of surgical therapy over medical therapy.[15–17] Individual complications have prompted some gastroenterologists to be cautious about recommending antireflux surgery, however.[18–22] A real "medical versus surgical" mentality exists. Most "review" articles are one-sided discussions touting only the advantages of medical or surgical therapy for GERD. However, our patients are best served by a balanced approach to the treatment of their chronic GERD. As we integrate information from nearly 10 years of laparoscopic antireflux surgery, it should not be surprising that our basic approach to the surgical management of

GERD, including the indications, contraindications, preoperative evaluation, and even the surgical procedures themselves are different now than in even the early laparoscopic era. For example, antireflux surgery was rarely offered to patients with uncomplicated GERD who were responsive to medical therapy. We now know that these patients have the best surgical outcomes.

Pathophysiology

The most important aspect of the pathophysiology of GERD is the competency of the antireflux barrier.[23] Factors contributing to its integrity include the lower esophageal sphincter (LES) pressure, the presence or absence of a hiatal hernia, and the occurrence of transient LES relaxations. LES pressure less than 6 mm Hg, LES length less than 2 cm, and intra-abdominal length less than 1 cm are strongly associated with GERD. The crural diaphragm contributes substantially to the integrity of the LES. When patients have a hiatal hernia, the crural diaphragm and the LES are displaced from each other, and consequently the sphincter is less competent. The most common pathophysiologic event at the time of a reflux episode is a transient LES relaxation. Of lesser importance, poor esophageal clearance and delayed gastric emptying may contribute to the severity of GERD. Antireflux surgery is the only available therapy that reliably increases LES pressure and LES length, decreases the frequency of transient LES relaxations, and corrects the hiatal hernia. Several studies show that antireflux surgery may improve esophageal motility and speed gastric emptying.[1,24]

Surgical Procedures

The classic operation is a Nissen fundoplication.[25] In this operation, the fundus is fully mobilized; specifically, the short gastric blood vessels are disconnected, or "taken down," from the fundus. A 1.0 to 1.5 cm plication is made using the fundus to wrap around the distal esophagus. Three sutures are usually placed, securing the wrap to the stomach and the esophagus. The hiatal hernia is reduced and the diaphragmatic crurae are closed. Many surgeons sew the fundoplication to the diaphragm to prevent it from moving postoperatively. This is often done over a large dilator to prevent the wrap from being too tight. There have been reports of perforations, however, which have led some experienced surgeons to abandon this part of the procedure.[25]

The Rosetti modification of a Nissen fundoplication is similar to the Nissen procedure with the exception that the short gastric blood vessels are not taken down. The Toupet fundoplication is also similar to the Nissen procedure, with the exception that it is a 180- to 270-degree wrap rather than a 360-degree wrap. The Collis-Nissen gastroplasty is the operation that should be performed in patients with a shortened esophagus.[26-29] This is particularly more common in patients with Barrett's esophagus and esophageal strictures. In this operation, the proximal stomach is ligated, creating additional length in the esophagus, a so-called neo-esophagus, in addition to performance of a fundoplication.

Surgical Results

Carlson and Frantzides[10] reviewed the surgical literature on more than 10,000 patients in the 1990s. The success rate, defined by Visick I or II was more than 90%, and the average length of follow-up for published series was less than 2 years.

Patients with GERD suffer from a poor quality of life. After laparoscopic fundoplication, the quality of life improves and becomes comparable to that of healthy individuals. Quality of life, as assessed by the Medical Outcomes Short Form-36 (SF-36), shows that patients with severe GERD have an extremely low quality of life, equivalent to a control population with congestive heart failure. Several studies show that after antireflux surgery these scores consistently increase to the scores of a control population of healthy volunteers.[11,12]

Numerous studies demonstrate the efficacy of antireflux surgery.[1-14] At USC Medical Center in Los Angeles, 100 patients were followed for an average of 21 months.[8] Ninety-six percent of patients had a good outcome, and 71% were completely free of symptoms. Only 3 patients were back on medical therapy. The condition of 2 patients was worsened by the procedure. Dysphagia was present in only 2 patients up to a year after surgery. Clinically significant complications occurred in 4 patients. The study was limited to patients with positive 24-hour pH study findings and "typical" symptoms of GERD. This is study is noteworthy because these patients are the ideal candidates for antireflux surgery. Additionally, the surgeons in this study were highly skilled and very experienced. Consequently, these are probably the best results that one could hope for.

Our ideas on the long-term durability of laparoscopic antireflux surgery come from a handful of studies with at least 5 years of follow-up. Longer term follow-up data are provided by the Mayo Clinic in Jacksonville for 171 of 291 patients who underwent a laparoscopic Nissen fundoplication at a mean of 6.4 years after surgery.[9] Again, 96% were satisfied with their results between 5 and 8 years later, 6% had symptoms of chest pain, 6% had heartburn, and 6% had regurgitation. Twenty percent of the patients had abdominal bloating, 12% had diarrhea, 27% reported some difficulty swallowing, and 7% required esophageal dilation.

Only 14% of the patients in the Mayo Clinic study were back on medical therapy after 5 to 8 years. However, most of the patients taking proton pump inhibitors (PPIs) are free of heartburn or have normal pH levels, suggesting that they are actually taking the medications for other reasons.[30] A study of 312 patients showed that many of the so-called postfundoplication sequelae are present before surgery.[31] In this study, antireflux surgery actually decreased the symptoms of heartburn, epigastric pain, regurgitation, bloating, dysphagia, odynophagia, nausea, vomiting, diet restriction, nocturnal coughing, and wheezing. In contrast, there was a significant increase in inability to belch, diarrhea, and passage of flatus.

Surgical Costs

Antireflux surgery should decrease health care utilization.[32] A retrospective matched cohort study of Tennessee Medicaid patients compared the costs of medical and surgical treatment for GERD in 1996; 7502 people had at least two encounters with a diagnosis of GERD.[33] Patients who had fundoplication (135) were compared to 250 randomly selected persons who were medically treated. Surgically treated patients used more GERD-related outpatient resources in the 3 months before the operation, particularly physician visits and diagnostic testing. The mean number of inpatient days for the fundoplication procedure was 3.2. Surgical treatment led to a 64% reduction in GERD medication use, with no increase in the use of other medical services in the following year.

Comparisons of Medical and Surgical Therapies

A review of six randomized trials and three cohort studies from 1966 through 1999 showed improved objective outcomes in five of six randomized trials and in two of three cohort studies after surgical therapy as compared with medical treatment.[34] Subjective outcomes—symptoms and patient satisfaction—were also more common among surgical patients in all but one study that assessed them.

The two largest published studies are the Veterans Administration (VA) Cooperative Study and the Nordic study, both of which demonstrated the marked superiority of surgical therapy.[15–17] The Veterans study enrolled patients with complicated GERD in the mid-1980s. It showed that surgical therapy was markedly superior to medical therapy of the era, histamine-2 receptor blockers and metoclopramide. Another trial enrolled 310 patients with erosive esophagitis, 155 randomized to continuous omeprazole therapy and 155 to open antireflux surgery. At both 3 and 5 years of follow-up, there were far more treatment failures among patients who were randomized to omeprazole treatment. However, the protocol also allowed dose adjustment in patients allocated to omeprazole therapy to either 40 or 60 mg daily in case of symptom recurrence. If this is considered, the failure rates still remained in favor of surgery, although the difference was not quite statistically significant. Quality of life assessment revealed values within normal ranges in both therapy arms during the 5 years.

There is little doubt that successful antireflux surgery corrects the underlying pathophysiology, improves symptoms, normalizes quality of life scores, reduces health care utilization, and appears as good or better than medical therapy in large comparative trials (Table 1).

Surgical Concerns

There are two reasons to be generally opposed to antireflux surgery. First, medical therapy is safe, effective, and well tolerated.[35] Second, surgical therapy is associated with serious, albeit infrequent, complications (Table 2). Even the most positive published surgical series mentions a small number of complications. For example, Peters reported a 96% improvement rate in the patients' primary symptom, yet 2 % of the patients were worse as a result of the surgery.[8] The results from less ex-

	Follow-Up, Years	Medical Therapy, %	Surgical Therapy, %
TABLE 1. Summary of Randomized, Long-Term Comparisons of Medical and Surgical Therapy			
Study			
Spechler[15]*			
GRACI score[†]	2	88	78[§]
Spechler[37]			
GRACI score (off medication)	10.6	96	84[§]
GRACI score (on medication)	10.6	83	78
Taking medication	10.6	92	62[§]
Lundell[17]‡			
In remission	5	42	58[§]

*Medical therapy was without PPIs.
[†]GRACI score indicates activity of reflux symptoms; lower scores are better.
[‡]Lundell calculated success rates based on patients taking omeprazole 20 mg/day. Success rates were still in favor of antireflux surgery when the omeprazole dose was raised to 20–40 mg/day, although the difference was no longer statistically significant.
[§]Statistically significant difference.

TABLE 2. Complication Rates Accumulated From Pooled Data	
Complication	Rate, %
Early	
Pnemothorax	1.0
Perforation	0.78
Gastrointestinal bleeding	0.75
Pneumonia	0.57
Pulmonary embolus	0.17
Mortality	0.08
Late	
Bloating	9.41
Reflux	3.47
Dysphagia	2.51
Need for revision	2.77

Adapted from Carlson MA, Frantzides CT: Complications and results of primary minimally invasive antireflux procedures: a review of 10,735 reported cases. J Am Coll Surg 193:428–439, 2001.

perienced centers are predictably worse. A recent study showed only a 57% satisfaction rate, with 67% of the patients developing new symptoms, such as difficulty swallowing or bloating. Additionally, 6.7% of the patients needed a repeat operation in less than 1 year.[36]

High-quality long-term data are scarce. Carlson showed that nearly all data available for review have a follow-up of less than 2 years.[10] In this review of more than 10,000 patients, the perioperative complication rate was around 5%, with a mortality rate of 0.08%. The need for reoperation ranged from 2% to 6% and was actually increasing toward the end of the 1990s. Long-term results from highly specialized centers suggest a satisfaction rate of 93%.[9] However, 14% of the patients are back on medication, and many patients have some gastrointestinal symptom. Again, the same results may not apply to less experienced centers.[37,38] A recently published study from the Veterans Administration showed that 62% of patients undergoing surgery required medications for heartburn after 10 to 13 years.[37] Given the safety and efficacy of PPI therapy, a surgical complication rate greater than 0% may be considered unacceptable. To summarize the feelings of the antisurgery congregation, "An esophagus disabled by an inappropriate or dysfunctional fundoplication wrap is a terrible price to pay for control of acid reflux."[19]

The two large, randomized series showing superior results with antireflux surgery can also be interpreted as being in favor of medical therapy.[15–17] The Nordic study randomized 310 patients with erosive esophagitis to omeprazole therapy or to open antireflux surgery. At both 3 and 5 years of follow-up, surgical therapy was far superior to omeprazole 20 mg daily. However, this difference disappeared when patients were allowed to adjust the dose of the omeprazole, which is the standard of care. There were no significant differences in costs or quality of life measures.[39,40] The initial report on the VA Cooperative Study showed marked superiority of surgical therapy over medical therapy.[15] However, follow-up for at least 10 years on the 247 patients in this trial showed no significant differences between the groups in the grade of esophagitis, frequency of treatment of esophageal stricture and subsequent antireflux operations, SF-36 standardized physical and mental component scale scores, and overall satisfaction with antireflux therapy.[37] More than 60% of the surgically treated patients were taking medical therapy. Interestingly, survival was decreased significantly in the surgical group as compared with the medical treatment group, largely because of deaths from heart disease. Nearly half of the patients in this study had Barrett's esophagus at the time of enrollment, yet there was no significant difference between groups in incidence of esophageal cancer after 10 to 13 years.

Given the safety of PPI therapy, one must wonder whether even the small risk of surgery is worthwhile in patients with uncomplicated GERD that responds to medical therapy. Complicated GERD is no longer an automatic indication for antireflux surgery; in fact, it may be a contraindication in patients who are doing well with medical therapy.

Keys to Success

Patient Selection

The gastroenterologist should be confident not only that the patient has GERD but also that the primary symptoms are related to reflux. The cases of patients with typical symptoms, such as heartburn and regurgitation, or endoscopic evidence of esophagitis are usually relatively straightforward. The cases of patients with nonerosive reflux disease and atypical reflux symptoms, such as cough, laryngitis, chest pain, or asthma, can be more complicated. In these patients, an incomplete response to PPI therapy may be due not to poor control of the reflux but to other factors involved in the patient's discomfort. Historically, we have reserved surgery for patients with refractory symptoms. We now know that the best predictor of a good surgical outcome is success with medical therapy.

Numerous studies show that medical or surgical therapy improves, but does not always relieve, the symptoms of chest pain, asthma, chronic cough, and hoarseness.[41–48] Symptom relief may be incomplete for several reasons.[23] First, these patients have heightened sensitivity to many different stimuli in the esophagus. Consequently, small amounts of acid could trigger discomfort in these patients. Complete symptom relief may be accomplished only by elimination of gastroesophageal reflux; this is rarely possible, even with the best medical or surgical therapy. Second, atypical symptoms of gastroesophageal reflux are often multifactorial in origin. Patients with chest pain may have cardiac disease, microvascular angina, musculoskeletal discomfort, or psychological problems. Many asthmatic patients have multiple potential trigger factors for bronchospasm, besides acid reflux. Patients with laryngitis or chronic cough may have other problems as well, including allergies, viral infections, or voice abuse. In one study, heartburn was relieved by fundoplication in 93% of patients, compared with only 56% of patients with atypical symptoms.[42]

Success with medical therapy was the only thing that predicted a successful surgical outcome. The success of antireflux surgery will parallel that of intensive medical treatment with high dose PPIs. The only possible exception is in asthmatic patients.[21,49] There are no comparative trials, but the results of several studies on antireflux surgery in asthmatic patients are impressive. Seven of nine patients who required daily oral corticosteroids for asthma were able to discontinue this treatment entirely after successful antireflux surgery.[44] In patients with a partial response to medical therapy, repeated ambulatory pH monitoring may be of benefit in separating the true medical failures from those patients with refractory atypical symptoms from other causes.[50]

Historically, antireflux surgery has been recommended for patients with refractory or complicated disease. However, the results of antireflux surgery in these patients are not as good. Patients with Barrett's esophagus generally have the poorest surgical success rates, ranging from 40% to 92%.[51–62] Two studies show that the need to repeat the operation is more likely in patients with Barrett's esophagus (6–8 %) compared to controls (about 2%).[59,63] Three published reports suggest that surgical therapy may decrease the development of dysplasia and esophageal cancer.[54–56] This is largely based on the fact that cancer rates in these studies are lower than expected. However, two studies show comparable data for patients in surveillance programs on PPI therapy.[64–65] Barrett's esophagus should not be considered an indication for surgery with the hope of decreasing the risk of the development of esophageal cancer.[60,61,66]

Gastroesophageal reflux disease can lead to esophageal stricture by causing chronic fibrosis and scarring in response to prolonged esophageal acid exposure. But some authors have suggested that nonsteroidal anti-inflammatory agents play a role in stricture formation.[67] Medical therapy with PPIs markedly improves dysphagia and lessens dilation requirements in up to 94% of patients.[68,69] Successful antireflux surgery decreases the need for further dilation as well. However, stricture patients generally have poorer surgical success rates than patients with uncomplicated disease; ranging from 70% to 91%.[70–73] While there are no comparative studies, it would appear that therapy with a PPI and intermittent dilation is as good as or better than surgical therapy.

Elderly patients seem to do fairly well with this operation.[74,75] However, some patients have a type III (mixed) paraesophageal herniation, in which the stomach is not only in the chest but above the lower esophageal sphincter. This is more common in elderly patients. The symptoms may be unusual but are generally postprandial heartburn, regurgitation, dysphagia, or chest pain.[76] There is little information on the medical management of this situation, but generally it is not successful. Surgical results in this situation are reasonably good. However, the morbidity rate is much higher because of the age and general state of health of the patients with this problem.[77–79]

Not surprisingly, patients with psychiatric disorders, anxiety, neurosis, or aerophagia have more problems after antireflux surgery.[80–82]

Pre-operative Evaluation

All patients considering antireflux surgery should undergo esophagogastroduodeuoscopy.[83] The finding of esophageal erosions, ulcers, or a columnar lined esophagus in a patient with typical reflux symptoms is fairly specific for GERD. The clinician should note the length of the esophagus and the size of the hiatal hernia. This information is complimentary to the findings of a barium swallow in the evaluation of patients with complicated disease. The need to do esophageal manometry has recently been questioned.[84–85] It is probably no longer necessary to tailor the operation based on esophageal motility testing.[86–89] However, esophageal dysmotility may reflect more severe disease and may help identify patients with a shortened esophagus. Esophageal manometry is useful to identify the rare patient with achalasia, whose symptoms of heartburn, regurgitation, and dysphagia are mistaken for GERD. Before we abandon preoperative esophageal manometry, we need to consider that many gastroenterologists and surgeons may wish that they had one in the up to 27% of patients with postoperative dysphagia.

Ambulatory esophageal pH monitoring is particularly useful in patients with atypical reflux symptoms or in cases in which the diagnosis is not certain. Repeated ambulatory pH monitoring while the patient is on medical therapy may be of benefit in patients with refractory atypical symptoms to document whether the acid reflux is truly refractory. Symptomatic gastric abnormalities are seen in only 1% to 2% of patients.[83] Gastric function testing should be done selectively in patients with signs or symptoms of gastric disease, such as nausea, vomiting, abdominal pain, severe gastritis, or gastroduodenal ulceration/erosion without evidence of *Helicobacter pylori* infection or nonsteroidal antiinflammatory drug use.

The preoperative evaluation should also focus on identifying patients with a shortened esophagus. These patients may require an esophageal lengthening procedure, such as a Collis-Nissen gastroplasty, as part of the antireflux operation.[26,27] A patient may be suspected to have esophageal shortening if he or she has Barrett's esophagus or an esophageal stricture, a 5 cm or larger hiatal hernia, or proximal location of the LES on esophageal manometry.

Operation Selection

It is assumed that patients undergoing laparoscopic surgery have comparable success rates at lower costs, with lower rates of morbidity and mortality compared to patients undergoing the open procedure.[90] However, two studies bring into question whether this is a good idea. A total of 5502 antireflux operations were performed in Finland between January 1987 and January 1996, with 43 fatal or life-threatening complications.[91] The serious complication rate was twice as high in the patients undergoing laparoscopic fundoplication as in those undergoing open fundoplication. One multicenter randomized trial to compare laparoscopic to open Nissen fundoplication had to be terminated early because of the high incidence of complications, mostly dysphagia in the laparoscopic group.[92] This study has been criticized because the surgeons were less experienced with the laparoscopic approach. However, this is precisely the point of the critics of surgery: The results of surgery are not as good in less experienced hands. Another randomized study showed no difference between open and laparoscopic fundoplication after 6 months.[93]

Several studies show that there is little difference in the results with different operations.[89,94–96] However, long-term results suggest that the Nissen procedure is more durable than the Toupet.[97–99] The Toupet fundoplication has been recommended for patients with esophageal dysmotility. However, several recent studies show that, in experienced hands, the dysphagia rate after either a Nissen or a Toupet fundoplication is low and not related to preoperative esophageal motility findings.[84,86–88,100,101] The Rosetti modification of a Nissen fundoplication is similar to the Nissen procedure, with the exception that the short gastric blood vessels are not taken down. Again, there are conflicting data, but the short-term dysphagia rate following this operation appears to be unacceptably high.[102–106]

The Collis-Nissen gastroplasty is the operation that should be performed in patients with a shortened esophagus.[27–29] This is more likely to occur in patients with poor esophageal motility or in those with GERD complications, such as strictures, esophagitis, and Barrett's esophagus. A shortened esophagus occurs in as many as 10% to 15% of patients undergoing antireflux surgery. However, only about 3% will require an esophageal lengthening procedure. Most patients will do well with extensive mobilization of the fundus and esophagus. While this decision is made at the time of surgery, it is useful for the surgeon to be prepared for this possibility.

Surgeon Selection

The estimated learning curve to perform this operation laparoscopically is in the neighborhood of 20 procedures.[107] However, the learning curve to recognize the need to perform advanced procedures, such as a laparoscopic Collis-Nissen gastroplasty and then actually do it well is probably much greater and may be in the range 200 to 400 procedures.[108] As stated earlier, a patient can be suspected to have esophageal shortening if he or she has Barrett's esophagus or an esophageal stricture, a 5 cm or larger hiatal hernia, or proximal location of the LES on esophageal manometry. Many patients with these features can be managed at the time of surgery with extensive mobilization of the fundus and esophagus, but Collis-Nissen gastroplasty is necessary in about 3% of patients. This is a technically more demanding operative procedure. The consistently lower rates of success in patients with complicated GERD having antireflux surgery may be related to poor recognition of the need to do this operation and poor technique in performing it. As we move forward, the most important preoperative responsibility of the gastroenterologist may be to identify the 10% to 15% of patients who may have a shortened esophagus and then directing them to a surgeon capable of both recognizing the need to perform a laparoscopic Collis-Nissen gastroplasty and doing it well.

Postoperative Problems

The approach to post-fundoplication symptoms is not difficult. Postoperative symptoms can be divided into two categories, recurrent or new.[108,109] Recurrent symptoms after surgery suggest that the surgery simply did not work. New postoperative symptoms suggest a complication at the time of surgery. On the other hand, the surgical management of these problems is very complex. The success rates for repeat operations are in the 75% to 85% range, with a morbidity rates in the range of 20% to 30%, and a mortality rate of greater than 1%.[63,110-117] Conservative management, if successful, is always preferable to a repeat operation. The decision to redo a fundoplication should not be taken lightly, and the reoperation should probably be done in centers with tremendous experience in these matters.

Fundoplication Assessment

The most important postoperative observation is whether the fundoplication is intact.[118–121] One must remember that the goal of the operative procedure is to fully mobilize the fundus and use it for the plication around the distal esophagus. When the fundus is fully mobilized, it will relax with the LES upon swallowing.[122] If the fundus is tethered to another abdominal structure, or if any part of the fundoplication includes stomach that does not relax, the patient will have dysphagia. This is much more likely to occur if the fundoplication is too long, in the wrong position, or oriented incorrectly. The keys to recognizing the integrity of the fundoplication are the length, orientation, and location of the fundoplication. Typically, a fundoplication is 1.0 to 1.5 cm in length. The folds of the fundoplication should be parallel to the diaphragm. An endoscopist can crudely evaluate this by comparing the direction of the folds with the distance marker on the endoscope on the retroflexed view. Usually, there should be no stomach above the wrap. Gastric folds above the wrap, directly above, or alongside suggest a poor fundoplication. If present, this may interfere with relaxation of the fundus, leading to dysphagia.

Recurrent Postoperative Symptoms

There are two reasons for a patient to have the same symptoms postoperatively: either the surgery was ineffective or the original diagnosis was incorrect. If the surgery simply did not work, the postoperative symptoms would be the same. Alternatively, there is no reason to believe that a patient will improve if the preoperative symptoms were not related to reflux in the first place. An incorrect original diagnosis is much more likely in patients who had no response to medical therapy preoperatively, especially those with atypical reflux symptoms. The initial approach to a patient with the same postoperative symptoms would be an empiric trial with a PPI for 1 or 2 months, which is frequently helpful.[123] If the patient cannot stop taking the PPI without relapse of symptoms, it may be reasonable to simply continue the medical therapy. One may consider a surgical revision if chronic PPI therapy is required. However, given the high morbidity and mortality rates associated with second operations, this should be discouraged. If there is no improvement with this empiric therapy, further evaluation will be needed. Assessment of the fundoplication should be made in these patients by a barium swallow test or an endoscopic examination. Certainly, if a second surgery is contemplated, a pH study must be performed to document the presence of reflux, especially if the patient has atypical GERD or if fundoplication looks good.

New Postoperative Symptoms

The major new postoperative symptom is dysphagia. Dysphagia in the early postoperative period is very common. In fact, most patients are on soft diets for the first few weeks. Patients who are unable to drink liquids after 2 weeks or eat solid foods after 6 weeks should be evaluated. The most important predictive factor in the management of postoperative dysphagia is the integrity of the fundoplication. A barium swallow test and endoscopic examination are complimentary in the assessment of the integrity of the wrap. The barium swallow test is better at looking at the length of the fundoplication, whereas the endoscopic examination is better for assessing the location and orientation. If the fundoplication should be short (1–2 cm), parallel to the diaphragm, and at the top of the stomach, dilation therapy followed by watchful waiting will help the great majority of patients. The use of large dilators, 46 to 54 French, is very safe.[118,124] There are conflicting reports on the use of the 3.0 cm pneumatic balloons. Early reports suggested poor success with a risk of perforation.[125] However, a recent study showed improvement in 9 of 16 patients with postfundoplication dysphagia.[126] If the fundoplication is not intact, if it is too long or is twisted, or if gastric folds are seen above the wrap (directly above or alongside), surgical revision is usually necessary.

Another new problem is the so-called "gas-bloat" syndrome. It is difficult to define the gas-bloat syndrome. Impairment of belching after antireflux surgery is fairly common. Consequently, nearly all patients have a bloating sensation that can last several months. This probably should not be considered the gas-bloat syndrome. Interestingly, several studies suggest that that bloating is a common preoperative symptom. The diagnosis of gas-bloat syndrome should probably be reserved for those patients who cannot belch at all or for those who feel disabled by the gas discomfort. Fortunately, this condition is very rare. The cause is unknown. One of the theories is that preoperative aerophagia persists postoperatively. The impairment of belching may keep more air in the intestine, giving rise to the bloating symptoms. However, patients with gas-bloat syndrome do not necessarily have more intestinal gas.[127] More likely, some patients may experience some degree of vagal nerve injury at the time of their fundoplication, which leads to the sensation of bloating.[109] Management of the gas-bloat syndrome includes trying anti-gas agents and decreasing the ingestion of gas-forming foods. Prokinetic agents may be of benefit, although there are limited data on this. There are reports of a few patients who underwent a surgical revision or esophageal dilation with improvement, but for the most part these treatments are ineffective and cannot be routinely recommended.

One of the most difficult postoperative problems is the management of the patient with vagal nerve injury. The post-fundoplication incidence of mild, transient nausea, bloating, or diarrhea is in the 10% to 15% range.[1,128] It suggests, although it is hard to prove, that minor, self-limited trauma may be quite common. Rarely, patients have a profound injury causing nausea, vomiting, and diarrhea. These patients should also have an endoscopic examination to rule out an easily treatable cause of the nausea, such as peptic ulcer disease. A gastric emptying study should be done to document that gastroparesis is present. The management of post-fundoplication nausea is no different than the treatment of other causes of nausea and includes maintenance of adequate hydration and nutrition as well as use of antiemetics and prokinetic agents. When severe, these can be the most difficult complications to handle.

Repeat Surgery

Patients who fail antireflux surgery may need to be considered for a second operation.[108] Prior to surgical revision, a barium swallow test and an endoscopic examination should be done to evaluate the integrity of the fundoplication. If there is a problem with the wrap, surgical revision is often necessary. Esophageal motility testing should be done to make sure the esophageal peristalsis is still satisfactory. Impaired esophageal motility may develop after inadequate surgery by creating a relative obstruction at the level of the lower esophageal sphincter. Patients with gastric symptoms may benefit from gastric function testing, such as a nuclear medicine gastric emptying study, or gastric acid analysis to rule out problems below the diaphragm that may have contributed to the surgical complication or developed as a result of the surgery. Ambulatory pH monitoring may be required to document that the postoperative symptoms are indeed related to reflux, especially if the symptoms are atypical or if the wrap looks good. The published success rates of 75% to 85% for a second operation come from tertiary care centers.[63,110–117] In many of these series, 30% to 40% of the second operations included alternative procedures, such as esophageal lengthening procedures, gastric drainage, vagotomy, biliary diversion procedures, or an esophageal resection. Hunter et al[63] achieved an ultimate success rate of 93% by revising the fundoplication again on 11 of their 100 patients.[63] In this study, the need for a repeat operation was four times as likely for a patient undergoing a repeat operation as for a patient with uncomplicated GERD undergoing a first operation. The success rate of a simple revision in less experienced hands would probably be much lower. Success rates of further operations are even lower, reported as 85% for second operations, 66% for third operations, and 42% for more than three operations.[112] The prereoperative evaluation and management should probably be done in centers with a great deal of experience in these matters

Endoscopic Therapy

The four basic types of endoscopic therapy are endoscopic suturing, radiofrequency ablation, injection therapy, and bulking procedures. There is a great deal of appeal to the idea of having a safe, simple, effective outpatient procedure for the millions of American suffering from GERD; however, there is a remarkable amount of cynicism about these therapies.[129] It did not help that the Food and Drug Administration (FDA) approved two devices more than a year before any human data were published. One FDA-approved suturing system has had no data published even in abstract form. There have been at least two deaths associated with these procedures. For the most part, major insurers refuse to pay for these procedures because they are "experimental." Perhaps the greatest reason to be skeptical is that the currently available therapies are already pretty good.[130] It is almost unthinkable that any endoscopic therapy will be as effective as PPIs or laparoscopic antireflux surgery. Consequently, the ultimate role of this type of therapy is entirely unknown.[131] However, the complexity of these procedures, coupled with mediocre long-term results, has limited our early experience with these treatments.

The endoscopic suturing procedure is relatively complex. Basically, an oroesophageal overtube is placed. The EndoCinch device (CR Bard, Inc, Murray Hill, NJ) is attached to the end of a standard endoscope. It is advanced through the overtube and past the squamocolumnar junction. The device is juxtaposed to the mucosa on the gastric side of the gastroesophageal junction. Applying suction, a fold of tissue is aspirated into the cavity of the sewing capsule. A stitch can then be advanced through the tissue. The suturing capsule is withdrawn with a metal tilt-tag attached to the suture to ensure retrieval. The device is reloaded with the same suture. The suturing system is reintroduced to the location of the previous stitch. Using rotation of the endoscope, placement of the next stitch is made adjacent to the first. Withdrawal of the suturing system is followed by traction on both suture ends until the redundant loop has been eliminated. Now, tying a half-hitch outside the patient and passing it with a knot pusher secures the plication. A suture cutter is introduced to divide the suture strands above the knot. Recently, a new device has been developed to clip the suture, rather than tie the knots.

This has greatly decreased the time involved in this part of the procedure. The above steps are repeated to create two to four plications. Plications may be placed at several levels and in several lines of orientation. Early results show improvement in heartburn severity, heartburn frequency, and regurgitation in 47 patients after 6 months.[132] One patient had a self-contained suture perforation that was successfully treated with antibiotics. Unpublished data on more than 1200 patients shows that there have been no significant, irreversible complications. Centers with significant experience have impressive initial success rates.[133,134] However, 2-year follow-up data on the original patients shows that only 25% were off all antireflux therapy.[135] A new suturing device (Wilson-Cook Medical, Winston-Salem, NC) looks far less complex and does not require an overtube. No published or unpublished data are available on this FDA-approved device.

Radiofrequency has been used to treat the uvula in patients with sleep apnea, as well as benign prostatic hypertrophy, spinal disk disease, and cardiac arrhythmias. In this procedure, a Stretta catheter is passed orally to the level of the cardioesophageal junction. This is a 65 cm long, 6 mm diameter shaft with a central balloon. The balloon is inflated to position the instrument. There are four 5.5 NiTi needle electrodes attached to the catheter, and these can be deployed into the muscular layer of the lower esophagus. Radiofrequency is applied to functionally heat the water molecules in the esophageal muscle. A thermocoupling device monitors the temperature in the tissue and will shut off when a critical (predetermined) temperature is achieved. An irrigation system is available to protect the esophageal mucosa. This procedure is performed at several levels between 2 cm above and 2 cm below the LES and requires a four-channel power source to deliver the energy. The instrument must have the ability to monitor the temperature and must have automatic shut-off capability. There is no need for an overtube. The average procedure time is just less than an hour. Histologically, the collagen contracts, leading to remodeling of the cardioesophageal junction and nerve ablation. Both types of injury are probably necessary for success. The mucosa is thickened at the level of the LES. The neural ablation probably results in fewer transient LES relaxations. There is minimal mucosal damage. In the original trials, there is improvement in heartburn scores after 6 and 12 months.[136,137] After 6 months, 87% of patients were able to discontinue PPIs, and 70% were off PPIs after 1 year. There were improvements in mental and physical scores on the SF-36. No significant procedure-related complications occurred in this study. Pooled data suggest that the early major complication rate including, death, perforation, sepsis, and gastrointestinal bleeding was around 1%. Recently, with experience and better instruction, the complication rate appears to dropping to around 0.1%. An unpublished sham study showed that 34 patients randomized to the Stretta procedure had less heartburn than patients who received sham therapy. However, it must be noted that there were no differences between the groups with regard to PPI requirements and pH monitoring results.[138]

Submucosal injection of polymethyl methacrylate (PMMA; Plexiglas) microspheres into the lower esophageal folds decreased the severity of symptoms and acid reflux in 10 patients with GERD who were either refractory to or dependent on PPIs.[139] Endoscopic ultrasonography demonstrated the efficacy of implantation. A significant decrease in the symptom severity score and mean total time with esophageal pH less than 4 was noted after the implantation of PMMA ($P < 0.05$). Seven of 10 patients were taking no medication after PMMA implantation. There were no serious procedure-related complications.

Enteryx (Boston Scientific Corp, Natick, MA) is a chemically inert, noncarcinogenic, hypoallergenic, nonantigenic, radiopaque compound that is available in a liquid organic state but will become solid upon hydration (or placement in tissue). It is already being used in the treatment of arteriovenous malformations, peripheral vascular disease, and hypervascular head and neck cancers. It can be injected into the LES under fluoroscopic and endoscopic guidance. The endoscopist can ensure that the injection is indeed into the muscular layer, as a ring will appear at the LES on the radiograph. This ring will persist as long as the material is in the LES. Multicenter studies are underway in several countries, including the United States. Preliminary data suggest short-term improvement in symptom scores of over 80% with virtually no significant complications.[140]

The Gatekeeper-Reflux Repair System (Medtronic, Inc, Minneapolis, MN) involves the placement of polyacrylonitrile-based hydrogel (HYPAN) prostheses in the region of the lower esophageal sphincter to prevent reflux. HYPAN is one of the least reactive polymers when compared to silicone, polyethylene, and polytetrafluoroethylene. It is hydrophilic and will swell within 6 hours of placement. Preliminary data suggest that this procedure can be done safely,[141] but there are virtually no effectiveness data to date.

There are at least two systems in development that actually grasp the lower esophageal sphincter area and irreversibly suture or clamp this area. The NDO plicator (Mansfield, MA) places a single transmural plication near the gastroesophageal junction under direct endoscopic visualization. Theoretically, this serosa-to-serosa union accentuates and restores the valvular mechanism of the gastroesophageal junction. Preliminary data on six patients suggest that it is safe and effective for up to 6 months.[142]

If endoscopic therapy is to make an impact on the management of patients with GERD, well-designed clinical trials will need to demonstrate that these procedures are successful, safe, and easy to perform.

Key Points: Surgical and Endoscopic Treatment of Gastroesophageal Reflux Disease

- ⟳ There is absolutely no evidence to advocate either medical or surgical therapy as the single best therapy. The decision to perform antireflux surgery must be individualized to the patient.
- ⟳ All patients taking long-term medical therapy for GERD should receive advice on the safety and wisdom of staying on that therapy, as well as information on antireflux surgery.
- ⟳ Fundoplication should be considered in three circumstances: (1) individuals who are intolerant of PPI therapy because of side effects, (2) patients who are poorly responsive to PPI therapy, and (3) when a patient desires a permanent solution to be free of the need to take medications.
- ⟳ Patients must be warned about the potential suboptimal results, including the frequent need for medication within a few years of having the procedure as well as the small but real possibility of becoming worse after the operation. Even in experienced hands, 1% to 2% of patients are worse after the procedure.
- ⟳ A careful preoperative evaluation to ensure that the patient's symptoms are reflux-related and that the right operative procedure is performed will offer the patient the best opportunity for success.
- ⟳ Widespread use of endoscopic therapy for GERD is probably still several years away.
- ⟳ The best endoscopic therapy is yet to be determined, but it will need to be safe, effective, and easy to use.

Suggested Reading

1. Hunter JG, Trus TL, Branum GD, et al: A physiologic approach to laparoscopic fundoplication for gastroesophageal reflux disease. Ann Surg 223:673–685, 1996.
2. DeMeester TR, Bonavina L, Albertucci M: Nissen fundoplication for gastroesophageal reflux disease: evaluation of primary repair in 100 consecutive patients. Ann Surg 204:9–20, 1986.
3. Trus TL, Laycock WS, Branum G, et al: Intermediate follow-up of laparoscopic antireflux surgery. Am J Surg 171:32–35, 1996.

4. Weerts JM, Dallemagne B, Hamoir E, et al: Laparoscopic Nissen fundoplication: detailed analysis of 132 patients. Surg Laparosc Endosc 3:359–364, 1993.
5. Hinder RA, Filipi CJ, Wetscher G, et al: Laparoscopic Nissen fundoplication is an effective treatment for gastroesophageal reflux disease. Ann Surg 20:472–481, 1994.
6. Jamieson GG, Watson DI, Britten-Jones R, et al: Laparoscopic Nissen fundoplication. Ann Surg 220:137–145, 1994.
7. Hinder RA: Surgical therapy for GERD: selection of procedures, short- and long-term results. J Clin Gastroenterol 30(3 Suppl):S48–50, 2000.
8. Peters JH, DeMeester TR, Crookes P, et al: The treatment of gastroesophageal reflux disease with laparoscopic Nissen fundoplication: prospective evaluation of 100 patients with "typical" symptoms. Ann Surg 228:40–50, 1998.
9. Bammer T, Hinder RA, Klaus A, Klingler PJ: Five- to eight-year outcome of the first laparoscopic Nissen fundoplications. J Gastrointest Surg 5:42–48, 2001.
10. Carlson MA, Frantzides CT: Complications and results of primary minimally invasive antireflux procedures: a review of 10,735 reported cases. J Am Coll Surg 193:428–439, 2001.
11. Trus TL, Laycock WS, Waring JP, et al: Improvement in quality of life measures after laparoscopic antireflux surgery. Ann Surg 229:331–336, 1999.
12. Kamolz T, Bammer T, Wykypiel H Jr, et al: Quality of life and surgical outcome after laparoscopic Nissen and Toupet fundoplication: one-year follow-up. Endoscopy 32:363–368, 2000.
13. Booth MI, Jones L, Stratford J, Dehn TC: Results of laparoscopic Nissen fundoplication at 2–8 years after surgery. Br J Surg 89:476–481, 2002.
14. Mobius C, Stein HJ, Feith M, et al: Quality of life before and after laparoscopic Nissen fundoplication. Surg Endosc 15:353–356, 2001.
15. Spechler SJ: Comparison of medical and surgical therapy for complicated gastroesophageal reflux disease in veterans. N Engl J Med 326:786–792, 1992.
16. Lundell L, Miettinen P, Myrvold HE, et al: Long-term management of gastro-oesophageal reflux disease with omeprazole or open antireflux surgery: results of a prospective, randomized clinical trial. Eur J Gastroenterol Hepatol 12:879–887, 2000.
17. Lundell L, Miettinen P, Myrvold HE, et al: Continued (5-year) followup of a randomized clinical study comparing antireflux surgery and omeprazole in gastroesophageal reflux disease. J Am Coll Surg 192:172–179, 2001.
18. Hookman P, Barkin JS: Surgical complications of laparoscopic fundoplication for gastroesophageal reflux disease: call for reevaluation of surgical criteria. Am J Gastroenterol 95:3305–3308, 2000.
19. Hogan WJ, Shaker R: Life after antireflux surgery. Am J Med 108(Suppl 4a):181S–191S, 2000.
20. Lind T: Changing surgical principles for gastro-oesophageal reflux disease: Is laparoscopic fundoplication justified in the light of surgical complications? Eur J Surg Suppl 585:31–33, 2000.
21. Kahrilas PJ: Management of GERD: medical versus surgical. Sem Gastrointest Dis 12:3–15, 2001.
22. Low DE: Surgery for hiatal hernia and GERD: Time for reappraisal and a balanced approach? Surg Endosc 15:913–917, 2001.
23. Wo JM, Waring JP: Medical therapy of gastroesophageal reflux and management of esophageal strictures. Surg Clin North Am 77:1041–1062, 1997.
24. Farrell TM, Richardson WS, Halkar R, et al: Nissen fundoplication improves gastric motility in patients with delayed gastric emptying. Surg Endosc 15:271–274, 2001.
25. Hunter JG, Champion JK: Laparoscopic Nissen fundoplication. In Toouli J, Gossot

D, Hunter JG (eds): Endosurgery. New York, Churchill Livingston, 1996, pp 305–314.

26. Awad ZT, Mittal SK, Roth TA, et al: Esophageal shortening during the era of laparoscopic surgery. World J Surg 25:558–561, 2001.

27. Horvath KD, Swanstrom LL, Jobe BA: The short esophagus: pathophysiology, incidence, presentation, and treatment in the era of laparoscopic antireflux surgery. Ann Surg 232:630–640, 2000.

28. Swanstrom LL, Marcus DR, Galloway GQ: Laparoscopic Collis gastroplasty is the treatment of choice for the shortened esophagus. Am J Surg 171:477–481, 1996.

29. Ferguson MK: Pitfalls and complications of antireflux surgery: Nissen and Collis-Nissen techniques. Chest Surg Clin North Am 7:489–509, 1997.

30. Lord RV, Kaminski A, Oberg S, et al: Absence of gastroesophageal reflux disease in a majority of patients taking acid suppression medications after Nissen fundoplication. J Gastrointest Surg 6:3–9, 2002.

31. de Beaux AC, Watson DI, O'Boyle C, Jamieson GG: Role of fundoplication in patient symptomatology after laparoscopic antireflux surgery. Br J Surg 88:1117–1121, 2001.

32. Romagnuolo J, Meier MA, Sadowski DC: Medical or surgical therapy for erosive reflux esophagitis: cost-utility analysis using a Markov model. Ann Surg 236:191–202, 2002.

33. Holzman MD, Mitchel EF, Ray WA, Smalley WE: Use of healthcare resources among medically and surgically treated patients with gastroesophageal reflux disease: a population-based study. J Am Coll Surg 192:17–24, 2001.

34. Allgood PC, Bachmann M: Medical or surgical treatment for chronic gastrooesophageal reflux? A systematic review of published evidence of effectiveness. Eur J Surg 166:713–721, 2000.

35. Klinkenberg-Knol EC, Festen HP, Jansen JB, et al: Long-term treatment with omeprazole for refractory reflux esophagitis: efficacy and safety. Ann Intern Med 121:161–167, 1994.

36. Vakil N, Shaw M, Kirby R: Clinical effectiveness of laparoscopic fundoplication in a U.S. community. Am J Med 114:1–5, 2003.

37. Spechler SJ, Lee E, Ahnen D, et al: Long-term outcome of medical and surgical therapies for gastroesophageal reflux disease: follow-up of a randomized controlled trial. JAMA 285:2331–2338, 2001.

38. Rantanen TK, Halme TV, Luostarinen ME, et al: The long term results of open antireflux surgery in a community-based health care center. Am J Gastroenterol 94:1777–1781, 1999.

39. Lundell L, Dalenback J, Janatuinen E, et al: Comprehensive 1-year cost analysis of open antireflux surgery in Nordic countries. Br J Surg 85:1002–1005, 1998.

40. Myrvold HE, Lundell L, Miettinen P, et al: The cost of long term therapy for gastrooesophageal reflux disease: a randomised trial comparing omeprazole and open antireflux surgery. Gut 49:488–494, 2001.

41. Richardson WS, Trus TL, Wo JM, et al: Atypical symptoms do not improve to the same extent as typical symptoms after laparoscopic fundoplication in gastroesophageal reflux patients [abstract]. Gastrointest Endosc 43:A433, 1996.

42. So JB, Zeitels SM, Rattner DW: Outcomes of atypical symptoms attributed to gastroesophageal reflux treated by laparoscopic fundoplication. Surgery 124:28–32, 1998.

43. Ekstrom T, Johansson KE: Effects of anti-reflux surgery on chronic cough and asthma in patients with gastro-oesophageal reflux disease. Respir Med 94:1166–1170, 2000.

44. Spivak H, Smith CD, Phichith A, et al: Asthma and gastroesophageal reflux: fundo-

plication decreases need for systemic corticosteroids. J Gastrointest Surg 3:477–482, 1999.

45. Klaus A, Swain JM, Hinder RA: Laparoscopic antireflux surgery for supraesophageal complications of gastroesophageal reflux disease. Am J Med 111(Suppl 8A):202S–206S, 2001.

46. Allen CJ, Anvari M: Gastro-oesophageal reflux related cough and its response to laparoscopic fundoplication. Thorax 53:963–968, 1998.

47. Lindstrom DR, Wallace J, Loehrl TA, et al: Nissen fundoplication surgery for extraesophageal manifestations of gastroesophageal reflux (EER). Laryngoscope 112:1762–1765, 2002.

48. Allen CJ, Anvari M: Preoperative symptom evaluation and esophageal acid infusion predict response to laparoscopic Nissen fundoplication in gastroesophageal reflux patients who present with cough. Surg Endosc 16:1037–1041, 2002.

49. Kahrilas PJ: Maximizing outcome of extraesophageal reflux disease. Am J Manag Care 6(16 Suppl):S876–882, 2000.

50. Katzka DA, Paoletti V, Leite L, Castell DO: Prolonged ambulatory pH monitoring in patients with persistent gastroesophageal reflux disease symptoms: testing while on therapy identifies the need for more aggressive anti-reflux therapy. Am J Gastroenterol 91:2110–2113, 1996.

51. Peters JH: The surgical management of Barrett's esophagus. Gastroenterol Clin North Am 26:647–668, 1997.

52. Csendes A, Braghetto I, Burdiles P, et al: Long-term results of classic antireflux surgery in 152 patients with Barrett's esophagus: clinical, radiologic, endoscopic, manometric, and acid reflux test analysis before and late after operation. Surgery. 126:645–657, 1998.

53. DeMeester TR, Attwood SE, Smyrk TC, et al: Surgical therapy in Barrett's esophagus. Ann Surg 212:528–540, 1990.

54. McDonald ML, Trastek VF, Allen MS, et al: Barretts's esophagus: does an antireflux procedure reduce the need for endoscopic surveillance? J Thorac Cardiovasc Surg 111:1135–1138, 1996.

55. Ortiz A, Martinez de Haro LF, Parrilla P, et al: Conservative treatment versus antireflux surgery in Barrett's oesophagus: long-term results of a prospective study. Br J Surg 83:274–278, 1996.

56. Katz D, Rothstein R, Schned A, et al: The development of dysplasia and adenocarcinoma during endoscopic surveillance of Barrett's esophagus. Am J Gastroenterol 93:536–541, 1998.

57. Farrell TM, Smith CD, Metreveli RE, et al: Fundoplication provides effective and durable symptom relief in patients with Barrett's esophagus. Am J Surg 178:18–21, 1999.

58. DeMeester TR: Antireflux surgery in the management of Barrett's esophagus. J Gastrointest Surg 4:124–128, 2000.

59. Yau P, Watson DI, Devitt PG, et al: Laparoscopic antireflux surgery in the treatment of gastroesophageal reflux in patients with Barrett esophagus. Arch Surg 135:801–805, 2000.

60. Jamieson GG, France M, Watson DI: Results of laparoscopic antireflux operations in patients who have Barrett's esophagus. Chest Surg Clin of North Am 12:149–155, 2002.

61. Ye W, Chow WH, Lagergren J, et al: Risk of adenocarcinomas of the esophagus and gastric cardia in patients with gastroesophageal reflux diseases and after antireflux surgery. Gastroenterology 121:1286–1293, 2001.

62. Hofstetter WL, Peters JH, DeMeester TR, et al: Long-term outcome of antireflux surgery in patients with Barrett's esophagus. Ann of Surg 234:532–538, 2001.

63. Hunter JG, Smith CD, Branum GD, et al: Laparoscopic fundoplication failures: patterns of failure and response to fundoplication revision. Ann Surg 230:595–604, 1999.
64. Drewitz DJ, Sampliner RE, Garewal HS: The incidence of adenocarcinoma in Barrett's esophagus: a prospective study of 170 patients followed 4.8 years. Am J Gastroenterol 92:212–215, 1997.
65. O'Connor JB, Falk GW, Richter JE: The incidence of adenocarcinoma and dysplasia in Barrett's esophagus: report on the Cleveland Clinic Barrett's Esophagus Registry. Am J Gastroenterol 94:2037–2042, 1999.
66. Shaheen NJ, Bozymski EM: Does antireflux surgery alter the natural history of Barrett's esophagus? Am J Gastroenterol 94:11–12, 1999.
67. Kim SL, Hunter JG, Wo JM, et al: NSAIDs, aspirin, and esophageal strictures: are over-the-counter medications harmful to the esophagus? J Clin Gastroenterol 29:32–34, 1999.
68. Marks RD, Richter JE, Rizzo J, et al: Omeprazole versus H2-receptor antagonists in treating patients with peptic stricture and esophagitis. Gastroenterology. 106:907–915, 1994.
69. Smith PM, Kerr GD, Cockel R, et al: A comparison of omeprazole and ranitidine in the prevention of recurrence of benign esophageal stricture. Gastroenterology. 107:1312–1318, 1994.
70. Stirling MC, Orringer MB: The combined Collis-Nissen operation for esophageal reflux strictures. Ann Thorac Surg 45:148–157, 1988.
71. Ritter MP, Peters JH, DeMeester TR, et al: Treatment of advanced gastroesophageal reflux disease with Collis gastroplasty and Belsey partial fundoplication. Arch Surg 133:523–528, 1998.
72. Spivak H, Farrell TM, Trus T, et al: Laparoscopic fundoplication for dysphagia and peptic esophageal strictures J Gastrointest Surg 2:555–560, 1998.
73. Klingler PJ, Hinder RA, Cina RA, et al: Laparoscopic antireflux surgery for the treatment of esophageal strictures refractory to medical therapy. Am J Gastroenterol 94:632–636, 1999.
74. Trus TL, Mauren SJ, Katz EM, et al: Laparoscopic antireflux surgery in the elderly. Am J Gastroenterol 93:351–353, 1998.
75. Khajanchee YS, Urbach DR, Butler N, et al: Laparoscopic antireflux surgery in the elderly. Surg Endosc 16:25–30, 2002.
76. Wo JM, Branum GD, Hunter JG, et al: Clinical presentation and natural history of type III (mixed) paraesophageal hernia. Am J Gastroenterol 91:914–916, 1996.
77. Dahlberg PS, Deschamps C, Miller DL, et al: Laparoscopic repair of large paraesophageal hiatal hernia. Ann Thorac Surg 72:1125–1129, 2001.
78. Velanovich V, Karmy-Jones R: Surgical management of paraesophageal hernias: outcome and quality of life analysis. Digest Surg 18:432–437, 2001.
79. Terry M, Smith CD, Branum GD, et al: Outcomes of laparoscopic fundoplication for gastroesophageal reflux disease and paraesophageal hernia. Surg Endosc 15:691–699, 2001.
80. Velanovich V, Karmy-Jones R: Psychiatric disorders affect outcomes of antireflux operations for gastroesophageal reflux disease. Surg Endosc 15:171–175, 2001.
81. Kamolz T, Bammer T, Pointner R: The effects of laparoscopic antireflux surgery on GERD patients with concomitant anxiety disorders. Surg Endosc 16:1247, 2002.
82. Kamolz T, Bammer T, Granderath FA, Pointner R: Comorbidity of aerophagia in GERD patients: outcome of laparoscopic antireflux surgery. Scand J Gastroenterol 37:138–143, 2002.
83. Waring JP, Hunter JG, Oddsdottir M, et al: The preoperative evaluation of patients considered for laparoscopic antireflux surgery. Am J Gastroenterol 90:35–37, 1995.

84. Fibbe C, Layer P, Keller J, et al: Esophageal motility in reflux disease before and after fundoplication: a prospective, randomized, clinical, and manometric study. Gastroenterology 121:5–14, 2001.

85. Castell DO: Esophageal manometry prior to antireflux surgery: required, preferred, or even needed? Gastroenterology 121:214–216, 2001.

86. Rydberg L, Ruth M, Abrahamsson H, Lundell L: Tailoring antireflux surgery: a randomized clinical trial. World J Surg 23:612–618, 1999.

87. Oleynikov D, Eubanks TR, Oelschlager BK, Pellegrini CA: Total fundoplication is the operation of choice for patients with gastroesophageal reflux and defective peristalsis. Surg Endosc 16:909–913, 2002.

88. Booth M, Stratford J, Dehn TC: Preoperative esophageal body motility does not influence the outcome of laparoscopic Nissen fundoplication for gastroesophageal reflux disease. Dis Esophagus 15:57–60, 2002.

89. Zornig C, Strate U, Fibbe C, et al: Nissen vs Toupet laparoscopic fundoplication. Surg Endosc 16:758–766, 2002.

90. Sandbu R, Hallgren T: The economics of laparoscopic antireflux operations compared with open surgery. Eur J Surg Suppl 585:37–39, 2000.

91. Rantanen TK, Salo JA, Sipponen JT: Fatal and life-threatening complications in antireflux surgery: analysis of 5,502 operations. Br J Surg 86:1573–1577, 1999.

92. Bais JE, Bartelsman JF, Bonjer HJ, et al: Laparoscopic or conventional Nissen fundoplication for gastro-oesophageal reflux disease: randomised clinical trial. Lancet 355:170–174, 2000.

93. Wenner J, Nilsson G, Oberg S, et al: Short-term outcome after laparoscopic and open 360 degrees fundoplication: a prospective randomized trial. Surg Endosc 15:1124–1128, 2001.

94. Watson DI, Jamieson GG, Pike GK, et al: Prospective randomized double-blind trial between laparoscopic Nissen fundoplication and anterior partial fundoplication. Br J Surg 86:123–130, 1999.

95. Pessaux P, Arnaud JP, Ghavami B, et al: Laparoscopic antireflux surgery: comparative study of Nissen, Nissen-Rossetti, and Toupet fundoplication. Surg Endosc 14:1024–1027, 2000.

96. O'Boyle CJ, Watson DI, Jamieson GG, et al: Division of short gastric vessels at laparoscopic nissen fundoplication: a prospective double-blind randomized trial with 5-year follow-up. Ann Surg 235:165–170, 2002.

97. Farrell TM, Archer SB, Galloway KD, et al: Heartburn is more likely to recur after Toupet fundoplication than Nissen fundoplication. Am Surg 66:229–236, 2000.

98. Fernando HC, Luketich JD, Christie NA, et al: Outcomes of laparoscopic Toupet compared to laparoscopic Nissen fundoplication. Surg Endosc 16:905–908, 2002.

99. Klapow JC, Wilcox CM, Mallinger AP, et al: Characterization of long-term outcomes after Toupet fundoplication: symptoms, medication use, and health status. J Clin Gastroenterol 34:509–515, 2002.

100. Heider TR, Farrell TM, Kircher AP, et al: Complete fundoplication is not associated with increased dysphagia in patients with abnormal esophageal motility. J Gastrointest Surg 5:36–41, 2001.

101. Sato K, Awad ZT, Filipi CJ, et al: Causes of long-term dysphagia after laparoscopic Nissen fundoplication. J Soc Laparoendosc Surgeons 6:35–40, 2002.

102. Herron DM, Swanstrom LL, Ramzi N, Hansen PD: Factors predictive of dysphagia after laparoscopic Nissen fundoplication. Surg Endosc 13:1180–1183, 1999.

103. Hunter JG, Swanstrom L, Waring JP: Dysphagia after laparoscopic antireflux surgery: the impact of operative technique. Ann Surg 51–57, 1996.

104. Leggett PL, Bissell CD, Churchman-Winn R, Ahn C: A comparison of laparoscopic

Nissen fundoplication and Rossetti's modification in 239 patients. Surg Endosc 14:473–477, 2000.

105. Contini S, Zinicola R, Bertele A, et al: Dysphagia and clinical outcome after laparoscopic Nissen or Rossetti fundoplication: sequential prospective study. World J Surg 26:1106–1111, 2002.

106. Chrysos E, Tzortzinis A, Tsiaoussis J, et al: Prospective randomized trial comparing Nissen to Nissen-Rossetti technique for laparoscopic fundoplication. Am J Surg 182:215–221, 2001.

107. Watson DI, Jamieson GG, Baigrie RJ, et al: Laparoscopic surgery for gastrooesophageal reflux: beyond the learning curve. Br J Surg 83:1284–1287, 1996.

108. Waring JP: Postfundoplication complications: Prevention and management. Gastro Clin North Am 28:1007–1019, 1999.

109. Waring JP: Management of postfundoplication complications. Sem Gastrointest Dis 10:121–129, 1999.

110. Leonardi HK, Crozier RE, Ellis FH Jr: Reoperation for complications of the Nissen fundoplication. J Thorac Cardiovasc Surg 81:50–56, 1981.

111. Stein HJ, Feussner H, Siewert JR: Failure of antireflux surgery: causes and management strategies. Am J Surg 171:36–40, 1996.

112. Little AG, Ferguson MK, Skinner DB: Reoperation for failed antireflux operations. J Thorac Cardiovasc Surg 92:667–672, 1986.

113. Siewert JR, Stein HJ, Feussner H: Reoperations after failed antireflux procedures. Ann Chir Gynecol 84:122–128, 1995.

114. Rieger NA, Jamieson GG, Britten-Jones R, Tew S: Reoperation after failed antireflux surgery. Brit J Surg 81:1159–1161, 1994.

115. Stirling MC, Orringer MB: Surgical treatment after the failed antireflux surgery. J Thorac Cardiovasc Surg 92:667–672, 1986.

116. Ellis FH Jr, Gibb SP, Heatley GJ: Reoperation after failed antireflux surgery. Eur J Cardiothorac Surg 10:25–31, 1996.

117. Hinder RA, Klingler PJ, Perdikis G, Smith SL: Management of the failed antireflux operation. Surg Clin North Am 77:1083–1098, 1997.

118. Wo JM, Trus TL, Richardson WS, et al: Evaluation and management of post-fundoplication dysphagia. Am J Gastroenterol 91:2318–2322, 1996.

119. Johnson DA, Younes Z, Hogan WJ: Endoscopic assessment of hiatal hernia repair. Gastrointest Endosc 52:650–659, 2000.

120. Jailwala J, Massey B, Staff D, et al: Post-fundoplication symptoms: the role for endoscopic assessment of fundoplication integrity. Gastrointest Endosc 54:351–356, 2001.

121. Hainaux B, Sattari A, Coppens E, et al: Intrathoracic migration of the wrap after laparoscopic Nissen fundoplication: radiologic evaluation. AJR 178:859–862, 2002.

122. Peters JH, DeMeester TR: Indications, benefits and outcome of laparoscopic Nissen fundoplication. Dig Dis Sci 14:169–79, 1996.

123. Pashankar D, Blair GK, Israel DM: Omeprazole maintenance therapy for gastroesophageal reflux disease after failure of fundoplication. J Ped Gastroenterol Nutr 32:145–149, 2001.

124. Malhi-Chowla N, Gorecki P, Bammer T, et al: Dilation after fundoplication: timing, frequency, indications, and outcome. Gastrointest Endosc 55:219–223, 2002.

125. Ellingson TL, Kozarek RA, Gelfand MD, et al: Iatrogenic achalasia. J Clin Gastroenterol 20:96–99, 1995.

126. Gaudric M, Sabate JM, Artru P, et al: Results of pneumatic dilatation in patients with dysphagia after antireflux surgery. Br J Surg 86:1088–1091, 1999.

127. Smith D, King NA, Waldron B, et al: Study of belching ability in antireflux surgery patients and normal volunteers. Br J Surg 78:32–35, 1991.

128. Swanstrom L, Wayne R: Spectrum of gastrointestinal symptoms after laparoscopic fundoplication. Am J Surg 167:538–541, 1994.
129. Hogan WJ: Endoscopic treatment modalities for GERD: technologic score or scare? Gastrointest Endosc 53:541–545, 2001.
130. Hogan WJ: Response to letter. Gastrointest Endosc 55:301–302, 2002.
131. Lehman GA: Endoscopic and endoluminal techniques for the control of gastroesophageal reflux: are they ready for widespread clinical application? Gastrointest Endosc 52:808–811, 2001.
132. Filipi CJ, Lehman GA, Rothstein RI, et al: Transoral, flexible endoscopic suturing for treatment of GERD: a multicenter trial. Gastrointest Endosc 53:416–422, 2001.
133. Velanovich V, Ben-Menachem T, Goel S: Case-control comparison of endoscopic gastroplication with laparoscopic fundoplication in the management of gastroesophageal reflux disease: early symptomatic outcomes. Surg Laparosc, Endosc Percutan Techn 12:219–223, 2002.
134. Raijchman I, Ben-Menachem T, Reddy G, et al: Symptomatic response to endoluminal gastroplication (ELGP) in patients with gastroesophageal reflux disease: a multicenter experience [abstract]. Gastrointest Endosc 53:AB74, 2001.
135. Rothstein RI, Pohl H, Grove M, et al. Endoscopic gastric plication for the treatment of GERD: two year results [abstract]. Am J Gastroenterol 96:S53, 2001.
136. Triadafilopoulos G, DiBaise JK, Nostrant TT, et al: Radiofrequency energy delivery to the gastroesophageal junction for the treatment of GERD. Gastrointest 53:407–415, 2001.
137. Triadafilopoulos G, DiBaise JK, Nostrant TT, et al: The Stretta procedure for the treatment of GERD: 6 and 12 month follow-up of the U.S. open label trial. Gastrointest Endosc 55:149–156, 2002.
138. Corley DA, Katz P, Wo J, et al: Radiofrequency energy to the gastroesophageal junction for the treatment of GERD: a randomized sham-controlled, multicenter clinical trial [abstract]. Gastrointest Endosc 55:AB100, 2002.
139. Feretis C, Benakis P, Dimopoulos C, et al: Endoscopic implantation of Plexiglas (PMMA) microspheres for the treatment of GERD. Gastrointest Endosc 53:423–426, 2001.
140. Johnson DA, Aisenberg J, Cohen L, et al: Enteryx, an injectable treatment for GERD: multicenter results [abstract]. Am J Gastroenterol 97:S12, 2002.
141. Fokkens P, Costamagna G, Gabbriella A, et al: Endoscopic augmentation of the lower esophageal sphincter for the treatment of GERD: multicenter study of the gatekeeper reflux repair system [abstract]. Gastrointest Endosc 55:AB90, 2002.
142. Chuttani R, Sud R, Sachdev G et al: Endoscopic full-thickness plication for GERD: final results of human pilot study [abstract]. Gastrointest Endosc 55:AB258, 2002.
143. Richardson WS, Hunter JG, Waring JP: Laparoscopic antireflux surgery. Sem Gastrointest Dis 8;100–110, 1997.

Gastroesophageal Reflux Disease in Children

*Qian Yuan, M.D., Ph.D.,
and Harland S. Winter, M.D.*

Gastroesophageal reflux (GER) is defined as the passage of gastric contents into the esophagus and is a normal physiologic process that is common in infancy. *Regurgitation* is the passage of refluxed gastric contents into the oral pharynx, and *vomiting* refers to expulsion of refluxed gastric contents from the mouth. Vomiting is the most common manifestation of GER in infancy, and in most healthy infants all symptoms resolve by 24 months of life. Gastroesophageal reflux disease (GERD) refers to conditions resulting from GER that may be as mild as intermittent heartburn to potentially life-threatening conditions such as severe asthma or apnea. Because GER in most infants usually resolves, symptomatic GER in infants younger than 1 year of age should be distinguished from GER in children older than 2 years of age. Clinicians and families should understand that GER is most commonly a normal physiologic event; however, when episodes are prolonged or excessively frequent, GERD may develop.

Epidemiology

Gastroesophageal reflux is common in infancy but declines in prevalence after the first year of life. A cross-sectional survey demonstrated that the prevalence of at least one episode per day of regurgitation was 50% in children 0 to 3 months of age, reached a peak of 67% at 4 months, and decreased to 5% of children 10 to 12 months of age.[1] A similar pattern was observed for children with more frequent episodes of regurgitation occurring at least four times per day. GER resolved in most children by 1 year of age, without recurrence of symptoms at a 1 year follow-up.[2] These findings support the belief that GER in most infants is a physiologic, self-limited condition that does not recur later in life.

Symptoms of heartburn and regurgitation seem to increase as children get older. Heartburn and regurgitation is reported in 1.8% and 2.3%, respectively, of children 3 to 9 years of age[3] and increases to 5.2% and 8.2% in children 10 to 17 years of age. By adulthood, the prevalence of heartburn and/or acid regurgitation was reported to be 19.8%.[4] Although prospective studies have not been performed in children as they get older, there are studies suggesting that the prevalence of GERD increases with age. Whether children older than 2 years with persistent reflux become adults with complications of GERD remains to be determined. At this time, there are no population-based studies to assess the incidence of GER or GERD in the pediatric population.

Mechanisms of Gastroesophageal Reflux

Antireflux Barrier

The lower esophageal sphincter (LES) constitutes the major barrier to acid reflux. The LES is a specialized region of smooth muscle that is contracted in the resting state. In the neonate, the sphincter length is about 1.5 cm and is located about 2 cm above the level of the diaphragm. In healthy adults, this specialized region of the esophagus is about 3 cm in length. As the cardia of the stomach grows, the LES becomes located at the level of the diaphragm. The crus of the diaphragm also contributes to preventing acid reflux by contracting during inspiration and increasing the high-pressure barrier in the region of the LES. Other anatomic components of the antireflux barrier include the phrenoesophageal ligament, which anchors the distal esophagus to the crural diaphragm and the angle of His.[5] These anatomic factors in the normal child contribute to the development of competency of the LES as the infant matures.

Transient Relaxation of the Lower Esophageal Sphincter

Transient relaxation of the LES, or a sudden decrease in LES pressure to the level of intragastric pressure that is unrelated to swallowing,[6] is the most frequent mechanism causing GER in children and adults.[7] Transient relaxations are usually accompanied by inhibition of the esophageal body and crural diaphragm and are of relatively longer duration than relaxation triggered by a swallow.[6] This inappropriate relaxation of LES tone allows gastric contents to enter the esophagus and exposes the esophageal mucosa to acidic gastric contents.

Esophageal Capacitance

Several factors contribute to GER in infants. A shorter esophagus, the small capacity of the esophagus, and recumbent posture (lack of gravity) increase the likelihood that refluxed material in the infant will fill the esophagus and overflow into the pharynx. Because of these factors, infants are more likely than adults to regurgitate or vomit when gastric contents empty from the stomach into the esophagus. At birth, the esophagus is approximately 11 cm in length and has a diameter of 5 mm. By adulthood, the esophagus is usually 24 to 30 cm in length, with lateral and anterior-posterior diameters of about 30 and 19 mm, respectively.[8] These increased dimensions result in increased capacitance of the organ and provide a larger reservoir for regurgitated food.

Airway Protective Mechanism

Aspiration, one of the complications of GERD, is the result of the failure of a number of protective barriers and responses that prevent refluxed gastric contents from entering the airway. These protective mechanisms include the barrier of the upper esophageal sphincter (UES), esophageal-glottal closure reflex, apnea, pharyngeal clearance, cough, and airway clearance of aspirated materials.[9] Distension of the upper esophagus can result in different responses, depending on amount of material that is regurgitated. The UES contracts if the refluxate volume is small, but when the refluxate is larger, vagal stimulation may lead to vocal cord closure, central apnea, and UES relaxation. The UES relaxation allows entry of gastric contents into the pharynx, which is then followed by a swallow to clear the pharynx. This process permits normal respiration to resume without aspiration. Any neuromuscular disorder of this complex sequence will increase the risk of aspiration. Normally, a cough expels small volumes of refluxate that may enter the larynx; bronchoconstriction prevents aspirated material from reaching the alveolar spaces. In the neonate, these protective mechanisms are not well developed. During a barium swallow, barium observed in the upper airway of a newborn may not be predictive of a neuromuscular disorder; however, aspirated contrast material in older children is more ominous.

Pathogenic Factors in Gastroesophageal Reflux Disease

Gastroesophageal reflux disease is a multifactorial disorder. Although transient LES relaxation, increased intra-abdominal pressure caused by straining, reduced esophageal capacitance, and decreased gastric compliance may all contribute to GERD, the role of gastric emptying in this process remains controversial.[10,11] The squamous epithelium of the esophagus has intrinsic defense mechanisms that protect against acid injury[12]; however, in adults with nonerosive reflux disease, a widening of the gap junctions between adjacent epithelial cells observed on electronic microscopy of distal esophageal mucosa[13] may be the harbinger of more serious histologic changes related to gastric acid and pepsin.[14] Vagal reflexes and impaired airway protection mechanisms may be responsible for airway complication of GER.

Decreased esophageal acid clearance mechanisms during sleep may lead to prolonged acid contact with the esophageal mucosa.[15] In the recumbent position, gravity and salivation are of little help to clear acid. Adults with nocturnal reflux symptoms have greater impairment of health-related quality of life than adults with nonnocturnal reflux symptoms.[16] Recumbent reflux episodes lasting longer than 5 minutes were predictive of erosive mucosal damage in adult GERD patients.[17] The significance of nocturnal GER is less well studied in pediatric patients than in adults. In children with GER, prolonged esophageal pH monitoring detected acid reflux during sleep in 21 of 22 children with endoscopy-confirmed esophagitis and recurrent lower respiratory tract symptoms, whereas GER was detected only in 8 of 19 children without esophagitis but with recurrent lower respiratory tract symptoms.[18]

Putative Genetic Predisposition for Gastroesophageal Reflux Disease

Familial clustering occurs for complications of GERD such as hiatal hernia, Barrett's esophagus, and esophageal adenocarcinoma in adults and in children.[19,20] Concordance for GER is higher in monozygotic twins than in dizygotic twins.[21] These observations suggest a genetic link, but although a locus on chromosome 13q14 was proposed for severe pediatric GERD phenotype,[22] the results have been questioned for technical reasons.[23] A locus on chromosome 9q22–9q31 was recently proposed in infants with esophagitis.

Clinical Manifestations

Mild reflux that does not compromise health, growth, or well-being occurs in many infants in the first year of life. These infants, often referred to as "happy spitters," develop normally, do not have excessive irritability, and exhibit no symptoms of respiratory disease. Vomiting or regurgitation is the most common manifestation of GER in these infants. The common presentation to the pediatrician of uncomplicated GER is effortless, painless vomiting in a thriving child with normal growth. GERD may develop in some children who manifest symptoms of weight loss or poor weight gain (failure to thrive), excessive irritability, anemia, hematochezia, and arching of the back during feedings. In rare situations, infants with GER may develop apparent life-threatening events (ALTE) or recurrent pneumonia. These serious problems in the infant younger than 6 months of age are rarely related solely to GERD and raise the specter of other global problems, such as central nervous system disease, cardiopulmonary disease, or mitochondrial disorders.

In the older preschool-aged children, GER may manifest as intermittent vomiting or an ill-defined sensation of epigastric or retrosternal discomfort. Older children are more likely to have an adult-type pattern of recurrent heartburn or regurgitation, with re-swallowing of gastric contents. Esophagitis in children may manifest as dysphagia or food impaction without evidence for a stricture. In younger children or older children who have had GER prior to the acquisition of language, refusal to eat solids or preference for only liquids may be the only symptoms of underlying GERD. Rarely, esophageal pain causes stereotypical repetitive stretching and arching movements that are mistaken for atypical seizures or a dystonic reaction (Sandifer's syndrome). More severe inflammation may cause chronic blood loss with anemia or hematemesis. Chronic inflammation, especially in the child with impaired clearance of regurgitated material into the esophagus, may result in Barrett's esophagus. The development of a columnar-lined esophagus is rare in children but may occur in children with severe spasticity from cerebral palsy, in children with repaired esophageal atresia, or in children with Down syndrome. These children have in common impaired esophageal motility and symptoms that begin prior to the development of language.

Diagnosis

Diagnostic tests are frequently performed in children suspected of having GER or GERD. Studies may document the presence of GER, complications of GERD, causal relationships between GER and symptoms such as cough or apnea, or disease improvement or resolution with medical or surgical therapy. In general, diagnostic tests can been divided into the following categories: (1) tests to quantify reflux, such as intraesophageal pH monitoring, scintigraphy, and intraluminal esophageal impedance; (2) assessment of inflammation by esophagogastroduodenoscopy and biopsy; (3) tests to assess conditions associated with GERD, such as scintigraphy, which measures gastric emptying, and esophageal manometry, which measures lower esophageal sphincter pressure and esophageal motility; and (4) measurements of disease activity using symptom assessment questionnaires or quality-of-life tools.

History and Physical Examination

In most infants and children with GER symptoms, a thorough history and physical examination is sufficient to suspect a diagnosis of GER. Most children with GERD have normal physical examination findings, but those with Sandifer's syndrome may exhibit unusual posturing that may be confused with a dystonic reaction or a seizure. The amount and frequency of each feeding, as ascertained by history-taking, may lead to a diagnosis of overfeeding, especially in the infant whose weight percentile greatly exceeds the height percentile. Observing the technique used to burp the infant should be part of the physical examination. Some parents need instruction in the proper positions for burping. Placing the infant over the shoulder or face down in the lap is often effective. Gentle rubbing of the back may help eliminate gas that is trapped in the stomach. GER that begins after 6 months of age is not physiologic and should prompt investigation for underlying causes. Similarly, fever, lethargy, hepatosplenomegaly, abdominal tenderness, abdominal distension, or neurologic symptoms such as seizures should raise concerns about serious illnesses associated with GER. Head growth is a critical aspect of the evaluation of any child with GER. Either macrocephaly or microcephaly may indicate a neurologic cause for GER. Children with GERD whose growth is delayed may be losing calories required to maintain a normal rate of growth but also may have an underlying metabolic abnormality contributing to growth delay. If the vomiting is forceful, bilious, or bloody, concern should be raised immediately about the possibility of obstruction or mucosal ulceration. Because of the length of the bowel in the infant, upper gastrointestinal bleeding most often manifests with hematochezia. Irritability or colic is very common in the first 2 months of life. Irritability that persists beyond 3 months or is associated with feeding raises the possibility of GERD. Assessment of a trial of acid suppression may be beneficial in establishing this diagnosis.

Most infants younger than 6 months of age with GER who have normal growth, no evidence of gastrointestinal blood loss, and no pulmonary symptoms do not develop GERD as they get older. However, any child who continues to regurgitate after 18 to 24 months of age or has any of the clinical warning signs, should be evaluated for other disorders or complications of GERD.

Upper Gastrointestinal Radiography

Upper gastrointestinal (or barium contrast) radiography cannot discriminate between physiologic and nonphysiologic GER episodes. The brief duration of the upper gastrointestinal series may result in false-negative findings, whereas the frequent occurrence of nonpathologic reflux results in false-positive findings. Therefore, barium contrast studies are not reliable diagnostic tests for GERD. However, an upper gastrointestinal series is useful for ruling out anatomic disorders that may manifest with GERD. In an infant with recurrent vomiting, contrast radiography can detect an esophageal or antral web, malrotation, or pyloric stenosis. If pyloric stenosis is suspected, ultrasonography is the diagnostic test of choice. Disorders of esophageal motility, such as achalasia, may also be detected, although young children with early achalasia may not have a dilated esophagus or the typical beaking seen in older patients. In an infant or a child with recurrent pneumonia, aspiration may be detected during the barium swallow. In neonates, small amounts of aspiration occur frequently and are not associated with serious problems. Aspiration is rare in the otherwise neurologically intact child, but a laryngeal cleft or tracheoesophageal fistula may be suspected in the otherwise normal child with recurrent pneumonia. Complications of GER, such as esophageal stricture or severe esophagitis, occasionally are detected by barium contrast radiography.

pH Monitoring

Intraesophageal pH monitoring is used clinically to assess the relationship between symptoms and GER by measuring the frequency and duration of acid reflux episodes to determine esophageal acid exposure. Patients with delayed acid clearance may be at increased risk for complications of GER. This test cannot detect non-acidic reflux episodes. Patients with an apparent life-threatening event or aspiration pneumonia may have brief reflux episodes that trigger the response but are within the range of "normal" GER. Esophageal pH monitoring is useful for detecting apnea only if performed simultaneously with measurement of respiration and chest wall movement.

An alternative to esophageal pH monitoring via nasal catheter is a catheter-free pH monitoring system called Bravo. A small capsule containing a radiotransmitter is clipped endoscopically onto the wall of the distal esophagus. The capsule can monitor pH for up to 48 hours and transmits data to a device that can be worn on the patient's belt. Over time, the capsule detaches from the esophageal wall and passes spontaneously through the gastrointestinal tract. There are currently no data on the use of this system in pediatric patients.

Esophagogastroduodenoscopy

Esophagogastroduodenoscopy enables visualization and biopsy of the esophageal epithelium. Children require sedation or general anesthesia for this procedure. Visually, one can determine the presence and severity of esophagitis, stricture, and Barrett's esophagus, and histologically, one can diagnose eosinophilic or infectious esophagitis. The presence of inflammation in the esophagus most commonly suggests peptic injury, whereas inflammation in the stomach or duodenum may support other conditions, such as food allergy or allergic gastroenteritis. Grading systems for the severity of erosive esophagitis, such as the Los Angeles classification,[24] have not yet been validated in pediatric patients. In children, there is a poor correlation between endoscopic appearance and histopathology. Therefore, esophageal biopsy is recommended when diagnostic endoscopy is performed.[25] In general, esophagogastroduodenoscopy is not useful for establishing the diagnosis of extra-esophageal manifestations of GERD.

Scintigraphy

The role of nuclear scintigraphy in the evaluation of pediatric GERD is unclear. A nuclear scan can detect reflux of nonacidic as well as acidic gastric contents and can provide information about gastric emptying. Refluxed gastric contents that are aspirated can be detected by scanning the lungs. However, a lack of standardized techniques and the absence of age-specific normative data limit the value of scintigraphy. Because this test is limited to observations in the immediate postprandial period, its value in assessing episodes of GERD is limited.

Multiple Intraluminal Electrical Impedance Measurement

Multiple intraluminal electrical impedance measurement is a pH-independent test that can detect acidic and nonacidic GER.[26] In infants, nonacidic GER has been suspected to be associated with respiratory symptoms.[25] Multiple intraluminal electrical impedance measurement has limited current clinical application because there are no well-defined normal values for pediatric age groups and ambulatory equipment is not yet available.

Empiric Therapy as a Diagnostic Test

The rationale for empiric therapy in adults with GERD is well accepted,[27] but there are no evidence-based studies in children to support the use of empiric trials. Nevertheless, standards of practice have established monitoring response to acid suppression as evidence of peptic-related disease. In pediatric patients, the decision to proceed to empiric therapy is supported by many considerations. GERD in most children is not associated with complications such as stricture or Barrett's esophagus. When the presenting symptoms are typical of GERD and there is no evidence for another disease that may manifest with vomiting, the diagnosis of GERD can be based on the history, and further diagnostic investigation is unlikely to alter initial management. If symptoms are caused by acid, most patients will respond to treatment with acid suppression.[25] Empiric therapy has not been validated for specific symptoms in pediatric patients, although the benefit of empiric treatment trials with omeprazole has been reported in adults with cough, heartburn, noncardiac chest pain, and dyspepsia. The concern with empiric trials in children is that patients who are at risk for developing complications of GERD may have intermittent symptoms in the early phases of the disease. Treatment may obscure the diagnosis of slow progression over many years.

Differential Diagnosis

Some of the disorders that manifest with recurrent vomiting and may mimic GERD[25] are listed in Table 1. Allergy, anatomic abnormalities, and renal and central nervous system diseases are among the many disorders that may have vomiting or regurgitation as the presenting symptoms. Laboratory studies, including complete blood count, electrolyte and blood urea nitrogen measurement, and review of newborn screening for metabolic disorders may be relevant to the evaluation of the newborn. An upper gastrointestinal series is recommended to evaluate anatomy in the infant with criteria predictive of GERD, listed earlier. Other diagnostic tests should be guided by the clinical presentation.

In many children, symptoms of GERD may be caused by a reaction to dietary protein, commonly termed "food allergy." Many of these chil-

TABLE 1. Differential Diagnosis of Vomiting in Infants and Children	
Systems	**Conditions**
Gastrointestinal	Pyloric stenosis
	Malrotation
	Intermittent intussusception
	Achalasia
	Gastroparesis
	Gastroenteritis
Infectious	Sepsis
	Meningitis
	Urinary tract infection
Neurologic	Hydrocephalus
	Subdural hematoma
	Intracranial hemorrhage
Renal	Obstructive uropathy
	Renal insufficiency
Metabolic	Galactosemia
	Fructose intolerance
	Urea cycle defects
Others	Congestive heart failure
	Dietary protein intolerance
	Lead poisoning

dren have histologic changes in the esophagus. In addition to GER, the differential diagnosis of esophagitis should include eosinophilic esophagitis and food allergy or intolerance. In patients with reflux symptoms unresponsive to appropriate acid suppression, the presence of numerous intraepithelial eosinophils may be a clue that the symptoms are related to specific foods[28] or allergy.[29,30] Intraepithelial eosinophils in the esophagus have been considered a marker for injury from acid reflux, and their presence correlates with abnormal esophageal acid clearance.[31] However, eosinophilia is not specific for GER. An endoscopic indication of eosinophilic esophagitis is a furrowed, occasionally ringed appearance of the esophageal mucosa, without erosions or other mucosal breaks. This pattern is also called *felinization*.[32] Histologic criteria for reflux esophagitis were defined in a study of 35 infants aged 2 weeks to 24 months with symptomatic GER. If the biopsy reveals extensive eosinophilia, for example, more than 20 intraepithelial eosinophils per high-power microscopic field, an allergic condition or idiopathic esophagitis, rather than GER, should be considered.[33]

Complications

Esophagitis and Barrett's Esophagus

In a series of 402 patients (1.5 to 25 years of age) who were admitted to the hospital and underwent esophagogastroduodenoscopy, erosive esophagitis was reported in 34.6% of children (mean age, 9.7 years) with GERD.[34] These children were neurologically normal and without congenital esophageal anomalies, but the percentage of children with erosive disease is significantly higher than that observed in outpatient populations. Nevertheless, the prevalence of erosive esophagitis seems to increase with age in the pediatric population. There is concern among clinicians that if esophageal inflammation caused by GER is untreated, stricture may form. Esophageal stricture was reported in 1.5% and Barrett's esophagus was suspected in 2.7% of pediatric patients in this cohort.[34] However, intestinal metaplasia or dysplasia was not seen in any biopsy samples. In a separate study, Barrett's esophagus was estimated in only 0.02% of children undergoing endoscopy, most of whom had risk factors for severe GERD (e.g., congenital esophageal anomalies, cerebral palsy).[36]

Asthma

Children with asthma likely represent a heterogeneous group of patients, and bronchospasm may have identifiable precipitants, which differ among subgroups of patients. Some children may wheeze in response to inhaled or ingested allergens; others may have respiratory distress in response to GER or viral infection. GER may not be a primary cause of asthma, although up to 50% of asthmatic children may have esophagitis,[18,37] GER likely exacerbates asthma by increasing airway hyperreactivity, either by causing microaspiration of acidic refluxate into the bronchial tree or via a vagally mediated esophagobronchial reflux. GER symptoms are common in children with asthma. The reported prevalence rates in 13 case series ranged from 25% to 75%.[25] About 50% of children with persistent asthma and abnormal esophageal pH study findings have no or minimal GER symptoms, including vomiting, regurgitation, and heartburn.

The association between nocturnal GER and asthma remains controversial. A potential association has been suggested in adult patients with asthma, and 24-hour esophageal pH monitoring has documented significantly more acid reflux during sleep in asthmatic adults than in nonasthmatic adults.[38] In children, some studies support this association,[39,40] whereas others do not.[41] Treatment trials with proton pump inhibitors or histamine-2 receptor antagonists in asthma patients with nocturnal symptoms have produced mixed results. In adults, omeprazole has been reported to improve nocturnal asthma symptoms[42] or have no effect.[43] In studies involving adults[44] and children,[45] ranitidine has produced modest effects.

Data from four case series reporting on 168 pediatric patients with asthma showed that clinical improvement or reduced dosages of bronchodilator and anti-inflammatory medications occurred in 63% of patients treated with conservative management (positional therapy and thickened formula), cisapride, and ranitidine.[45–48] Results from studies on adults have suggested that the duration of therapy is important, and aggressive acid suppression for at least 3 months may be necessary to reduce respiratory symptoms.

In six case series of asthmatic children who underwent antireflux surgery ($n = 258$), clinical improvement (decreased frequency and severity of asthmatic attacks) and reduced dosages of bronchodilator and anti-inflammatory medications occurred in 85%.[25] It appears that the children all have severe persistent asthma requiring intensive steroid therapy before surgery, and the diagnosis of GER was most often confirmed by esophageal pH studies. Failure of antireflux medical therapy did not preclude a favorable response to antireflux surgery.

To assess the clinical response to controlling GER, a 3-month trial of effective acid suppressive therapy may be administered to children in whom symptoms of asthma and GER coexist, or in infants and toddlers with chronic vomiting or regurgitation and recurrent episodes of cough and wheezing.[25] Outcome variables (e.g., frequency of GER or asthma symptoms, symptom scores, changes in spirometry measurements) should be determined prior to initiating therapy and then monitored during therapy. In patients with persistent asthma in whom GER symptoms are absent, esophageal pH monitoring is beneficial in select patients who are more likely to benefit from antireflux therapy. Children with radiographic evidence of recurrent pneumonia, nocturnal asthma more than once a week, or dependency on oral corticosteroids or high-dose inhaled corticosteroids are more at risk to have GERD and asthma. If pH studies in this population of children show an increased frequency or duration of esophageal acid exposure, a trial of prolonged antireflux medical therapy may be beneficial in establishing the association. Again, outcome variables should be determined prior to initiating therapy and then monitored during therapy.

Aspiration

Chronic pulmonary aspiration occurs when airway protective mechanisms are defective or overwhelmed and the lungs are contaminated with pharyngeal and/or gastric contents. The extent of pulmonary injury depends on the frequency, quantity, and composition of the aspirate. The sequelae of aspiration include interstitial lung disease, pulmonary fibrosis, acid aspiration pneumonitis, and aspiration pneumonia with pleural effusion. Aspiration is more common in children with neurologic disorders, who often have impaired airway protective mechanisms, than in other children with GER symptoms. Because of oropharyngeal incoordination, these children may also aspirate during swallowing. Distinguishing reflux from aspiration may be difficult. In most children, aspiration pneumonitis resolves spontaneously. Bacterial pneumonia, reflecting the anaerobic flora in the mouth, occurs in about 20% to 45% of patients who aspirate gastric contents. This may occur as early as 2 days but usually develops within 1 week of aspiration. In about 10% of patients, a fulminant course ensues, with progressive respiratory failure in 24 to 48 hours.

Specific tests to detect aspiration are limited in sensitivity and may be difficult to interpret because small amounts of aspiration may occur without ill effect. One test consists of obtaining macrophages by pulmonary lavage during flexible bronchoscopy and staining for milk-derived lipid. Lipid-filled vacuoles may be observed in the cytoplasm; the presence of large numbers of lipid-laden macrophages is suggestive of pulmonary aspiration.[49] However, considerable overlap in lipid content exists between normal control subjects, patients with other causes of pulmonary disease, and patients with a history consistent with aspiration.[25] In addition, bronchoscopy with pulmonary lavage cannot distinguish between aspiration due to GER and aspiration during swallowing. The quantity of lipid-laden macrophages is thought to be important in establishing a diagnosis, but to date no system of measuring the extent of lipid infiltration has been found to be clinically useful. The higher the value on a lipid-laden alveolar macrophage score[35] or lipid-laden macrophage index,[49] the greater the likelihood of chronic pulmonary aspiration. Nevertheless, studies have shown considerable overlap in results between patients with and without aspiration.

A barium esophagram and upper gastrointestinal series may be useful when respiratory complications of GER are suspected. Although not as sensitive or specific as other tests, they can rule out potential anatomic causes, such as an antral web or malrotation. Anatomic abnormalities are important to consider in the pediatric population. Nuclear scintigraphy offers some advantages over contrast radiography as diagnostic tool. Labeling saliva with technetium-99m and scanning over the upper airway may identify aspiration that is not associated with GERD. This test, termed a *salivogram,* may be the only way to distinguish between aspiration with GER and aspiration without GER.

Upper Airway Symptoms

Laryngeal inflammation in children may be caused by minute amounts of subglottic acid exposure. A fiberoptic laryngoscopic evaluation is preferable to dual-level esophageal pH monitoring and can distinguish posterior laryngeal inflammation from isolated laryngomalacia or other airway abnormalities, such as a laryngeal cleft. pH probe testing often is not sensitive enough to detect the small amounts of acid that may reflux into the airway. Laryngitis is manifested by hoarseness in verbal children and by a hoarse cry in nonverbal children. There are limited data on the association between GER and chronic laryngeal symptoms, such as cough and hoarseness.[50] There are no randomized placebo-controlled treatment trials to evaluate antireflux therapy in adults or children with GER-related laryngeal symptoms. Uncontrolled case series in children have demonstrated symptomatic improvement, but high doses of acid suppression medications are often required. Studies in adults suggest that a therapeutic trial must be prolonged (longer than 3 months) to adequately assess therapy.

Extraesophageal Complications

The causal relationship between GER and a number of extraesophageal complications, including dental erosion, recurrent sinusitis and otitis media, has not been definitively studied in the pediatric population.[2,52–55] There are no reported studies on the association between otitis media and GER, but otalgia has been associated with GER and was reported to improve with antireflux treatment.[56] Randomized placebo-controlled trails are needed to determine the etiologic role of GER in these conditions, and appropriate diagnostic testing is needed to enable pediatric practitioners to practice evidence-based medicine.[57]

Apparent Life-Threatening Event

An apparent life-threatening event (ALTE) is defined as an episode in an infant that is frightening to the observer and characterized by a combination of apnea, change in color (e.g., cyanosis, pallor, rubor), change in muscle tone (limpness, stiffness), or choking and gagging that requires intervention by the caregiver. An ALTE may be caused by a number of different conditions, including cardiac disease, upper airway obstruction, central nervous system disorder, infection, GER, and intentional suffocation. The prevalence of recurrent regurgitation or emesis in infants with ALTE is thought to be between 60% to 70%,[25] and abnormal esophageal pH studies have been demonstrated in 40% to 80% of infants. Studies in unselected patients with ALTE, however, failed to demonstrate a convincing temporal relationship between acid reflux and apnea or bradycardia. Children often had apneic episodes unrelated to GER episodes. GER may be the underlying cause in as many as 20% of infants with infantile apnea,[58] however, the range of duration of normal acid clearance in infants younger than 1 year of age is so great that most infants with pathologic reflux fall within this range. Even finding greater than normal acid reflux does not establish a causal relationship in infants with apnea.[59,60] Apnea related to reflux usually occurs when the infant is awake, supine, and fed within the past hour.[25] It appears to be obstructive (with persistence of respiratory effort) rather than central (absence of respiratory effort), and may occur in infants with no history of regurgitation.[61] Esophageal pH monitoring is useful to determine a temporal association between acid reflux and ALTE only if performed simultaneously with measurement of respiration and chest wall movement. In managing children with ALTE and GER, the effectiveness of antireflux therapy has not been adequately studied. Therapeutic options include thickened feedings, prokinetic therapy, and acid suppression. Since many infants improve with maturation, antireflux surgery should be reserved for infants in whom a definitive association with reflux can be established.

Management

Conservative Management

In an infant with uncomplicated GER, parental education, reassurance, and anticipatory guidance are recommended. Management options include thickening of formula and possibly a 1- or 2-week trial of a hypoallergenic formula. Thickening of formula has been shown to decrease regurgitation, increase sleep time, and reduce crying time.[62] In the United States, thickening is usually achieved with the addition of rice cereal to formula. If an infant formula has a caloric density of 20 kcal per ounce, the addition of 1 tablespoonful of rice cereal per ounce of formula increases the caloric density to about 34 kcal per ounce.[25] Commercially available ready-to-feed thickened formulas can be purchased. Pharmacotherapy usually is not recommended for the "happy spitter" who is otherwise thriving. If symptoms do not improve by 18 to 24 months of age, further diagnostic evaluation is recommended.

Management in the Neurologically Compromised Child

Gastroesophageal reflex with or without aspiration occurs frequently in neurologically impaired children, especially those with mental retardation,[63,64] cerebral palsy, spasticity, tetraplegia,[65,66] and hydrocephalus.[67] GER in neurologically impaired children is a challenge, because the child may not communicate his or her discomfort. These children appear to be at a higher risk for erosive esophagitis and are often resistant to standard medical treatment.[67,68] Surgical options include fundoplication and esophagogastric disconnection.[69] Antireflux surgery is effective in controlling GER but has been associated with a high risk of complications, including recurrent GER after fundoplication, and the need for reoperations.[70–72] The possibility of aspiration increases in these children after fundoplication because they may not be able to empty their esophagus as well with a wrap. Antireflux surgery should be avoided in children with neurologic deficits who preoperatively exhibit symptoms caused by activation of the emetic reflex, such as pallor, sweating, retching, and forceful vomiting.[73]

Pharmacotherapy

The goal of pharmacotherapy for GER is to control symptoms, promote healing, and prevent complications by reducing exposure of the esophagus or respiratory tract to acid refluxate. The two major pharmacotherapies for GERD include acid suppression and prokinetic agents.

Acid Suppressants. Antacids neutralize gastric acid and are commonly used for the short-term relief of intermittent GER symptoms in children and adolescents. Although there appears to be little risk to this therapy, supportive evidence is lacking. In infants, treatment with aluminum-containing antacids may significantly increase plasma aluminum levels and cause constipation.[74] Magnesium-containing antacids are more likely to cause diarrhea in infants. Because more convenient and safe alternatives are available, chronic antacid therapy is generally not recommended. Surface agents include sodium alginate and sucralfate gel. Sucralfate also is an aluminum complex, and potential adverse effects of excess aluminum in infants and children need to be considered.

Histamine-2 Receptor Antagonists (H₂RAs). H₂RAs suppress gastric acid secretion of the parietal cell by inhibiting the binding of histamine to specific (histamine-2) receptors on the luminal surface. Activation of these receptors by histamine stimulates the parietal cell to secrete acid by triggering a sequence of intracellular events that lead to activation of the hydrogen/potassium adenosine triphosphatase (H^+, K^+-ATPase). H^+, K^+-ATPase is the final step in acid production and is also known as the proton pump.

Results from two randomized placebo-controlled trials evaluating H₂RAs in children with reflux esophagitis showed that cimetidine treatment had a significant positive impact on healing of esophagitis.[75,76] There is important pediatric information in the approved label for both Pepcid (famotidine) and Zantac (ranitidine). Pepcid is indicated for use in pediatric patients 1 to 16 years of age with GERD with or without esophagitis. Recent changes encompassed labeling for patients younger than 1 year of age. Zantac is indicated for use in pediatric patients aged 1 month to 16 years for the treatment of GERD and erosive esophagitis. Recent labeling changes encompassed extension of the age range to include 0 to 1 month. Pediatric information is not provided in the approved labels for Axid (nizatidine) or Tagamet (cimetidine). The North American Society for Pediatric Gastroenterology, Hepatology, and Nutrition (NASPGHAN) recommended dosages of H₂RA for use in infants and children are listed in Table 2,[25] along with recommended dosages

TABLE 2.	Pharmacotherapy for Gastroesophageal Reflux Disease in the Pediatric Population	
Medication	**Dose in Infants and Children**	**Dose in Adults**
H₂RA		
Cimetidine	40 mg/kg/day divided tid or qid	1600 mg/day
Famotidine	1 mg/kg/day divided bid	20 or 40 mg bid
Nizatidine	10 mg/kg/day divided bid	150 mg bid or 300 mg HS
Ranitidine	5–10 mg/kg/day divided tid	150 mg bid-qid
PPI		
Lansoprazole	15 mg qd (body weight ≤30 kg) or 30 mg qd (>30 kg)	15 or 30 mg qd
Omeprazole	10 mg qd (body weight <20 kg) or 20 mg (≥20 kg) *or* 1.0 mg/kg/day qd or divided bid	20 mg qd
Esomeprazole	Not available	20 or 40 mg qd
Pantoprazole	Not available	40 mg qd
Rabeprazole	Not available	20 mg qd
H₂RA = histamine-2 receptor antagonist; PPI = proton pump inhibitor		

in adults with GERD. As a class, H_2RAs appear to have a good safety profile and are well tolerated. Commonly reported adverse effects and precautions with these medications are listed in Table 3.[25]

Proton Pump Inhibitor. The enzyme H^+, K^+-ATPase, or the proton pump, is present in the canalicular membrane of gastric parietal cells, where it secretes hydrochloric acid and hydrogen ion (H^+) in exchange for potassium ion (K^+). H^+,K^+-ATPase inhibitors, or proton pump inhibitors (PPIs), cross the membrane of parietal cells and accumulate in the secretory canaliculus. In an acidic environment, PPIs are converted to an activated form (sulfenamide), and the activated PPI binds to and inhibits active proton pumps. PPIs are most effective when the parietal cell is stimulated to secrete acid in response to a meal.

Data are limited on PPI pharmacology in infants and children. Pharmacokinetic and pharmacodynamic properties of lansoprazole and omeprazole have been studied in children,[77–80] but no randomized placebo-controlled trials of PPIs in infants or children have been reported to date. A randomized controlled study comparing omeprazole and high-dose ranitidine demonstrated comparable effectiveness in reducing symptoms and improving histopathology in 25 infants and children with

TABLE 3.	Side Effects of Histamine-2 Receptor Antagonists (H_2RAs) and Proton Pump Inhibitors (PPIs)			
Medications	**Headache, Dizziness, Nausea**	**Constipation, Diarrhea**	**Skin Rash**	**Others**
H_2RAs				
Cimetidine	yes	no	yes	Gynecomastia, neutropenia, thrombocytopenia, agranulocytosis, bradycardia
Famotidine	yes	yes	no	
Nizatidine	yes	yes	no	Anemia, urticaria
Ranitidine	yes	yes	yes	Thrombocytopenia, elevated liver transaminases, fatigue, irritability
PPIs				
Omeprazole	yes	yes	yes	Vitamin B_{12} deficiency, abdominal pain
Lansoprazole	yes	yes	no	Elevated liver transaminases, abdominal pain, proteinuria, angina, hypotension
Esomeprazole	yes	diarrhea only	no	Gastritis, abdominal pain, respiratory infection
Pantoprazole	yes	diarrhea only	no	Abdominal pain
Rabeprazole	yes	diarrhea only	no	Abdominal pain

esophagitis.[81] It should be noted that this study used a relatively low omeprazole dose (40 mg/1.73/m²) and a very high ranitidine dose (20 mg/kg). In reported series of children with esophagitis refractory to H₂RA and other treatments, omeprazole and lansoprazole have been shown to be more effective. The efficacy of other PPIs (esomeprazole, pantoprazole, rabeprazole) in the pediatric population has not yet been reported.

The safety and effectiveness of Prevacid (lansoprazole) has been established in patients aged 1 to 11 years for the treatment of symptomatic GERD and erosive esophagitis. The safety and effectiveness of Prilosec (omeprazole) has been established in patients aged 2 to 16 years for acid-related gastrointestinal diseases, including the treatment of symptomatic GERD, treatment of erosive esophagitis, and maintenance of healing of erosive esophagitis. Pediatric information is not provided in the approved labels for Aciphex (rabeprazole), Nexium (esomeprazole), or Protonix (pantoprazole).

The recommended omeprazole dosage in the NASPGHAN guideline was 1.0 mg/kg every day or divided into twice-a-day dosing.[25] The recommended Prilosec dose is 10 mg/day if body weight is less than 20 kg and 20 mg/day if weight is 20 kg or greater. The recommended Prevacid dosage for the treatment of symptomatic GERD and erosive esophagitis is 15 mg every day for up to 12 weeks if body weight is 30 kg or less and 30 mg every day for up to 12 weeks if weight is greater than 30 kg. The available information on pediatric dosing for PPIs is listed in Table 2. Pediatric dosing information for esomeprazole, pantoprazole, and rabeprazole is currently not available.

The PPIs are available in capsule (esomeprazole, lansoprazole, omeprazole), tablet (pantoprazole, rabeprazole), and packet granule (lansoprazole) formulations. In addition, lansoprazole is available as a strawberry-flavored oral suspension. In Canada, omeprazole is available as a multiple unit pellet system formulation. For patients who have difficulty swallowing capsules or tablets, one option is to open a capsule or packet granules and sprinkle the intact granules or pellets on applesauce. Alternatively, a PPI capsule can be emptied in water or juice, but should not be chewed. **Optimal effectiveness is achieved when the PPI is administered one half-hour before breakfast so that peak plasma concentrations coincide with the meal.**[25] If there is a second daily dose, it is best administered one half-hour before the evening meal.

The safety profiles of PPIs in the pediatric population have not been well studied. Reported adverse effects are listed in Table 3.[77]

Two approaches to acid-reducing therapy have been described. A step-down approach, currently favored by many practitioners, starts with a PPI as a first-line acid-suppression treatment. After improvement is achieved and maintained with a PPI, the patient is switched to an

H_2RA. In contrast, a step-up approach begins treatment with an H_2RA. If there is an inadequate response, treatment is switched to a PPI. If the response remains inadequate, an increase in PPI dose is the next step. There are no published studies comparing these strategies in children.

Prokinetic Agents. The rationale for prokinetic therapy in the treatment of GERD is based on evidence that such medications enhance esophageal peristalsis and accelerate gastric emptying.[25] The only prokinetic agent that has been shown to effectively reduce esophageal acid exposure in children is cisapride, a mixed serotonergic agonist. However, cisapride has been withdrawn and is available in the United States only through a limited-access program to patients for whom other antireflux therapies are ineffective. Studies evaluating bethanechol, a direct cholinergic agonist, and domperidone, a dopamine antagonist available in Canada, have been few and have reported mixed results.[25] There is only one randomized controlled trial evaluating bethanechol,[82] and none evaluating domperidone in children with GER. Studies with erythromycin have suggested that its prokinetic effects on the gastrointestinal tract occur at doses lower than those used to treat infection.[83] Erythromycin has been evaluated in various pediatric populations, but there is no randomized controlled trial in children with GER. The efficacy of metoclopramide, an antidopaminergic agent, has been evaluated in a randomized controlled trial in children with GER. Esophageal pH improvement was reported in one of six trials and clinical improvement in one of four trials. Use of metoclopramide has been hampered by a high incidence of adverse events, including central nervous system side effects.

The safety profiles of bethanechol and metoclopramide have limited their use for treatment of GERD in adults.[84] Bethanechol at 25 mg four times a day has been associated with significant abdominal cramping, blurred vision, fatigue, and urinary urgency,[84] and bethanechol is contraindicated in patients with hyperthyroidism, bronchial asthma, and other conditions. The adverse effect with domperidone such as prolactinemia occurred in 10% to 15% of adult patients, and other minor side effects, including dry mouth, skin rash, headache, diarrhea, and restlessness, have occasionally been reported.[84] Adverse effects associated with metoclopromide include central nervous system complications, such as parkinsonian reactions and tardive dyskinesia, which may be irreversible. Strict limitation of dose is important to prevent extrapyramidal adverse effect. Irritability and sleep disturbances may result from even a relatively low dose of metoclopramide (0.1 mg/kg Qid).

Antireflux Surgery

The objectives of antireflux surgery are to restore the intra-abdominal portion of the esophagus, approximate diaphragmatic cruae, and reduce hiatal hernia when present. Fundoplication, which is the wrapping of the fundus around the LES, is commonly performed by the Nissen method (a 360-degree wrap). The results of pediatric series of laparoscopic fundoplication suggest that outcome and complication rates are similar to those with the open procedure, but the hospital stay is shortened.[85]

Candidates for antireflux surgery include children with GERD who have failed medical therapy and have a complication of GERD. Postoperative morbidity is higher in pediatric patients with neurologic impairment, esophageal atresia, and chronic pulmonary disease. Symptoms associated with activation of the emetic reflex (pallor, sweating, retching, forceful vomiting) have been identified as predictors of failure of antireflux surgery in neurologically impaired children with GER symptoms.[73]

In one study of 12 children aged 0.5 to 13 years, the effect of antireflux surgery on mechanisms underlying GER was studied.[86] One month after laparoscopic Nissen fundoplication, continuous manometric evaluation was performed for an hour before and after the administration of apple juice. There was a significant postprandial increase in basal LES pressure, compared with a decrease in preoperative values. In addition, there was significant residual LES pressure at the nadir of swallow-induced LES relaxation and no significant changes on the motility of the esophageal body. These findings were similar to effects reported in children who underwent open Nissen fundoplication and in adults.

Complete relief of symptoms has been reported in 57% to 92% of children with GERD who undergo antireflux surgery.[25] The rate of mortality related to the operation ranged from 0% to 4.7%, and unrelated mortality rates from comorbid conditions were 0% to 21%. Overall complication rates of 2.2% to 45% have been reported. Commonly reported complications include dumping syndrome, gas-bloat syndrome, small-bowel obstruction, and wrap breakdown.[25,87,88] Up to 19% of patients may require reoperation.

Newer and Investigational Approaches to Antireflux Therapy

Several new therapeutic approaches to antireflux treatment have been developed, including endotherapies that have been approved by the Food and Drug Administration, investigational endoscopic techniques to enhance the antireflux barrier, and investigational pharmacologic agents. Both endoscopically guided delivery of radiofrequency energy (Stretta) and endoscopic sewing devices (EndoCinch) have been approved by the Food and Drug Administration. The role of these outpatient procedures in antireflux management is not yet defined, and long-term effects are largely unknown.[89] These approaches have not been evaluated in pediatric patients. Investigational endoscopic techniques also include the injection of polymers at the gastroesophageal junction.[90,91] A number of investigational agents are being evaluated to inhibit transient LES relaxations, including cholecystokinin-A antagonists, anticholinergic agents, nitric oxide synthase inhibitors, somatostatin, serotonin type 3-receptor antagonists, and γ-aminobutyric acid-B agonists, such as baclofen.[92–94] None of these therapies have been reported in the pediatric population.

Key Points: Gastroesophageal Reflux Disease in Children

- GER in the vast majority of children younger than 1 year of age resolves without sequelae. However, when GERD begins after the age of 2 years, concerns are raised that this could be the early manifestation of disease that will develop as the child gets older.
- Children with neuromuscular disorders, including esophageal dysmotility, are at an increased risk to develop complications of GERD.
- GERD in the pediatric population should be considered to be part of a continuum that includes all ages.
- We do not have sufficient knowledge to understand all the factors that contribute to strictures, Barrett's esophagus, and adenocarcinoma in this clinical setting. Fortunately, these complications are rare in the pediatric population.
- The question remains whether early diagnosis and effective treatment in childhood will modify the course of disease in the adults. Studies are needed in the pediatric population to answer this question.

Suggested Reading

1. Nelson SP, Chen EH, Syniar GM, et al: Prevalence of symptoms of gastroesophageal reflux during infancy: a pediatric practice-based survey. Pediatric Practice Research Group. Arch Pediatr Adolesc Med 151:569–572, 1997.
2. Nelson SP, Chen EH, Syniar GM, et al: One-year follow-up of symptoms of gastroesophageal reflux during infancy. Pediatric Practice Research Group. Pediatrics 102:E67, 1998.
3. Nelson SP, Chen EH, Syniar GM, et al: Prevalence of symptoms of gastroesophageal reflux during childhood: a pediatric practice-based survey. Pediatric Practice Research Group. Arch Pediatr Adolesc Med 154:150–154. 2000.
4. Locke GR 3rd, Talley NJ, Fett SL, et al: Prevalence and clinical spectrum of gastroesophageal reflux: a population-based study in Olmsted County, Minnesota. Gastroenterology 112:1448–1456, 1997.

5. Mittal RK, Balaban DH: The esophagogastric junction. N Engl J Med 336:924–932, 1997.

6. Mittal RK, Holloway RH, Penagini R, et al: Transient lower esophageal sphincter relaxation. Gastroenterology 109:601–610, 1995.

7. Kawahara H, Dent J, Davidson G: Mechanisms responsible for gastroesophageal reflux in children. Gastroenterology 113:399–408, 1997.

8. Weaver T: Anatomy and Embryology. Philadelphia, BC Decker, 1991.

9. Lang IM, Medda BK, Shaker R: Mechanisms of reflexes induced by esophageal distension. Am J Physiol Gastrointest Liver Physiol 281:G1246–1263, 2001.

10. Omari TI, Barnett CP, Benninga MA, et al: Mechanisms of gastro-oesophageal reflux in preterm and term infants with reflux disease. Gut 51:475–479, 2002.

11. Ewer AK, Durbin GM, Morgan ME, et al: Gastric emptying in preterm infants. Arch Dis Child Fetal Neonatal Ed 71:F24–27, 1994.

12. Orlando RC: Mechanisms of reflux-induced epithelial injuries in the esophagus. Am J Med 108(Suppl 4a):104S-108S, 2000.

13. Tobey NA, Carson JL, Alkiek RA, et al: Dilated intercellular spaces: a morphological feature of acid reflux–damaged human esophageal epithelium. Gastroenterology 111:1200–1205, 1996.

14. Dent J: Gastro-oesophageal reflux disease. Digestion 59:433–445, 1998.

15. Orr WC, Robinson MG, Johnson LF: Acid clearance during sleep in the pathogenesis of reflux esophagitis. Dig Dis Sci 26:423–427, 1981.

16. Farup C, Kleinman L, Sloan S, et al: The impact of nocturnal symptoms associated with gastroesophageal reflux disease on health-related quality of life. Arch Intern Med 161:45–52, 2001.

17. Orr WC, Allen ML, Robinson M: The pattern of nocturnal and diurnal esophageal acid exposure in the pathogenesis of erosive mucosal damage. Am J Gastroenterol 89:509–512, 1994.

18. Baer M, Maki M, Nurminen J, et al: Esophagitis and findings of long-term esophageal pH recording in children with repeated lower respiratory tract symptoms. J Pediatr Gastroenterol Nutr 5:187–190, 1986.

19. Orenstein SR, Shalaby TM, Barmada MM, et al: Genetics of gastroesophageal reflux disease: a review. J Pediatr Gastroenterol Nutr 34:506–510, 2002.

20. Locke GR 3rd, Talley NJ, Fett SL, et al: Risk factors associated with symptoms of gastroesophageal reflux. Am J Med 106:642–649, 1999.

21. Cameron AJ, Lagergren J, Henriksson C, et al: Gastroesophageal reflux disease in monozygotic and dizygotic twins. Gastroenterology 122:55–59, 2002.

22. Hu FZ, Preston RA, Post JC, et al: Mapping of a gene for severe pediatric gastroesophageal reflux to chromosome 13q14. JAMA 284:325–334, 2000.

23. Orenstein SR, Shalaby TM, Finch R, et al: Autosomal dominant infantile gastroesophageal reflux disease: exclusion of a 13q14 locus in five well characterized families. Am J Gastroenterol 97:2725–2732, 2002.

24. Lundell LR, Dent J, Bennett JR, et al: Endoscopic assessment of oesophagitis: clinical and functional correlates and further validation of the Los Angeles classification. Gut 45:172–180, 1999.

25. Rudolph CD, Mazur LJ, Liptak GS, et al: Guidelines for evaluation and treatment of gastroesophageal reflux in infants and children: recommendations of the North American Society for Pediatric Gastroenterology and Nutrition. J Pediatr Gastroenterol Nutr 32(Suppl 2):S1–31, 2001.

26. Wenzl TG: Investigating esophageal reflux with the intraluminal impedance technique. J Pediatr Gastroenterol Nutr 34:261–268, 2002.

27. DeVault KR, Castell DO. Updated guidelines for the diagnosis and treatment of gas-

troesophageal reflux disease. The Practice Parameters Committee of the American College of Gastroenterology. Am J Gastroenterol 94:1434–1442, 1999.

28. Kelly KJ, Lazenby AJ, Rowe PC, et al: Eosinophilic esophagitis attributed to gastroesophageal reflux: improvement with an amino acid-based formula. Gastroenterology 109:1503–1512, 1995.

29. Iacono G, Carroccio A, Cavataio F, et al: Gastroesophageal reflux and cow's milk allergy in infants: a prospective study. J Allergy Clin Immunol 97:822–827, 1996.

30. Walsh SV, Antonioli DA, Goldman H, et al: Allergic esophagitis in children: a clinicopathological entity. Am J Surg Pathol 23:390–396, 1999.

31. Winter HS, Madara JL, Stafford RJ, et al: Intraepithelial eosinophils: a new diagnostic criterion for reflux esophagitis. Gastroenterology 83:818–823, 1982.

32. Bousvaros A, Antonioli DA, Winter HS: Ringed esophagus: an association with esophagitis. Am J Gastroenterol 87:1187–1190, 1992.

33. Black DD, Haggitt RC, Orenstein SR, Whitington PF: Esophagitis in infants: morphometric histological diagnosis and correlation with measures of gastroesophageal reflux. Gastroenterology 98:1408–1414, 1990.

34. El-Serag HB, Bailey NR, Gilger M, et al: Endoscopic manifestations of gastroesophageal reflux disease in patients between 18 months and 25 years without neurological deficits. Am J Gastroenterol 97:1635–1639, 2002.

35. Ahrens P, Noll C, Kitz R, et al: Lipid-laden alveolar macrophages (LLAM): a useful marker of silent aspiration in children. Pediatr Pulmonol 28:83–88, 1999.

36. Hassall E: Co-morbidities in childhood Barrett's esophagus. J Pediatr Gastroenterol Nutr 25:255–260, 1997.

37. Shapiro GG, Christie DL: Gastroesophageal reflux in steroid-dependent asthmatic youths. Pediatrics 63:207–212, 1979.

38. Sontag SJ, O'Connell S, Khandelwal S, et al: Effect of positions, eating, and bronchodilators on gastroesophageal reflux in asthmatics. Dig Dis Sci 35:849–856, 1990.

39. Martin ME, Grunstein MM, Larsen GL: The relationship of gastroesophageal reflux to nocturnal wheezing in children with asthma. Ann Allergy 49:318–322, 1982.

40. Davis RS, Larsen GL, Grunstein MM: Respiratory response to intraesophageal acid infusion in asthmatic children during sleep. J Allergy Clin Immunol 72:393–398, 1983.

41. Hughes DM, Spier S, Rivlin J, et al: Gastroesophageal reflux during sleep in asthmatic patients. J Pediatr 102:666–672, 1983.

42. Kiljander TO, Salomaa ER, Hietanen EK, et al: Gastroesophageal reflux in asthmatics: a double-blind, placebo-controlled crossover study with omeprazole. Chest 116:1257–1264, 1999.

43. Ford GA, Oliver PS, Prior JS, et al: Omeprazole in the treatment of asthmatics with nocturnal symptoms and gastro-oesophageal reflux: a placebo-controlled cross-over study. Postgrad Med J 70:350–354, 1994.

44. Ekstrom T, Lindgren BR, Tibbling L: Effects of ranitidine treatment on patients with asthma and a history of gastro-oesophageal reflux: a double blind crossover study. Thorax 44:19–23, 1989.

45. Gustafsson PM, Kjellman NI, Tibbling L: A trial of ranitidine in asthmatic children and adolescents with or without pathological gastro-oesophageal reflux. Eur Respir J 5:201–206, 1992.

46. Andze GO, Brandt ML, St Vil D, et al: Diagnosis and treatment of gastroesophageal reflux in 500 children with respiratory symptoms: the value of pH monitoring. J Pediatr Surg 26:295–299, 1991.

47. Berquist WE, Rachelefsky GS, Kadden M, et al: Gastroesophageal reflux-associated recurrent pneumonia and chronic asthma in children. Pediatrics 68:29–35, 1981.

48. Tucci F, Resti M, Fontana R, et al: Gastroesophageal reflux and bronchial asthma: prevalence and effect of cisapride therapy. J Pediatr Gastroenterol Nutr 17:265–270, 1993.

49. Nussbaum E, Maggi JC, Mathis R, et al: Association of lipid-laden alveolar macrophages and gastroesophageal reflux in children. J Pediatr 110:190–194, 1987.

50. Bauer ML, Lyrene RK: Chronic aspiration in children: evaluation of the lipid-laden macrophage index. Pediatr Pulmonol 28:94–100, 1999.

51. Gumpert L, Kalach N, Dupont C, et al: Hoarseness and gastroesophageal reflux in children. J Laryngol Otol 112:49–54, 1998.

52. Dahshan A, Patel H, Delaney J, et al: Gastroesophageal reflux disease and dental erosion in children. J Pediatr 140:474–478, 2002.

53. O'Sullivan EA, Curzon ME, Roberts GJ, et al: Gastroesophageal reflux in children and its relationship to erosion of primary and permanent teeth. Eur J Oral Sci 106:765–769, 1998.

54. Phipps CD, Wood WE, Gibson WS, et al: Gastroesophageal reflux contributing to chronic sinus disease in children: a prospective analysis. Arch Otolaryngol Head Neck Surg 126:831–836, 2000.

55. El-Serag HB, Gilger M, Kuebeler M, et al: Extraesophageal associations of gastroesophageal reflux disease in children without neurologic defects. Gastroenterology 121:1294–1299, 2001.

56. Gibson WS Jr, Cochran W: Otalgia in infants and children: a manifestation of gastroesophageal reflux. Int J Pediatr Otorhinolaryngol 28:213–218, 1994.

57. Tolia V: Gastroesophageal reflux and supraesophageal complications: really true or ballyhoo? J Pediatr Gastroenterol Nutr 34:269–273, 2002.

58. Kahn A RE, Franco P, N'Duwimama M, Blum D: Apparently life-threatening events and apnea of infancy. In Beckerman R, Hunt C, eds: Respiratory Control Disorders in Infants and Children. Baltimore, Williams & Wilkins; 1992, p. 178–192.

59. Walsh JK, Farrell MK, Keenan WJ, et al: Gastroesophageal reflux in infants: relation to apnea. J Pediatr 99:197–201, 1981.

60. de Ajuriaguerra M, Radvanyi-Bouvet MF, Huon C, et al: Gastroesophageal reflux and apnea in prematurely born infants during wakefulness and sleep. Am J Dis Child 145:1132–1136, 1991.

61. Colletti RB, Christie DL, Orenstein SR: Statement of the North American Society for Pediatric Gastroenterology and Nutrition (NASPGN). Indications for pediatric esophageal pH monitoring. J Pediatr Gastroenterol Nutr 21:253–262, 1995.

62. Orenstein SR, Magill HL, Brooks P: Thickening of infant feedings for therapy of gastroesophageal reflux. J Pediatr 110:181–186, 1987.

63. Sondheimer JM, Morris BA: Gastroesophageal reflux among severely retarded children. J Pediatr 94:710–714, 1979.

64. Spitz L, Roth K, Kiely EM, et al: Operation for gastro-oesophageal reflux associated with severe mental retardation. Arch Dis Child 68:347–351, 1993.

65. Gustafsson PM, Tibbling L: Gastro-oesophageal reflux and oesophageal dysfunction in children and adolescents with brain damage. Acta Paediatr 83:1081–1085, 1994.

66. Ravelli AM, Milla PJ: Vomiting and gastroesophageal motor activity in children with disorders of the central nervous system. J Pediatr Gastroenterol Nutr 26:56–63, 1998.

67. Shteyer E, Rothman E, Constantini S, et al: Gastroesophageal reflux in infants with hydrocephalus before and after ventriculo-peritoneal shunt operation. Pediatr Neurosurg 29:138–141, 1998.

68. Wilkinson JD, Dudgeon DL, Sondheimer JM: A comparison of medical and surgical treatment of gastroesophageal reflux in severely retarded children. J Pediatr 99:202–205, 1981.

69. Danielson PD, Emmens RW: Esophagogastric disconnection for gastroesophageal reflux in children with severe neurological impairment. J Pediatr Surg 34:84–86, 1999.

70. Alexander F, Wyllie R, Jirousek K, et al: Delayed gastric emptying affects outcome of Nissen fundoplication in neurologically impaired children. Surgery 122:690–697, 1997.

71. Dedinsky GK, Vane DW, Black T, et al: Complications and reoperation after Nissen fundoplication in childhood. Am J Surg 153:177–183, 1987.

72. Subramaniam R, Dickson AP: Long-term outcome of Boix-Ochoa and Nissen fundoplication in normal and neurologically impaired children. J Pediatr Surg 35:1214–1216, 2000.

73. Richards CA, Milla PJ, Andrews PL, et al: Retching and vomiting in neurologically impaired children after fundoplication: predictive preoperative factors. J Pediatr Surg 36:1401–1404, 2001.

74. Tsou VM, Young RM, Hart MH, et al: Elevated plasma aluminum levels in normal infants receiving antacids containing aluminum. Pediatrics 87:148–151, 1991.

75. Cucchiara S, Gobio-Casali L, Balli F, et al: Cimetidine treatment of reflux esophagitis in children: an Italian multicentric study. J Pediatr Gastroenterol Nutr 8:150–156, 1989.

76. Simeone D, Caria MC, Miele E, et al: Treatment of childhood peptic esophagitis: a double-blind placebo-controlled trial of nizatidine. J Pediatr Gastroenterol Nutr 25:51–55, 1997.

77. Andersson T, Hassall E, Lundborg P, et al: Pharmacokinetics of orally administered omeprazole in children. International Pediatric Omeprazole Pharmacokinetic Group. Am J Gastroenterol 95:3101–3106, 2000.

78. Hassall E, Israel D, Shepherd R, et al: Omeprazole for treatment of chronic erosive esophagitis in children: a multicenter study of efficacy, safety, tolerability and dose requirements. International Pediatric Omeprazole Study Group. J Pediatr 137:800–807, 2000.

79. Faure C, Michaud L, Shaghaghi EK, et al: Lansoprazole in children: pharmacokinetics and efficacy in reflux oesophagitis. Aliment Pharmacol Ther 15:1397–1402, 2001.

80. Tran A, Rey E, Pons G, et al: Pharmacokinetic-pharmacodynamic study of oral lansoprazole in children. Clin Pharmacol Ther 71:359–367, 2002.

81. Cucchiara S, Minella R, Iervolino C, et al: Omeprazole and high dose ranitidine in the treatment of refractory reflux oesophagitis. Arch Dis Child 69:655–659, 1993.

82. Euler AR: Use of bethanechol for the treatment of gastroesophageal reflux. J Pediatr 96:321–324, 1980.

83. Curry JI, Lander TD, Stringer MD: Review article: erythromycin as a prokinetic agent in infants and children. Aliment Pharmacol Ther 15:595–603, 2001.

84. Ramirez B, Richter JE: Review article: promotility drugs in the treatment of gastro-oesophageal reflux disease. Aliment Pharmacol Ther 7:5–20, 1993.

85. Rothenberg SS: Experience with 220 consecutive laparoscopic Nissen fundoplications in infants and children. J Pediatr Surg 33:274–278, 1998.

86. Kawahara H, Imura K, Nakajima K, et al: Motor function of the esophagus and the lower esophageal sphincter in children who undergo laparoscopic nissen fundoplication. J Pediatr Surg 35:1666–1671, 2000.

87. Di Lorenzo C, Orenstein S: Fundoplication: friend or foe? J Pediatr Gastroenterol Nutr 34:117–124, 2002.

88. Samuk I, Afriat R, Horne T, et al: Dumping syndrome following Nissen fundoplication, diagnosis, and treatment. J Pediatr Gastroenterol Nutr 23:235–240, 1996.

89. Thiny MT, Shaheen NJ: Is Stretta ready for primetime? Gastroenterology 123:643–644, 2002.

90. Mason RJ, Crookes PF: Endoscopic antireflux procedures. Semin Laparosc Surg 8:265–271, 2001.
91. Mason RJ, Hughes M, Lehman GA, et al: Endoscopic augmentation of the cardia with a biocompatible injectable polymer (Enteryx) in a porcine model. Surg Endosc 16:386–391, 2002.
92. Holloway RH: Systemic pharmacomodulation of transient lower esophageal sphincter relaxations. Am J Med 111(Suppl 8A):178S-185S, 2001.
93. Zhang Q, Lehmann A, Rigda R, et al: Control of transient lower oesophageal sphincter relaxations and reflux by the GABA(B) agonist baclofen in patients with gastro-oesophageal reflux disease. Gut 50:19–24, 2002.
94. Cange L, Johnsson E, Rydholm H, et al: Baclofen-mediated gastro-oesophageal acid reflux control in patients with established reflux disease. Aliment Pharmacol Ther 16:869–873, 2002.

HOT TOPICS

Dyspepsia: The Spectrum of the Problem

chapter 16

Michael P. Jones, M.D.,
and Brian E. Lacy, M.D., Ph.D.

Dyspepsia refers to episodic or recurrent abdominal pain or discomfort thought to arise in the proximal gastrointestinal tract. The causes of dyspepsia are multiple and diverse and include structural disorders such as ulcers, cancer, gastritis, duodenitis, medications, infections, and metabolic disorders. Dyspepsia not caused by an organic or structural lesion is called functional (or *nonulcer*) *dyspepsia* and may result from abnormalities in gastric accommodation, visceral hypersensitivity, delayed gastric emptying, vagal nerve dysfunction, and psychological factors.

Dyspepsia is the most common problem encountered in gastroenterology practice[1] and accounts for 2% to 5% of primary care visits.[2] Although prevalence estimates vary, most studies suggest that nearly 25% of adults suffer dyspeptic symptoms at some point during the year. Dyspepsia is an important problem because it is associated with persistent symptoms, diminished quality of life, and high utilization of health care resources. Given the prevalence of this disorder, one would expect that there would be uniform agreement on how to define, evaluate, diagnose, and treat this problem in a cost-effective manner. Unfortunately, this is not the case.

In this introductory chapter, we hope to convey the challenges we all face in evaluating, diagnosing, and treating dyspepsia. This chapter begins by providing a definition that is useful and acceptable to all involved in the care and treatment of patients with dyspepsia. In addition, we discuss commonly used measurements of dyspepsia, review the prevalence and natural history of the disorder, define the economic costs of this disorder, and discuss how dyspepsia affects quality of life. Other chapters in this book focus on the causes of dyspepsia, cost-effective diagnosis, and treatment.

Dyspepsia: A Difficult Definition

Although many clinicians voice the notion that they "know dyspepsia when they see it," a precise, accepted definition of dyspepsia is critical because it affects how clinicians and researchers evaluate and treat these patients. Thus, if a patient is labeled as having gastroesophageal reflux disease (GERD), rather than dyspepsia, it would not only lower the reported prevalence of the disease, but would also alter data on response to treatment, because these patients may not respond as well to proton pump inhibitors. The lack of a standard, agreed-upon definition may explain large differences in the reported prevalence of the disorder, the natural history of the disorder, results of testing, and response to treatment.

Literally, *dyspepsia* means "bad digestion" (from the Greek terms *duis,* "bad," and *peptein,* "to digest"). More than 25 years ago, dyspepsia was first defined as abdominal or retrosternal pain, accompanied by symptoms of loss of appetite, nausea, vomiting, or jaundice.[3] Symptoms were thought to involve the upper gastrointestinal tract, but lower tract symptoms were not precluded from the definition. In addition, symptoms referable to the pancreaticobiliary system were allowed, and the chronicity of symptoms was not mentioned. In 1985, a position paper published by the American College of Physicians stated that dyspepsia should be defined as epigastric pain or discomfort with bowel habits remaining unchanged.[4,5] Thus, over time, the definition has evolved into one specifically involving the upper gastrointestinal tract. Symptoms compatible with irritable bowel syndrome (IBS) do not constitute dyspepsia using the Rome II criteria,[6] although in practice dyspepsia and IBS frequently coexist.[7,8]

Dyspeptic symptoms tend to be chronic, and the importance of chronicity has been emphasized by a number of authors.[9–11] Currently, diagnostic criteria require that symptoms be present for at least 12 weeks, which need not be consecutive, over the last 12 months.[6,12]

Symptoms allowable in the definition of dyspepsia have undergone modification over time as well. The presence of pain has remained constant, as has nausea, especially postprandial nausea. Vomiting may be present, although patients with predominant complaints of nausea and vomiting should be evaluated for gastroparesis. Postprandial fullness was suggested by Kahn and Greenfield[5] as an important characteristic to include, and belching and burping may also be present.[4] Symptoms that occur secondary to the ingestion of fatty foods have not stood the test of time, nor has the intriguing term *burbulence.*[13]

Although symptoms referable to the pancreaticobiliary system were originally included in the definition,[3] later definitions, including the Rome II criteria, have excluded patients with known pancreaticobiliary disease.[6,9]

In 1988, Colin-Jones and colleagues[14] first introduced the concept that dyspepsia should be broken down into separate categories. Dyspeptic symptoms could be thought of as reflux-like, ulcer-like, dysmotility-like (secondary to a motility disorder), or nonspecific in nature. This appeared to make remarkable sense, since it was apparent that patients with dyspepsia were a heterogeneous group. Patients with dyspepsia might have different symptoms, require different tests, and respond differently to treatment. However, several studies have shown that subdividing dyspepsia into different groups leads neither to more cost-effective testing nor to an improvement in treatment.[7,15] This issue is extensively addressed in later chapters.

Recent guidelines now exclude symptoms consistent with acid reflux from the broad heading of *dyspepsia.* Initially, these symptoms were included because many patients have both acid reflux disease and dyspeptic symptoms. It is also recognized that GERD may manifest as upper abdominal pain or discomfort in the absence of classic heartburn. Nevertheless, because heartburn appears to stand as its own clinical entity, patients with predominant heartburn symptoms are currently not described as having dyspepsia.

Uninvestigated and Functional Dyspepsia

In the evaluation of a patient with dyspepsia, it is important to first determine whether the patient has undergone previous investigation or not. Patients with new complaints or no previous investigation are categorized as having *uninvestigated dyspepsia.* Evaluation may disclose evidence for a structural disorder, such as an ulcer, cancer, or gallstones, which can then be specifically treated. Investigated patients not found to have an organic lesion to explain their symptoms are labeled as having *functional* (or *nonulcer*) *dyspepsia.*

Although several definitions are still employed for dyspepsia, we prefer to use the criteria outlined by the Rome II committee.[6] Thus, patients with functional dyspepsia should have complaints of abdominal pain or discomfort, thought to arise in the upper gastrointestinal tract, that has been present for at least 12 weeks, which need not be consecutive, over the last 12 months. There should not be any evidence of an organic disease process (biochemical, metabolic, endoscopic) that could explain the patient's symptoms. Patients may also have symptoms of postprandial nausea, epigastric fullness, bloating, belching, and even occasional vomiting. Patients who have predominant symptoms of classic heartburn (pyrosis, water brash, regurgitation), patients with abdominal complaints relieved by defecation (IBS), and patients with known pancreaticobiliary disease should be excluded from the definition. In addition, patients with predominant nausea, vomiting, and early satiety should be investigated for possible gastroparesis. However, patients may have dyspepsia (either uninvestigated, structural, or functional) and also have coexisting IBS, GERD, or pancreaticobiliary disorders.

Dyspepsia: A Common and Costly Problem

Epidemiology

It is generally estimated that dyspepsia accounts for 20% to 40% of gastroenterology consultations and 2% to 5% of primary care visits, although estimates of the prevalence of dyspepsia have varied.[1,2] These differences are largely attributable to variations in the population being surveyed and in the definition of dyspepsia used by the investigators. Additionally, population surveys querying for prevalence of dyspeptic symptoms produce estimates that are much higher than studies of patients seen in clinical practice. This is because only 20% to 25% of dyspeptic individuals seek care.[16] Dyspeptic patients who consult physicians are characterized by greater worry over serious illness or cancer, heightened levels of anxiety, depression, and illness behavior, and recent traumatic life events.[17–20] To be effective in the evaluation and management of these patients, clinicians must be attuned to these factors.

Available prevalence estimates of dyspepsia range from 12% to more than 45%, with an average estimate of about 25%.[2,21–24] Lifetime prevalence estimates range from about 40% to 60%.[25] Few studies have attempted to determine the incidence. Estimates range from 1% to 11.5%, with one study in the United States of 5.6% developing symptoms.[26–28] Although there is some degree of turnover in the dyspeptic population with time, many patients experience chronic symptoms. Jones showed that 74% of patients with dyspepsia continued to have symptoms over 2 years,[26] and Talley found that 86% reported similar symptoms over a 12 to 20-month period.[27]

Demographic and environmental factors show inconsistent associations with dyspepsia. Kay et al[29] studied the interactions of sex, age, body mass index, smoking, alcohol consumption, and psychic vulnerability and found that only psychic vulnerability was strongly related to dyspepsia.[29] Many studies demonstrate either conflicting results on the effects of demographic and environmental factors on dyspepsia or no association at all.

Economic Burden

The economic burden of dyspepsia is considerable but difficult to estimate. The best estimates of economic impact come from European studies; data in the United States is largely lacking. Logan and Delaney[18] report that at any one time, up to 4% of the population in the United Kingdom are thought to be taking prescribed drugs for dyspepsia, and that more than 10% of drug expenditure in primary care is for dyspepsia. These estimates do not include use of nonprescription medications.

Indirect costs in terms of lost wages and loss of productivity are also significant. A Swedish study estimated direct costs of dyspepsia to be approximately £26 million (~ US $38 million) annually for 8 million people. When indirect costs were included, total costs increased to about £280 million (almost US $410 million). This is largely attributed to the average of 26 more days of productivity lost by dyspeptic patients.[30]

Other recent data from a large cross-sectional survey in the United Kingdom suggest that dyspepsia may be costing society approximately £1 billion (US $1.46 billion) annually in indirect costs, with direct health care costs estimated to be £500 million (US $730 million).[31] Similar estimates exist for costs of diagnosis and management of dyspepsia in the United States.[32]

Quality of Life

Physicians tend to consider health problems in terms of symptoms and diseases, but the main determinant of whether an individual with dyspeptic symptoms seeks care has more to do with the personality of the individual than with digestive pathophysiology. Several studies demonstrate that dyspeptic consulters do not differ from dyspeptic nonconsulters with respect to symptom severity, but they do have greater anxiety, hypochondriasis, and an action-oriented coping style.[19,33] This is not the same as saying that dyspeptic symptoms are psychosomatic. It does mean that dyspeptic consulters seek care because their symptoms are more troubling to them than to the dyspeptic nonconsulter. In short, their symptoms have a greater impact on the quality of their lives.

Defining Quality of Life. Measurements of quality of life attempt to quantitate the patient experience to better understand and guide therapy. The World Health Organization defines quality of life as "not only the absence of disease and infirmity but also the presence of physical, mental and social well-being."[34] *Health-related quality of life* refers to how a medical condition impacts on the areas of life that make it worth living, including physical and emotional function.[35] Given the absence of hard physiologic end points in the evaluation and treatment of patients with functional digestive disorders, such as nonulcer dyspepsia, experts in the field have recommended the use of quality-of-life measures as primary outcomes in clinical trials.[36]

Measuring Quality of Life. Instruments to measure quality of life are derived from extensive interviews and focus groups that identify factors that accurately reflect well-being. Candidate factors are further studied to determine their validity, reliability, responsiveness, and coverage.[37] *Validity* refers to an instrument's ability to measure what it purports to measure. *Reliability* is the reproducibility of that measure. *Responsiveness* is the relationship between the changes in the score of the instrument with changes in the condition the instrument is seeking to measure. Finally, *coverage* is the spectrum of quality-of-life factors that the instrument measures.

Quality-of-life instruments may be generic or disease-specific. Generic measures are useful to measure and compare quality of life in patients with a wide variety of diseases. Generic measures suffer from the limitation that they may be insensitive for detecting small but clinically important changes in specific disease states. To avoid this limitation, disease-specific measures have been developed for a number of disorders, including dyspepsia. These instruments tend to be related to traditional clinical disease measures and may be more responsive than generic measures in specific situations.[35,37] The choice of generic or disease-specific measure depends on the question being asked and the population being studied. Often, studies include both a general and a disease-specific measure. Therapeutic trials often use disease-specific instruments as they seek to detect changes in quality-of-life with the greatest possible sensitivity. A variety of both general and disease-specific quality-of-life measures have been used in the evaluation of dyspepsia. These were recently reviewed and are summarized in Table 1.[38]

Quality of Life in Dyspeptic Patients. The quality of life in patients with dyspepsia is significantly poorer than that seen in healthy control subjects.[39–41] Figure 1 shows Psychological General Well-Being Index (PGWB) scores for a group of patients with nonulcer dyspepsia evaluated in our laboratory. Functional dyspeptic patients have general quality-of-life scores that are significantly lower than those of healthy control subjects and comparable to those of patients with GERD or gastroparesis. The same patients with nonulcer dyspepsia also completed the Nepean Dyspepsia' Index (NDI), which is a disease-specific quality-of-life measure. As shown in Figure 2, quality of life is significantly decreased for both the general and the disease-specific measure as compared with healthy control subjects ($P<0.0001$ for both PGWB and NDI).

The correlation of PGWB and NDI is modest, however ($r = -0.41$; $P < 0.0001$), which is attributable to two important points. First, all of these instruments measure quality of life in slightly different ways. This is particularly true when comparing general and disease-specific measures. Second, these instruments provide information regarding the correlation of quality of life in the disease state being studied. Correlation

TABLE 1. Quality of Life Measures Commonly Used in Dyspepsia

| Instrument | Domains/ Categories | Reliability | | Validity |
		Test-Retest	Internal Consistency	
Generic Measures				
SF-36	Physical functioning, bodily pain, role limitations–physical, social functioning, general mental health, role limitations–emotional, vitality, general health perception	r > 0.70	α = 0.70	Content Criterion Construct
Psychological General Well-Being Index (PGWB)	General health, positive well-being, self-control, vitality, depression, anxiety	r = 0.66	α > 0.90	Discriminant Concurrent
Sickness Impact Profile	Ambulation, mobility, body care and movement, social interaction, alertness, emotional behavior	r = 0.92	α = 0.94	Criterion Convergent Discriminant
Disease-Specific Measures				
Nepean Dyspepsia Index (NDI)	Tension/sleep, interference with daily living, eating/drinking, knowledge/control, work/study	r = 0.85–0.94	α = 0.85–0.95	Discriminant Convergent
Satisfaction with Dyspepsia Related Health Scale (SODA)	Severity of common symptoms, pain intensity, pain disability, satisfaction with dyspepsia-related health	ICC = 0.45–0.61	α = 0.74–0.93	Discriminant Convergent
Quality of Life in Reflux and Dyspepsia (QOLRAD)	Emotions; vitality, sleep, eating/drinking, physical/social functioning	NA	α = 0.97	Discriminant Convergent

r = Pearson correlation coefficient, ICC = intraclass correlation coefficient (poor: < 0.4; excellent: > 0.75), α = Chronbach's α coefficient (≥ 0.7 for clinical trials; ≥ 0.9 for individual assessment).

Adapted from Yacavone RF, Locke GR 3rd, Provenzale DT, Eisen GM: Quality of life measurement in gastroenterology: What is available? Am J Gastroenterol 96:285–297, 2001.

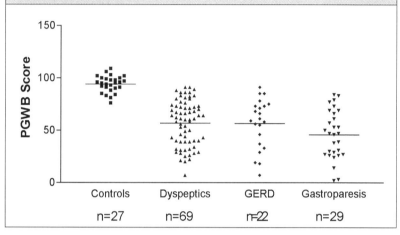

Figure 1. Quality of life in functional dyspepsia, gastroesophageal reflux disease (GERD), and gastroparesis patients compared with healthy control subjects. Psychological General Well-Being (PGWB) scores are significantly lower in all groups compared with controls ($P < 0.001$ for all). The groups do not differ significantly from one another.

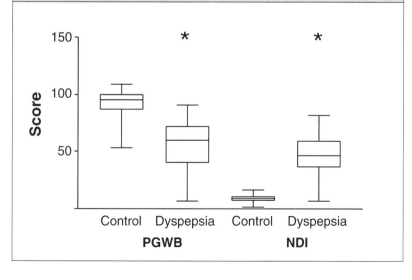

Figure 2. Comparison of general (PGWB) and disease-specific (NDI) quality of life in functional dyspepsia patients. Data are shown as box-whisker plot. The box represents the 25th to 75th percentiles, and the line in the box is the mean. The whiskers represent the range for each data set. Both instruments demonstrate significantly lower quality of life in dyspeptic patients compared with control subjects. PGWB = Psychological General Well-Being Index. NDI = Nepean Dyspepsia Index. *$P < 0.0001$ compared with controls.

does not imply causality. The interrelationship of psychosocial factors, principally anxiety, depression and somatization with dyspepsia is well documented but often clinically unrecognized.[42–45] The revised Symptom Checklist 90 (SCL-90R) is a self-administered instrument used to assess a variety of psychological constructs.[46] Results of SCL-90R for the same controls and dyspeptic patients reported above are shown in Figure 3. Compared with healthy controls, patients with functional dyspepsia demonstrate significantly greater levels of psychiatric distress both overall (data not shown) and on all subscales of the SCL-90R. The greatest differences are seen for somatization, depression, anxiety and obsessive-compulsive behavior.

Effects of Therapy on Quality of Life. While psychosocial issues can play an important role in functional dyspepsia, it is important to remember that dyspepsia is symptom with its own differential diagnosis. Accurate identification of the cause of a patient's dyspeptic symptoms may allow institution of effective therapy. This in turn can be reasonably expected to improve quality of life. For patients with peptic ulcer disease, both treatment with H_2-receptor antagonists and eradication of *Helicobacter pylori* result in decreased symptoms and improved quality of life.[47,48] Eradication of *H. pylori* in nonulcer dyspepsia does not

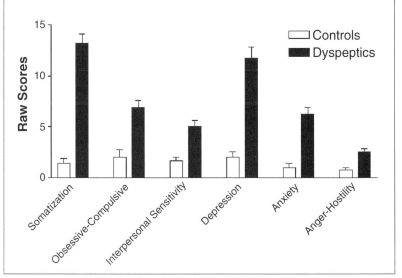

Figure 3. Selected SCL-90R subscale scores in healthy subjects and patients with functional dyspepsia. Differences between control subjects and dyspeptic patients are significant at $P < 0.01$ level for all subscales shown.

appear to confer any benefits in terms of symptom reduction or improvement in quality of life beyond placebo.[49] While acid suppression with proton pump inhibitors has been shown to produce statistically significant but clinically small improvements in patients with ulcer- or reflux-like dyspepsia, these changes were not associated with significant improvement in the Psychological General Well-Being Index.[50] While current options are quite limited, several studies have demonstrated improvement in quality of life in patients with nonulcer dyspepsia treated with prokinetic agents, chiefly cisapride.[51–53]

Conclusions. Quality of life is a clinically important and measurable end point in dyspepsia. A variety of instruments, both general and disease-specific are currently available. Quality of life is substantially reduced in patients with dyspepsia. Reduction of quality of life is attributable not only to dyspeptic symptoms themselves but also to comorbid conditions. In the case of nonulcer dyspepsia, psychosocial comorbidity may be substantial and should be sought. Effective relief of dyspeptic symptoms along with treatment of comorbid conditions results in improvement in quality of life.

Evaluating Dyspepsia

Dyspepsia is a symptom and not a diagnosis. A partial differential diagnosis of dyspepsia is shown in Table 2. Although important clues as to the causes of symptoms may be obtained from the history and examination, symptom patterns alone do not discriminate organic from functional disease.[54] In 50% to 60% of cases, no cause is identified, and patients are termed to have functional or nonulcer dyspepsia.[55,56]

TABLE 2.   Partial Differential Diagnosis of Dyspepsia
Nonulcer dyspepsia
Gastroesophageal reflux disease
Peptic ulcer disease
Medication-related: nonsteroidal anti-inflammatory drugs, antibiotics, iron, potassium supplements, digoxin
Carbohydrate malabsorption (lactose, fructose, sorbitol)
Cholelithiasis or choledocholithiasis
Chronic pancreatitis
Systemic disorders (diabetes, thyroid, parathyroid, hypoadrenalism, connective tissue disease)
Intestinal parasites
Abdominal malignancy (especially pancreatic and gastric cancer)
Chronic mesenteric ischemia

Evaluation of the Uninvestigated Dyspeptic Patient

Upper gastrointestinal endoscopy is the most commonly performed diagnostic study in patients with dyspepsia. It is recommended by the American College of Physicians and American Gastroenterological Association in the evaluation of patients with alarm symptoms (bleeding, anemia, weight loss, dysphagia, severe early satiety) or those who are refractory to, or relapse quickly after, an empiric trial of acid suppressive therapy.[4,55,57] While patients often worry that dyspeptic symptoms may be due to underlying malignancy, in Western society, esophageal and gastric cancer are quite uncommon in patients younger than 50 years of age. A retrospective study by Gillen et al[57] found that only 1 in 28,000 people younger than 55 were diagnosed with a malignancy of the upper gastrointestinal tract over a 5-year period.[58] Upper endoscopy identifies 33% to 80% of dyspeptic patients with an organic basis for their symptoms, most typically GERD and peptic ulcer disease.[15,58] Importantly, upper endoscopy, despite higher "buy-in" costs, results in overall lower health care costs as compared with empirical histamine-2 receptor antagonist (H_2RA) therapy and improves quality of life in patients with functional dyspepsia even if symptoms persist.[58,59]

Because a substantial number of dyspeptic patients have underlying peptic ulcer disease that can be cured by the eradication of *Helicobater pylori,* the strategy of testing patients with uninvestigated dyspepsia for *H. pylori* and treating those who are infected has become quite popular. Proponents have argued that this strategy eliminates ulcer disease and is cost saving.[55,60,61] The utility of this approach is obviously highly dependent on the prevalence of *H. pylori,* the prevalence of peptic ulcer disease, the degree to which eradication of *H. pylori* improves symptoms of functional dyspepsia, and the cost and availability of alternative management strategies.

The empiric use of antisecretory agents, particularly proton pump inhibitors, can be reasonably expected to provide relief in dyspeptic patients with GERD and peptic ulcer disease. Additionally, there is some suggestion that a subset of patients with ulcer-like functional dyspepsia will benefit from acid suppression as well.[62]

Evaluation of the Functional Dyspeptic Patient

In the majority of patients with dyspeptic complaints, either no cause of symptoms is found, or the patient fails empiric therapy. These patients are termed *functional dyspeptics,* and the cause of their symptoms remains speculative. However, today's functional disorder may be tomorrow's disease. As such, a variety of novel diagnostic modalities have been developed to further investigate dyspeptic symptoms. These tests are briefly described.

Gastric Emptying Scans. Solid-phase gastric emptying scans are delayed in 30% to 50% of patients with *nonulcer dyspepsia;* however, symptoms do not correlate with the degree of delayed gastric emptying.[63–67] Additionally, attempts to improve symptoms of dyspepsia by using prokinetic agents have fared poorly. This may well reflect the fact that gastric emptying scans provide only a crude measure of the elegant and sophisticated processes required to mix, grind, process, and empty an ingested meal.

Ultrasonography. Ultrasonography is used in some European academic centers as a reliable, noninvasive measurement of gastric emptying.[69] Ultrasonography is also useful in determining the size of the proximal stomach.[69,70] Gilja et al[71] found that after a soup meal, patients with functional dyspepsia were significantly more symptomatic than control subjects. Additionally, the proximal stomach was smaller in dyspeptic subjects than in control subjects. These results support the theory that patients with functional dyspepsia may suffer from abnormal gastric accommodation in response to a meal.

Endoscopic Ultrasonography. This technique has only recently been applied to the investigation of patients with dyspepsia. Compared with endoscopy and transabdominal ultrasonography, endoscopic ultrasonography appears to be less sensitive than endoscopy but more sensitive than transabdominal ultrasonography.[72,73] Endoscopic ultrasonography may play a role in the evaluation of patients with persistent dyspeptic symptoms and an otherwise unrewarding evaluation.

Electrogastrography. Normal gastric motility depends on the presence of intact, and functioning, electrical and muscular systems within the stomach. One proposed cause of dyspepsia is that it develops secondary to abnormalities of gastric myoelectrical activity. Electrical dysrhythmias have been associated with delayed gastric emptying and chronic nausea and vomiting.[74,75] Similar to electrocardiography, electrogastrography is a noninvasive technique that records gastric myoelectrical activity from surface electrodes on the abdominal wall. Electrogastrography has been used in a number of studies to assess gastric myoelectrical activity in patients with dyspepsia.

A number of investigators have reported that gastric dysrhythmias are more common in patients with functional dyspepsia than in healthy volunteers.[76–78] There are some data to suggest that dyspeptic patients with abnormal electrogastrographic findings are more likely to improve with prokinetics than dyspeptic patients with normal electrogastrographic findings.[79] While this is an encouraging observation, further study is needed before electrogastrography can be reasonably considered a useful tool in the clinical arena.

Gastric Barostat. The barostat is a device used to measure gastric physiology in vivo without interfering with gastric function. More specifically, it allows determination of gastric compliance and sensation. This is accomplished using a balloon passed into the upper stomach (usually orally) that is attached to an electronic pump that can infuse or withdraw air automatically, thereby allowing intragastric balloon pressure to remain constant, while changes in volume within the balloon are measured.

Studies using the barostat have shown that some patients with functional dyspepsia have less relaxation of the proximal stomach after a test meal than healthy volunteers. Additionally, these patients tend to have more complaints of nausea, bloating, early satiety, and abdominal pain during gastric distention than did volunteers.[80–82]

Several studies have called the significance of this finding into question. Mearin et al[83] reported that, although dyspeptic patients reported more symptoms during balloon distension, gastric compliance was not different between dyspeptic patients and control subjects.[84] These results were confirmed recently by Boeckxstaens et al in Amersterdam.[85] In this study, functional dyspeptic patients were significantly more symptomatic than healthy volunteers using the NDI, but differences in gastric compliance and accommodation were not seen.

In summary, some patients with functional dyspepsia have abnormal relaxation of the proximal stomach, which may account for symptoms of postprandial nausea and discomfort. Additionally, dyspeptic patients are often more sensitive to gastric distention, thus reinforcing the notion that many patients with functional dyspepsia suffer from visceral hypersensitivity.[85] However, visceral hypersensitivity is not present in all patients with functional dyspepsia and thus cannot account for all of the symptoms seen in this disorder.

Drink Tests. The invasive nature of barostat studies has led researchers to develop noninvasive diagnostic tests that can objectively measure gastric compliance and sensitivity. Various drink tests have been developed that use either water or nutritional drinks consumed in a timed manner. The amount of liquid ingested is measured, and symptoms of nausea, pain, bloating, and fullness are recorded. Several studies have noted that functional dyspeptic patients develop fullness at lower ingested volumes, and have more symptoms overall with ingestion, than do healthy control subjects.[40,86] However, correlation of volume to fullness with any symptom other than nausea has not been demonstrated, and the correlation of drink test volumes with other measures of gastric physiology has been poor.[39,40,84,86]

Single Photon Emission Computed Tomography Imaging. Single photon emission computed tomography imaging is a relatively new technology that can measure the size of different tissues or organs after the uptake of a radiolabeled material (e.g., ^{99m}Tc-pertechnetate). The material is taken up by the gastric mucosa, allowing an estimate of gastric volume that correlates well with measurements of intragastric volume made using a barostat.[87] When patients with nonulcer dyspepsia were compared to healthy volunteers, a reduction in postprandial volume was found in 41% of patients.[88] This finding is consistent with ultrasonography and barostat studies demonstrating that some patients with functional dyspepsia show impaired relaxation of the proximal stomach after a standard meal. Single photon emission computed tomography imaging is currently not widely available and is considered an investigational device.

Antroduodenal Manometry. In 1985, Malagelada and Stangehellini reported on 104 patients with functional dyspepsia who underwent antroduodenal manometry. A number of motility abnormalities were seen, with the most common finding being antral hypomotility. Unfortunately, there was no pattern of dysmotility that was specific for dyspepsia and there was no correlation of abnormal motility with symptoms. Similar findings have been reported by other investigators.[90,91]

Key Points: Dyspepsia

∞ Dyspepsia is a symptom and not a diagnosis.
∞ Dyspeptic symptoms may be caused by a variety of digestive and systemic disorders, which should be sought and treated as appropriate.
∞ In the majority of patients with dyspeptic symptoms, no cause will be found. These patients can be considered to have functional dyspepsia.
∞ While not associated with significant mortality, functional dyspepsia is associated with substantial, chronic use of health care resources, increased absenteeism, and decreased quality of life.
∞ A number of techniques have emerged or are emerging to evaluate digestive physiology and symptom generation in cases of functional dyspepsia. To date, such studies have demonstrated a number of physiologic aberrations, but none of these have been convincingly shown to be pathogenic.

Suggested Reading

1. Switz DM: What the gastroenterologist does all day: A survey of a state society's practice. Gastroenterology. 70:1048–1050, 1976.
2. Knill-Jones RP: Geographical differences in the prevalence of dyspepsia. Scand J Gastroenterol Suppl 182:17–24, 1991.
3. Horrocks JC, de Dombal FT: Computer-aided diagnosis of "dyspepsia". Am J Dig Dis 20:397–406, 1975.

4. Health and Public Policy Committee, American College of Physicians: Endoscopy in the evaluation of dyspepsia. Ann Intern Med 102:266–269, 1985.

5. Kahn KL, Greenfield S: The efficacy of endoscopy in the evaluation of dyspepsia: A review of the literature and development of a sound strategy. J Clin Gastroenterol 8:346–358, 1986.

6. Talley NJ, Stanghellini V, Heading RC, et al: Functional gastroduodenal disorders. Gut 45(Suppl 2):II37–42, 1999.

7. Agreus L, Svardsudd K, Nyren O, Tibblin G: Irritable bowel syndrome and dyspepsia in the general population: Overlap and lack of stability over time [see comments]. Gastroenterology 109:671–680, 1995.

8. Bortolotti M, Bolondi L, Santi V, et al: Patterns of gastric emptying in dysmotility-like dyspepsia. Scand J Gastroenterol 30:408–410, 1995.

9. Knill-Jones RP: A formal approach to symptoms in dyspepsia. Clin Gastroenterol 14:517–529, 1985.

10. Talley NJ, McNeil D, Piper DW: Discriminant value of dyspeptic symptoms: A study of the clinical presentation of 221 patients with dyspepsia of unknown cause, peptic ulceration, and cholelithiasis. Gut 28:40–46, 1987.

11. Thompson WG: Dyspepsia: Is a trial of therapy appropriate? [see comments]. Can Med Assoc J 153:293–299, 1995.

12. Penston JG, Pounder RE: A survey of dyspepsia in Great Britain. Aliment Pharmacol Ther 10:83–89, 1996.

13. Heatley RV, Rathbone BJ: Dyspepsia: A dilemma for doctors? Lancet 2:779–782, 1987.

14. Management of dyspepsia: report of a working party. Lancet 1:576–579, 1988.

15. Talley NJ, Weaver AL, Tesmer DL, Zinsmeister AR: Lack of discriminant value of dyspepsia subgroups in patients referred for upper endoscopy [see comments]. Gastroenterology 105:1378–1386, 1993.

16. Brown C, Rees WD: Dyspepsia in general practice. BMJ 300:829–830, 1990.

17. Lydeard S, Jones R: Factors affecting the decision to consult with dyspepsia: Comparison of consulters and non-consulters. J R Coll Gen Pract 39:495–498, 1989.

18. Logan R, Delaney B: ABC of the upper gastrointestinal tract: Implications of dyspepsia for the NHS. BMJ 323:675–677, 2001.

19. Cheng C, Hui WM, Lam SK: Coping style of individuals with functional dyspepsia. Psychosom Med 61:789–795, 1999.

20. Cheng C: Seeking medical consultation: Perceptual and behavioral characteristics distinguishing consulters and nonconsulters with functional dyspepsia. Psychosom Med 62:844–852, 2000.

21. Westbrook JI, Talley NJ: Empiric clustering of dyspepsia into symptom subgroups: A population-based study. Scand J Gastroenterol 37:917–923, 2002.

22. Westbrook JI, McIntosh JH, Talley NJ: The impact of dyspepsia definition on prevalence estimates: considerations for future researchers. Scand J Gastroenterol 35:227–233, 2000.

23. Dominitz JA, Provenzale D: Prevalence of dyspepsia, heartburn, and peptic ulcer disease in veterans. Am J Gastroenterol 94:2086–2093, 1999.

24. Locke GR 3rd: Prevalence, incidence and natural history of dyspepsia and functional dyspepsia. Baillieres Clin Gastroenterol 12:435–442, 1998.

25. Talley NJ: Scope of the problem of functional digestive disorders. Eur J Surg Suppl 582:35–41, 1998.

26. Jones R, Lydeard S: Dyspepsia in the community: A follow-up study. Br J Clin Pract 46:95–97, 1992.

27. Talley NJ, Weaver AL, Zinsmeister AR, Melton LJD: Onset and disappearance of gas-

trointestinal symptoms and functional gastrointestinal disorders. Am J Epidemiol 136:165–177, 1992.

28. Weir RD, Backett EM: Studies of the epidemiology of peptic ulcer in a rural community: prevalence and natural history of dyspepsia and peptic ulcer. Gut 9:75–83, 1968.

29. Kay L, Jorgensen T: Epidemiology of upper dyspepsia in a random population: Prevalence, incidence, natural history, and risk factors. Scand J Gastroenterol 29:2–6, 1994.

30. Moayyedi P: Helicobacter pylori test and treat strategy for young dyspeptic patients: New data. Gut 50(Suppl 4):iv47–50, 2002.

31. Moayyedi P, Mason J: Clinical and economic consequences of dyspepsia in the community. Gut 50(Suppl 4):iv10–12, 2002.

32. Fennerty MB: Use of antisecretory agents as a trial of therapy. Gut 50(Suppl 4):iv63–66, 2002.

33. Herschbach P, Henrich G, von Rad M: Psychological factors in functional gastrointestinal disorders: Characteristics of the disorder or of the illness behavior? Psychosom Med 61:148–153, 1999.

34. Constitution of the World Health Organization: Handbook of Basic Documents. Geneva: Palais des Nations, 1952.

35. Guyatt GH, Feeny DH, Patrick DL: Measuring health-related quality of life. Ann Intern Med 118:622–629, 1993.

36. Veldhuyzen van Zanten SJ, Talley NJ, Bytzer P, et al: Design of treatment trials for functional gastrointestinal disorders. Gut 45(Suppl 2):II69–77, 1999.

37. Eisen GM, Locke GR 3rd, Provenzale D: Health-related quality of life: A primer for gastroenterologists. Am J Gastroenterol 94:2017–2021, 1999.

38. Yacavone RF, Locke GR 3rd, Provenzale DT, Eisen GM: Quality of life measurement in gastroenterology: What is available? Am J Gastroenterol 96:285–297, 2001.

39. Maganti K, Ebert CC, Jones MP: Predictive value of symptoms in functional dyspepsia. Neurogastroenterol Motil 14:A439, 2002.

40. Jones MP, Hoffman S, Shah D, Ebert CC: The drink test: Observations from healthy controls and patients with functional dyspepsia. Am J Physiol 2002;in press.

41. Jones MP, Ebert CC, Hsu C, Howden CW: Predictive value of the water load test in nonulcer dyspepsia. Am J Gastroenterol 96:S59, 2001.

42. Kaplan DS, Masand PS, Gupta S: The relationship of irritable bowel syndrome (IBS) and panic disorder. Ann Clin Psychiatry 8:81–88, 1996.

43. Noyes R Jr, Cook B, Garvey M, Summers R: Reduction of gastrointestinal symptoms following treatment for panic disorder. Psychosomatics 31:75–79, 1990.

44. Blewett A, Allison M, Calcraft B, et al: Psychiatric disorder and outcome in irritable bowel syndrome. Psychosomatics 37:155–160, 1996.

45. Blanchard EB, Scharff L, Schwarz SP, et al: The role of anxiety and depression in the irritable bowel syndrome. Behav Res Ther 28:401–405, 1990.

46. Derogatis LR, Rickels K, Rock AF: The SCL-90 and the MMPI: A step in the validation of a new self-report scale. Br J Psychiatry 128:280–289, 1976.

47. Wilhelmsen I, Berstad A: Quality of life and relapse of duodenal ulcer before and after eradication of Helicobacter pylori. Scand J Gastroenterol 29:874–879, 1994.

48. Rampal P, Ruszniewski P, Boureau F, et al: Pain and quality of life in patients with acute duodenal ulcer treated with ranitidine. Aliment Pharmacol Ther 9:433–439, 1995.

49. Talley NJ, Vakil N, Ballard ED 2nd, Fennerty MB: Absence of benefit of eradicating Helicobacter pylori in patients with nonulcer dyspepsia. N Engl J Med 341:1106–1111, 1999.

50. Talley NJ, Meineche-Schmidt V, Pare P, et al: Efficacy of omeprazole in functional dyspepsia: Double-blind, randomized, placebo-controlled trials (the Bond and Opera studies). Aliment Pharmacol Ther 12:1055–1065, 1998.

51. Cutts TF, Abell TL, Karas JG, Kuns J: Symptom improvement from prokinetic therapy corresponds to improved quality of life in patients with severe dyspepsia. Dig Dis Sci 41:1369–1378, 1996.

52. Mones J, Adan A, Segu JL, et al: Quality of life in functional dyspepsia. Dig Dis Sci 47:20–26, 2002.

53. Abell TL, Cutts TF, Cooper T: Effect of cisapride therapy for severe dyspepsia on gastrointestinal symptoms and quality of life. Scand J Gastroenterol Suppl 195:60–63; discussion 63–64, 1993.

54. Bytzer P, Hansen JM, Schaffalitzky de Muckadell OB, Malchow-Moller A: Predicting endoscopic diagnosis in the dyspeptic patient: The value of predictive score models. Scand J Gastroenterol 32:118–125, 1997.

55. American Gastroenterological Association: Medical position statement: Evaluation of dyspepsia. Gastroenterology 114:579–581, 1998.

56. Fisher RS, Parkman HP: Management of nonulcer dyspepsia. N Engl J Med 339:1376–1381, 1998.

57. Gillen D, McColl KE: Does concern about missing malignancy justify endoscopy in uncomplicated dyspepsia in patients aged less than 55? [see comments]. Am J Gastroenterol 94:75–79, 1999.

58. Bytzer P, Hansen JM, Schaffalitzky de Muckadell OB: Empirical H_2-blocker therapy or prompt endoscopy in management of dyspepsia. Lancet 343:811–816, 1994.

59. Wiklund I, Glise H, Jerndal P, et al: Does endoscopy have a positive impact on quality of life in dyspepsia? Gastrointest Endosc 47:449–454, 1998.

60. Lam SK, Talley NJ: Report of the 1997 Asia Pacific Consensus Conference on the management of *Helicobacter pylori* infection. J Gastroenterol Hepatol 13:1–12, 1998.

61. Talley NJ, Lam SK, Goh KL, Fock KM: Management guidelines for uninvestigated and functional dyspepsia in the Asia-Pacific region: First Asian Pacific Working Party on Functional Dyspepsia. J Gastroenterol Hepatol 13:335–353, 1998.

62. Talley NJ, Meineche-Schmidt V, Pare P, et al: Efficacy of omeprazole in functional dyspepsia: Double-blind, randomized, placebo-controlled trials (the Bond and Opera studies). Aliment Pharmacol Ther 12:1055–1065, 1998.

63. Jian R, Ducrot F, Piedeloup C, et al: Measurement of gastric emptying in dyspeptic patients: Effect of a new gastrokinetic agent (cisapride). Gut 26:352–358, 1985.

64. Maes BD, Ghoos YF, Hiele MI, Rutgeerts PJ: Gastric emptying rate of solids in patients with nonulcer dyspepsia. Dig Dis Sci 42:1158–1162, 1997.

65. Perri F, Clemente R, Festa V, et al: Patterns of symptoms in functional dyspepsia: Role of *Helicobacter pylori* infection and delayed gastric emptying. Am J Gastroenterol 93:2082–2088, 1998.

66. Waldron B, Cullen PT, Kumar R, et al: Evidence for hypomotility in non-ulcer dyspepsia: A prospective multifactorial study. Gut 32:246–251, 1991.

67. Talley NJ, Verlinden M, Jones M: Can symptoms discriminate among those with delayed or normal gastric emptying in dysmotility-like dyspepsia? Am J Gastroenterol 96:1422–1428, 2001.

68. Bolondi L, Bortolotti M, Santi V, et al: Measurement of gastric emptying time by real-time ultrasonography. Gastroenterology 89:752–759, 1985.

69. Gilja OH, Detmer PR, Jong JM, et al: Intragastric distribution and gastric emptying assessed by three-dimensional ultrasonography. Gastroenterology 113:38–49, 1997.

70. Gilja OH, Hausken T, Odegaard S, Berstad A: Monitoring postprandial size of the proximal stomach by ultrasonography. J Ultrasound Med 14:81–89, 1995.

71. Gilja OH, Hausken T, Odegaard S, Berstad A: Three-dimensional ultrasonography of the gastric antrum in patients with functional dyspepsia. Scand J Gastroenterol 31:847–855, 1996.

72. Lee YT, Lai AC, Hui Y, et al: EUS in the management of uninvestigated dyspepsia. Gastrointest Endosc 56:842–848, 2002.

73. Sahai AV, Penman ID, Mishra G, et al: An assessment of the potential value of endoscopic ultrasound as a cost-minimizing tool in dyspeptic patients with persistent symptoms. Endoscopy 33:662–667, 2001.

74. Chen JD, Lin Z, Pan J, McCallum RW: Abnormal gastric myoelectrical activity and delayed gastric emptying in patients with symptoms suggestive of gastroparesis. Dig Dis Sci 41:1538–1545, 1996.

75. Koch KL: Gastrointestinal factors in nausea and vomiting of pregnancy. Am J Obstet Gynecol 185(5 Suppl):S198–203, 2002.

76. Cucchiara S, Bortolotti M, Colombo C, et al: Abnormalities of gastrointestinal motility in children with nonulcer dyspepsia and in children with gastroesophageal reflux disease. Dig Dis Sci 36:1066–1073, 1991.

77. Lin Z, Eaker EY, Sarosiek I, McCallum RW: Gastric myoelectrical activity and gastric emptying in patients with functional dyspepsia. Am J Gastroenterol 94:2384–2389, 1999.

78. Parkman HP, Miller MA, Trate D, et al: Electrogastrography and gastric emptying scintigraphy are complementary for assessment of dyspepsia. J Clin Gastroenterol 24:214–219, 1997.

79. Besherdas K, Leahy A, Mason I, et al: The effect of cisapride on dyspepsia symptoms and the electrogastrogram in patients with non-ulcer dyspepsia. Aliment Pharmacol Ther 12:755–759, 1998.

80. Coffin B, Azpiroz F, Guarner F, Malagelada JR: Selective gastric hypersensitivity and reflex hyporeactivity in functional dyspepsia [see comments]. Gastroenterology 107:1345–1351, 1994.

81. Salet GA, Samsom M, Roelofs JM, et al: Responses to gastric distension in functional dyspepsia. Gut 42:823–829, 1998.

82. Tack J, Piessevaux H, Coulie B, et al: Role of impaired gastric accommodation to a meal in functional dyspepsia. Gastroenterology 115:1346–1352, 1998.

83. Mearin F, Balboa A, Zarate N, et al: Placebo in functional dyspepsia: Symptomatic, gastrointestinal motor, and gastric sensorial responses. Am J Gastroenterol 94:116–125, 1999.

84. Boeckxstaens GE, Hirsch DP, Kuiken SD, et al: The proximal stomach and postprandial symptoms in functional dyspeptics. Am J Gastroenterol 97:40–48, 2002.

85. Tack J, Caenepeel P, Fischler B, et al: Symptoms associated with hypersensitivity to gastric distention in functional dyspepsia. Gastroenterology 121:526–535, 2001.

86. Boeckxstaens GE, Hirsch DP, Berkhout B, Tytgat GN: Is a drink test a valuable tool to study proximal study function? Gastroenterology 116:A960, 1999.

87. Bouras EP, Delgado-Aros S, Camilleri M, et al: SPECT imaging of the stomach: Comparison with barostat, and effects of sex, age, body mass index, and fundoplication. Single photon emission computed tomography. Gut 51:781–786, 2002.

88. Kim DY, Delgado-Aros S, Camilleri M, et al: Noninvasive measurement of gastric accommodation in patients with idiopathic nonulcer dyspepsia. Am J Gastroenterol 96:3099–3105, 2001.

89. Malagelada JR, Stanghellini V: Manometric evaluation of functional upper gut symptoms. Gastroenterology 88:1223–1231, 1985.

90. Di Lorenzo C, Hyman PE, Flores AF, et al: Antroduodenal manometry in children and adults with severe non-ulcer dyspepsia. Scand J Gastroenterol 29:799–806, 1994.

91. Wilmer A, Van Cutsem E, Andrioli A, et al: Ambulatory gastrojejunal manometry in severe motility-like dyspepsia: Lack of correlation between dysmotility, symptoms, and gastric emptying [see comments]. Gut 42:235–242, 1998.

A Cost-Effective Approach to Dyspepsia

chapter

17

Peter Bytzer, M.D., Ph.D.

No other decision area in gastroenterology has been more debated over the past decade than the role of endoscopy in dyspepsia. There are several reasons for this. First, clinicians confronted with a patient suffering from dyspepsia must deal with an extremely common disorder with a limited number of underlying causes. Additionally, there are various therapeutic options, which require a precise diagnosis. Finally, a well-established diagnostic "gold standard" (endoscopy) is widely available but competing diagnostic modalities exist that are either cheaper or more convenient. It is no wonder that this field has produced exciting new evidence during the past decade.

In a world of limited health-care resources, clinicians need to recognize the importance of health economics and the relevance of a cost-effectiveness approach in decision-making. Limited health care resources should be spent on strategies with a documented effect. Inefficient strategies should be abandoned so that the associated costs can be transferred to alternative programs with proven cost-effectiveness.

The purpose of a cost-effectiveness analysis is to correlate costs with health outcomes. Because these measures mean little by themselves, the cost-effectiveness of one strategy must be compared to that of a competing strategy to produce useful information. However, an economic evaluation is no more than an aid to decision making. Many difficult value judgments still have to be made before a plan of care can be implemented for each individual patient. Thus, the problem of managing patients with dyspeptic symptoms represents a perfect challenge in clinical decision-making, as evidenced by the vast number of decision analyses and clinical trials that have been published and debated over the last decade. The major controversy has been over the optimal management strategy for patients with dyspeptic symptoms who do not present with alarm symptoms suggestive of malignancy or complicated ulcerative disease. Is it safe to manage the patient empirically? Who should receive endoscopy? Is a strategy based on noninvasive *Helicobacter pylori* testing safe and cost-effective?

Dyspepsia: A Complex Problem

The percentage of consultations for dyspepsia in primary care varies between 1% and 4%,[1,2] and 5% to 9% of the population seek treatment for dyspepsia each year.[3] Symptoms suggestive of irritable bowel syndrome and reflux disease frequently overlap but do not form part of the dyspepsia definition. Surveys from primary care have shown that dyspeptic patients usually present with a multitude of different symptoms thought to emerge from the upper gastrointestinal tract and they rarely suffer just from epigastric pain as the sole symptom. Even so, it is useful to distinguish between dyspepsia (epigastric pain or discomfort) and gastroesophageal reflux disease (predominant heartburn) in clinical trials and other research areas.

Management Strategy Options

Very little is known about the factors that influence a primary care physician's decision to refer a patient for specialist evaluation. Even when the clinician suspects peptic ulcer disease, less than half of the patients are referred for confirmatory diagnosis.[2] Surprisingly, endoscopic diagnostic profiles for unselected patients in primary care[4,5] and for patients selected for endoscopy[6,7] differ only slightly. This suggests that either it is not possible to assess the risk for organic dyspepsia, or assessment does not play an important role in the decision to refer. As a consequence, many patients with organic dyspepsia due to peptic ulcer disease, gastroesophageal reflux, or even malignancy are managed empirically in primary care.

Identification of patients who require further investigation to rule out serious structural disease such as peptic ulcer disease or cancer is a key issue, since unaided clinical diagnosis is unreliable. The use of an age threshold (typically 45 to 50 years) and identification of alarm features, including weight loss, repeated vomiting, use of nonsteroidal anti-inflammatory drugs, signs of gastrointestinal bleeding, abdominal mass, and anemia, appears to be valid based on the limited evidence available.

All dyspepsia management strategies have been designed to reduce the number of endoscopic procedures. All strategies involve some form of initial screening for the purpose of selecting patients for further management. The traditional policy includes a trial of antisecretory medication to gauge symptomatic relief before deciding on a referral. A competing policy is based on noninvasive *H. pylori* screening, reserving endoscopy either for those patients whose test result is positive (test-and-scope strategy) or for those not responding to eradication therapy (test-and-treat strategy). A summary of various management strategies is presented in Table 1.

Watchful Waiting

Many dyspeptic patients present with mild symptoms of short duration,[2] and most dyspeptic conditions resolve spontaneously. Furthermore, the majority of patients seeking treatment for dyspepsia do not have serious underlying pathologic conditions, such as cancer or peptic ulcer disease. Thus, the strategy of watchful waiting, combined with reassurance, empirical over-the-counter remedies and lifestyle corrections, may be a valid option in many cases. Watchful waiting is used by many family physicians as an initial approach. Unfortunately, we have very limited clinical data comparing the watch-and-wait strategy with alternative strategies.

Clinical Diagnosis

Clinical judgment based on symptoms and demographic characteristics is not reliable as a basis for decisions about management in dyspeptic patients without alarm symptoms. Several clinical studies of patients referred for endoscopy or primary care patients have confirmed that unaided clinical diagnosis cannot be trusted.[6,8] The overall diagnostic accuracy in the published studies ranges from 24% to 65%. Diagnostic predictions made by family physicians and gastroenterologists do not differ in accuracy when tested against endoscopy as the gold standard.[9] The most valid predictions are those with a diagnosis of functional dyspepsia. However, when adjusting for the high prevalence of patients with functional dyspepsia (usually above 60%), family physicians may just as well toss a coin when trying to distinguish between patients with functional dyspepsia and patients with organic dyspepsia. Both family physicians and specialists will misclassify at least half of the ulcer patients and overlook one third of patients with serious pathologic condition.[9]

Classification by means of symptom complexes has been suggested to improve decision-making.[10] Such symptom grouping seems to be a poor predictor of the endoscopic diagnosis, however.[11,12]

Computer Algorithms

Despite the low predictive value of clinical judgment for diagnosis, simple variables such as symptoms, age, gender, and smoking habits offer a readily available form of stratification of dyspeptic patients. Much effort has been put into developing computer algorithms based on mul-

TABLE 1. Summary of Management Strategies for Dyspeptic Patients without Alarm Features

Strategy	Algorithm	Advantages	Disadvantages
Watchful waiting	Reassurance and/or lifestyle corrections combined with empirical over-the-counter remedies	Inexpensive	Not validated Will miss patients with organic disease Postpones endoscopy
Clinical diagnosis	Endoscopy reserved for those with a clinical suspicion of organic disease (e.g., peptic ulcer)	Inexpensive	Unreliable
Computer algorithms	Endoscopy reserved for those with a combination of features suggesting organic disease	Inexpensive	Not validated Unreliable
Empirical antisecretory therapy	Endoscopy reserved for those not responding to a short course of antisecretory medication and for those with early relapse after therapy	Provides prompt symptom relief for patients with acid-related disorders May rule out (coexisting) reflux disease	Postpones endoscopy Selection for endoscopy not improved
Helicobacter pylori test-and-treat	Endoscopy reserved for those not responding to *H. pylori* eradication therapy	Provides definitive therapy for patients with *H. pylori*-related disorders Validated in randomized trials against prompt endoscopy	May become irrelevant when the prevalence of infection and peptic ulcer disease declines
H. pylori test-and-scope	Endoscopy reserved for those testing positive for *H. pylori* infection	Saves endoscopies in areas with low *H. pylori* prevalence	Increases endoscopy referral rates in areas with high *H. pylori* prevalence Postpones eradication therapy
Prompt endoscopy	Endoscopy for all dyspeptic patients with symptoms severe enough to justify therapy	Diagnostic gold standard	Invasive Waiting lists Relatively expensive Insensitive test for reflux disease

tiple clinical and demographic criteria to help categorize these patients. Probabilistic models make use of multiple regression techniques to produce equations that show the likelihood of a diagnosis.

Most models have tried to identify patients at low risk of organic dyspepsia who might be safely managed without endoscopy.[8,13–17] Although they are theoretically attractive, these models have not gained wide acceptance in clinical practice for several reasons. First, the majority of published models do not meet the methodologic standards that are required before a clinical prediction rule can be adopted in practice. Next, and importantly, only a few scoring systems have been subjected to proper validation experiments, and the overall conclusions have been that these score models cannot be trusted outside the settings in which they were developed.

To become a valid decision support instrument in primary care, the scoring system must prove itself in those patients who are managed at the level between primary and secondary care (i.e., those patients who are *potential* candidates for a diagnostic endoscopy). In a Danish validation experiment, predictive score models to diagnose peptic ulcer or organic dyspepsia could not be safely applied to patients managed empirically in primary care.[17] Thus, score models to predict endoscopic diagnosis have not proved their value in the management of patients with dyspepsia.

Empirical Antisecretory Therapy

Empirical treatment is probably the most widely used approach for patients with dyspepsia. By starting with a short course of empirical antisecretory therapy, further diagnostic studies are delayed and patients with mild and self-limiting symptoms are not referred for endoscopy. The largest cost for primary care in most industrialized countries is prescribing for the treatment of dyspepsia. It has been estimated that up to 25% of all acid blockers are prescribed as part of empirical management of dyspeptic patients.

Economic considerations have been the major argument for favoring empirical antisecretory therapy over prompt endoscopy. According to this strategy, all patients with uninvestigated dyspepsia should receive a short course of an H_2-blocker or a proton pump inhibitor before deciding on referral for endoscopy. Only patients with continuing symptoms or early relapse should be investigated. The strategy has the obvious advantage of providing effective treatment and prompt symptom relief for those with acid-related disorders. For patients with functional dyspepsia, the advantage is less clear,[18,19] but at least the drugs are safe and usually without side effects.

Even though empirical treatment of undiagnosed cancer is not desirable, gastric and esophageal cancers are rare findings in dyspeptic patients without alarm symptoms. Most endoscopy centers report prevalence rates below 1% to 2%, and the risk is even lower among unselected patients in primary care.

Unfortunately, the outcome of empirical therapy has almost no diagnostic value in dyspeptic patients. This was demonstrated in a large randomized trial with a 1-year follow-up comparing prompt endoscopy to an empirical treatment strategy using H_2-blocker.[20] The empirical treatment strategy did not improve case selection for endoscopy, resulted in a paradoxical selection of a majority of patients with functional dyspepsia for endoscopy, and left many ulcer cases undiagnosed.[20,21]

The economic benefits of the empirical treatment strategy assume that investigations are not only postponed, but made permanently superfluous. However, decision analyses[22–25] and results from clinical trials and surveys[20,21,26] give conflicting evidence. Relapse rates of dyspeptic symptoms and cost of endoscopy are the important factors in cost-effectiveness analyses.[24] Compared to treatment guided by endoscopy, empirical treatment is not associated with fewer symptoms or a higher level of quality of life.[20] In areas where endoscopy is expensive, empirical management would be a more desirable approach.

Even though the symptomatic outcome of a therapeutic trial of an acid blocker in dyspeptic patients will not reliably predict or exclude ulcer disease, several studies suggest that a positive response to a short trial of a proton pump inhibitor may be a sensitive indicator of gastroesophageal reflux disease.[27,28] In patients with reflux and dyspepsia symptoms (epigastric pain or discomfort), a short course of a proton pump inhibitor may be valuable to exclude symptomatic gastroesophageal reflux. Some researchers have even argued that patients with functional dyspepsia who respond to acid suppression therapy suffer from nonerosive gastroesophageal reflux disease.[29] In the near future, when the incidence and prevalence of both *H. pylori* infection and peptic ulcer disease are very low, a strategy of empirical proton pump inhibitor therapy may be the most cost-effective and reasonable initial strategy in primary care.[25,30]

Helicobacter pylori–Based Strategies

Noninvasive *H. pylori* testing (i.e., fecal antigen testing or urea breath testing) has introduced a clinically relevant instrument to screen out dyspeptic patients before endoscopy. The *H. pylori*-based strategies rest on the following assumptions and observations: (1) Peptic ulcer disease is very rare in noninfected dyspeptic patients who do not take nonsteroidal anti-inflammatory drugs; (2) the probability of an ulcer in an infected dyspeptic patient is 30% to 55%[31,32]; and (3) gastric cancer is an extremely rare cause of dyspepsia in young patients (<45–55 years) who do not have warning symptoms such as weight loss and signs of bleeding.[33,34] Thus, the probability of an organic cause of dyspepsia in young, noninfected patients who do not have alarm features but use NSAIDs is very low.

The validity of the test-and-scope strategy has been evaluated in series of patients referred for endoscopy, and the test-and-treat strategy has been validated against competing strategies in large randomized trials.

The Test-and-Scope Strategy

In the test-and-scope strategy, endoscopy is limited to patients younger than 45 years of age who are *H. pylori* positive, are taking NSAIDs, or present with alarm symptoms (Fig. 1). Approximately 25% to 33% of the total number of endoscopies can be saved without overlooking serious pathology, as evidenced by a number of reports.[35] Importantly, almost no gastric cancer and very few ulcer patients will be missed.

The prevalence of *H. pylori* is critical when designing a management strategy which involves *H. pylori* testing. This has to do with the relationship between pretest probabilities and predictive values. The predictive value of a positive *H. pylori* test decreases when the prevalence of *Helicobacter* infection decreases and, as a consequence, the number of false-positive test results increases. In other words, the lower the prevalence of *H. pylori,* the less confident you should be with a positive test result. In most industrialized communities, *H. pylori* prevalence is decreasing rapidly and is probably not more than 25% in people younger than 45 years.[36] In this setting, a test-and-scope strategy will save many endoscopies without the risk of overlooking ulcers due to a very low false-negative rate. In high-prevalence areas, however, the strategy may lead to a paradoxical increase in referrals for endoscopy.

The studies published so far have not addressed the very important question about the relevance of a strategy that is applied posthoc, that is, after a decision of referral for endoscopy has been made. Since the endoscopic result is still the diagnostic gold standard, the strategy has only been tested postendoscopy. The validity of the strategy needs to be confirmed in the true target population, that is, the large group of dyspeptic patients in primary care who are potential candidates for endoscopy. Furthermore, because the attitude toward the eradication of *H. pylori* has changed over the last decade, the test-and-scope strategy has become irrelevant. This is because most clinicians would choose to offer eradication therapy to dyspeptic patients who test positive for *H. pylori,* irrespective of the outcome of a diagnostic endoscopy.

The Test-and-Treat Strategy

A management strategy based on serology *H. pylori* status was first proposed in 1989.[37] When applied in a primary care setting, a test-and-treat strategy of *H. pylori* testing (Fig. 2) followed by empirical eradication therapy for *H. pylori*–positive patients will probably be more attractive to patients, clinicians, and health care providers when compared to the test-and-scope strategy. The major strength of this strategy is that it identifies and treats the vast majority of patients with peptic ulcer disease, in contrast to all the other strategies besides prompt endoscopy. However, in *H. pylori* low prevalence areas, the test-and-treat strategy leads to overtreatment with eradication therapy due a low predictive value of a positive test.

Some decision analysis models[38,39] and randomized controlled trials[32,40–43] favor the test-and-treat strategy, which is associated with a reduction in endoscopy referral rate of at least 66%. The benefits of this strategy are attributable largely to the cure of peptic ulcer disease. However, recent data from the United States, Australia, and Europe have reported surprisingly low prevalence rates of *H. pylori* in ulcer patients.[44,45] Jyotheeswaran et al[46] reported that only 61% of 144 patients with duodenal ulcer, who had no history of NSAID use, were infected with *H. pylori*. These results, if confirmed, may have important consequences for the future management of dyspeptic patients. Specifically, if the proportion of idiopathic duodenal ulcer is higher than previously reported, the safety and the benefits of the test-and-treat strategy may be disputed.

The precise guidelines for the test-and-treat strategy need to be defined according to local conditions, with particular focus on *H. pylori*

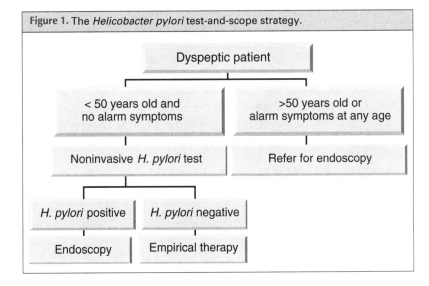

Figure 1. The *Helicobacter pylori* test-and-scope strategy.

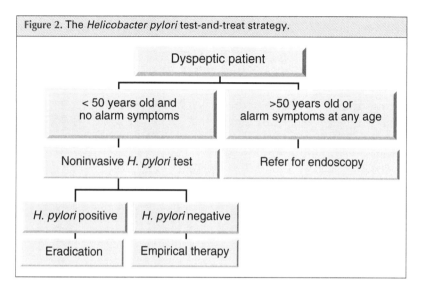

Figure 2. The *Helicobacter pylori* test-and-treat strategy.

and peptic ulcer prevalence rates. In view of the rapidly declining prevalence of *H. pylori* infection, the long-term effects of the policy should be monitored closely.

Diagnostic Endoscopy

Endoscopy is the gold standard investigation for dyspepsia and dyspepsia is the most common indication for the procedure. Endoscopic results reliably distinguish between patients with an organic cause of the symptoms (e.g., peptic ulcer disease, reflux esophagitis, or cancer) and those with functional complaints. Many practitioners have argued that the endoscopic result will not influence the clinical decision. The majority of dyspeptic patients have normal endoscopic findings and this has led many practitioners to question the usefulness and the cost-effectiveness of the procedure. Others have argued that the investment of diagnostic resources in endoscopy, while expensive in the short term, is likely to generate valuable information in identifying a management strategy that is most cost-effective over the long term.

Fear of gastric cancer is the main reason for considering endoscopy in patients older than 45 years of age with a recent onset of dyspeptic symptoms. Malignancy is an extremely rare finding in young dyspeptic patients. Additionally, a policy of prompt endoscopy in patients older than 45 or 50 has the potential to reduce mortality by increasing the proportion of early gastric cancers detected.[47] On the other hand, retrospective analyses suggest that the selection process should be based on the presence or absence of alarm symptoms rather than on arbitrary age thresholds.[48] Importantly, the incidence of gastric cancer is rapidly decreasing in the industrialized world. Thus, a general proposal to submit all dyspeptic patients over the age of 45 to endoscopy, with the purpose of diagnosing gastric cancer, may not be efficacious in the future.

Endoscopy has a definite impact on patient management. One study demonstrated unpredicted diagnostic and therapeutic consequences for one third of the endoscoped patients.[49] Even a negative endoscopic finding influences outcome, since management may be simplified and patients' anxiety may be relieved.[50,51]

A reliable endoscopic result presupposes that the patient is investigated while experiencing symptoms and without pretreatment with ulcer healing drugs.[52] With a typical waiting time of several weeks for endoscopy, patients usually start antisecretory therapy concurrently with referral for investigation. Furthermore, endoscopy is an insensitive tool in reflux disease and will demonstrate no mucosal abnormalities in up to two thirds of patients with impaired quality of life due to reflux symptoms.[53]

Cost-Effectiveness

The effectiveness of a management strategy in dyspepsia is difficult to appreciate in a single outcome variable; therefore, more complex measures are often applied. These include symptom relief, quality of life, and diagnostic abilities. Demonstrating the effectiveness of endoscopy in the management of dyspepsia requires showing that patients benefit from the procedure.[54] Many different outcome measures have been included in the analyses, and unfortunately there is no agreement on how to estimate effectiveness in dyspepsia. From the patient's perspective, relief of symptoms is a very relevant outcome measure and often the only estimate included. Quality of life is another important outcome when assessing the impact of a management strategy in a chronic condition. The diagnostic ability of a management policy is also an important outcome. Identifying and curing patients with *H. pylori*-associated ulcer disease should be a priority in any strategy, and the possibility of misclassification of ulcer patients and cancer patients should be analyzed. A particular problem is the choice of time frame over which costs and outcome are calculated. For a chronic or relapsing condition such as dyspepsia, long-term costs should be calculated, but this is not practical or achievable. Most studies have limited themselves to a 1-year time horizon. This is probably a conservative approach, and it almost certainly underestimates the benefits of *H. pylori* eradication.

The objective of this method is to identify the effect on resources of the analyzed strategies. The cost-effectiveness of the different policies is considerably affected by the cost of endoscopy. These costs can be quite arbitrary, since they are often reported as charges. They reflect not only resources used but also profit or losses to the institution and may, therefore, be inflated. Published costs for endoscopy differ widely, ranging from $53 in Germany to up to $1180 in the United States. Even within the same country, cost estimates published in the same year differ by up to 400%.[55] Cost estimates are usually much lower in European countries than in the United States. This is probably due to differences in the calculations and in the payer perspective used. Most U.S. estimates use a third-party payer perspective when reporting reimbursement charges.

Cost-effectiveness analyses in dyspepsia management are difficult to interpret and to compare because of a lack of uniformity in designing, measuring, and reporting costs and health-care related outcome. Based on strong evidence from randomized trials and on circumstantial evidence from decision analyses, the test-and-treat strategy appears to be cost-effective compared to early endoscopy. Furthermore, this strategy has the obvious advantage of offering prompt relief and long-term benefits to peptic ulcer patients, who should be given high priority in the management policies. Implementing a test-and-treat strategy in primary care will probably save the cost of endoscopies without harmful effects. However, in view of the rapidly declining prevalence of *H. pylori* infection in the Western world, the long-term effects of this policy should be monitored closely.

Key Points: Cost-Effective Approach to Dyspepsia

- ∞ Endoscopy is still the diagnostic gold standard in dyspeptic patients.
- ∞ If endoscopy is available with a short waiting time and is reasonably priced, patients with dyspepsia should be managed on the basis of a precise diagnosis obtained by endoscopy at an early stage before the onset of symptomatic treatment.
- ∞ This ideal situation is not generally available, and clinicians will probably still be divided on how and when endoscopy should be used.
- ∞ Today, most patients can be managed in primary care by an *H. pylori* test-and-treat algorithm and patients will not be referred unless eradication therapy and empirical proton pump inhibitor treatment trials have failed.
- ∞ Cost-effectiveness analyses in dyspepsia management are difficult to interpret and to compare; however, there is strong evidence that the test-and-treat strategy is cost-effective compared to prompt endoscopy.

Key Points (*Continued*)

∞ The test-and-treat strategy has the obvious advantage of offering prompt relief and long-term benefits to peptic ulcer patients.

∞ The rapidly declining prevalence of *H. pylori* infection in the Western world may soon make the test-and-treat policy irrelevant, and empirical proton pump inhibitor therapy may become the favored initial strategy.

Suggested Reading

1. Warndorff DK, Knottnerus JA, Huijnen LGJ, Starmans R: How well do general practitioners manage dyspepsia? J R Coll Gen Pract 39:499–502, 1989.
2. Heikkinen M, Pikkarainen P, Takala J, Julkunen R: General practitioners' approach to dyspepsia: Survey of consultation frequencies, treatment, and investigation. Scand J Gastroenterol 31:648–653, 1996.
3. Penston JG, Pounder RE: A survey of dyspepsia in Great Britain. Eur J Gastroenterol Hepatol 10:83–89, 1996.
4. Heikinnen M, Pikkarainen P, Takala J, Räsänen H, Julkunen R: Etiology of dyspepsia: Four hundred unselected consecutive patients in general practice. Scand J Gastroenterol 30:519–523, 1995.
5. Hansen JM: Dyspepsia in primary care: Clinical decision making and pharmacotherapy in non-organic dyspepsia. Scand J Gastroenterol 33:799–805, 1998.
6. Bytzer P, Hansen JM, Havelund T, et al: Predicting endoscopic diagnosis in the dyspeptic patient: The value of clinical judgement. Eur J Gastroenterol Hepatol 8:359–363, 1996.
7. Adang RP, Vismans JF-JFE, Talmon JL, et al: The diagnostic outcome of upper gastrointestinal endoscopy: Are referral source and patient age determining factors? Eur J Gastroenterol Hepatol 6:329–335, 1994.
8. Johannessen T, Petersen H, Kleveland PM, et al: The predictive value of history in dyspepsia. Scand J Gastroenterol 25:689–697, 1990.
9. Hansen JM, Bytzer P, The Danish Dyspepsia Study Group: The reliability of the unaided clinical diagnosis in dyspeptic patients in primary care. Gastroenterology 112:A140–A140, 1997.
10. Colin-Jones DG, Bloom B, Bodemar G, et al: Management of dyspepsia: Report of a working party. Lancet 1:576–579, 1988.
11. Talley NJ, Weaver AL, Tesmer DL, Zinsmeister AR: Lack of discriminant value of dyspepsia subgroups in patients referred for upper endoscopy. Gastroenterology 105:1378–1386, 1993.
12. Bytzer P, Hansen JM, Schaffalitzky de Muckadell OB: Symptom grouping in dyspepsia: Any predictive value? Scand J Gastroenterol 28(Suppl 197):28, 1993.
13. Davenport PM, Morgan AG, Damborough A, de Dombal FT: Can preliminary screening of dyspeptic patients allow more effective use of investigational techniques? BMJ 290:217–220, 1985.
14. Horrocks JC, de Dombal FT: Computer-aided diagnosis of "dyspepsia". Am J Dig Dis 20:397–406, 1975.
15. Crean GP, Card WI, Beattie AD, et al: 'Ulcer-like dyspepsia'. Scand J Gastroenterol 17(Suppl 79):9–15, 1982.

16. Mann J, Holdstock G, Harman M, et al: Scoring system to improve cost effectiveness of open access endoscopy. BMJ 287:937–940, 1983.

17. Bytzer P, Hansen JM, Schaffalitzky de Muckadell OB, Malchow-Møller A: Predicting endoscopic diagnosis in dyspeptic patients: The value of predictive score models. Scand J Gastroenterol 32:118–125, 1997.

18. Bytzer P, Talley NJ: Current indications for acid suppressants in dyspepsia. Baillieres Best Pract Res Clin Gastroenterol 15:385–400, 2001.

19. Wong WM, Wong BC, Hung WK, et al: Double blind, randomised, placebo controlled study of four weeks of lansoprazole for the treatment of functional dyspepsia in Chinese patients. Gut 51:502–506, 2002.

20. Bytzer P, Hansen JM, Schaffalitzky de Muckadell OB: Empirical H_2-blocker therapy or prompt endoscopy in management of dyspepsia. Lancet 343:811–816, 1994.

21. Brignoli R, Watkins P, Halter F: The OMEGA-project: A comparison of two diagnostic strategies for risk- and cost-oriented management of dyspepsia. Eur J Gastroenterol Hepatol 9:337–343, 1997.

22. Silverstein MD, Petterson T, Talley NJ: Initial endoscopy or empiric therapy with or without testing for *Helicobacter pylori* for dyspepsia: A decision analysis. Gastroenterology 110:72–83, 1996.

23. Ebell MH, Warbasse L, Brenner C: Evaluation of the dyspeptic patient: A cost-utility study. J Fam Pract 44:545–555, 1997.

24. Fendrick AM, Chernew ME, Hirth RA, Bloom BS: Alternative treatment strategies for patients with suspected peptic ulcer disease. Ann Intern Med 123:260–268, 1995.

25. Spiegel BM, Vakil NB, Ofman JJ: Dyspepsia management in primary care: A decision analysis of competing strategies. Gastroenterology 122:1270–1285, 2002.

26. Ryder SD, O'Reilly S, Miller RJ, et al: Long term acid suppressing treatment in general practice. BMJ 308:827–830, 1994.

27. Schindlbeck NE, Klauser AG, Voderholzer WA, Müller-Lissner SA: Empiric therapy of gastro-oesophageal reflux disease. Arch Intern Med 155:1808–1812, 1995.

28. Fass R, Ofman JJ, Gralnek IM, et al: Clinical and economic assessment of the omeprazole test in patients with symptoms suggestive of gastroesophageal reflux disease. Arch Intern Med 159:2161–2168, 1999.

29. Nyren O: Functional dyspepsia: Bye-bye to PPIs. Gut 51:464–465, 2002.

30. Ladabaum U, Chey WD, Scheiman JM, Fendrick AM: Reappraisal of non-invasive management strategies for uninvestigated dyspepsia: a cost-minimization analysis. Aliment Pharmacol Ther 16:1491–1501, 2002.

31. McColl KEL, El-Nujumi A, Murray L, et al: The *Helicobacter pylori* breath test: A surrogate marker for peptic ulcer disease in dyspeptic patients. Gut 40:302–306, 1997.

32. Heaney A, Collins JSA, Watson RGP, et al: A prospective randomised trial of a 'test and treat' policy versus endoscopy based management in young *Helicobacter pylori* positive patients with ulcer-like dyspepsia, referred to a hospital clinic. Gut 45:186–190, 1999.

33. Gillen D, McColl KEL: Does concern about missing malignancy justify endoscopy in uncomplicated dyspepsia in patients aged less than 55? Am J Gastroenterol 94:75–79, 1999.

34. Breslin NP, Thomson ABR, Bailey RJ, et al: Gastric cancer and other endoscopic findings in young patients with dyspepsia. Gut 46:93–97, 2000.

35. Bytzer P: Can noninvasive *Helicobacter pylori* testing save endoscopy? [editorial]. Endoscopy 29:649–651, 1997.

36. Agréus L, Engstrand L, Svärdsudd K, et al: *Helicobacter pylori* seropositivity among Swedish adults with and without abdominal symptoms: A population-based epidemiologic study. Scand J Gastroenterol 30:752–757, 1995.

37. Loffeld RJLF, Stobberingh E, Flendrig JA, et al: Diagnostic value of an immunoassay

to detect anti *Campylobacter pylori* antibodies in non-ulcer dyspepsia. Lancet i:1182–1185, 1989.

38. Ofman JJ, Etchason J, Fullerton S, Kahn KL, Soll AH: Management strategies for *Helicobacter pylori*-seropositive patients with dyspepsia: Clinical and economic consequences. Ann Intern Med 126:280–291, 1997.

39. Briggs AH, Sculpher MJ, Logan RPH, et al: Cost effectiveness of screening for and eradication of *Helicobacter pylori* in management of dyspeptic patients under 45 years of age. BMJ 312:1321–1325, 1996.

40. Lassen AM, Bytzer P, Schaffalitzky de Muckadell OB: *Helicobacter pylori* test and eradicate versus prompt endoscopy for management of dyspeptic patients: A randomised trial. Lancet 356:455–460, 2000.

41. Jones RH, Tait CL, Sladen G, Weston-Baker J: A trial of a test-and-treat strategy for *Helicobacter pylori* positive dyspeptic patients in general practice. Int J Clin Pract 53:413–416, 1999.

42. McColl KE, Murray LS, Gillen D, et al: Randomised trial of endoscopy with testing for *Helicobacter pylori* compared with non-invasive *H pylori* testing alone in the management of dyspepsia. BMJ 324:999–1002, 2002.

43. Chiba N, van Zanten SJ, Sinclair P, et al: Treating *Helicobacter pylori* infection in primary care patients with uninvestigated dyspepsia: The Canadian adult dyspepsia empiric treatment-*Helicobacter pylori* positive (CADET-Hp) randomised controlled trial. BMJ 324:1012–1016, 2002.

44. Bytzer P, Teglbjërg PS, Danish Ulcer Study Group: *Helicobacter pylori*-negative duodenal ulcers: Prevalence, clinical characteristics and prognosis. Results from a clinical trial with 2 year follow-up. Am J Gastroenterol 96:1409–1416, 2001.

45. Quan C, Talley NJ: Management of peptic ulcer disease not related to *Helicobacter pylori* or NSAIDs. Am J Gastroenterol 97:2950–2961, 2002.

46. Jyotheeswaran S, Shah AN, Jin HO, et al: Prevalence of *Helicobacter pylori* in peptic ulcer patients in Great Rochester, NY: Is empirical triple therapy justified? Am J Gastroenterol 93:574–578, 1998.

47. Hallissey MT, Allum WH, Jewkes AJ, Ellis DJ, Fielding JWL: Early detection of gastric cancer. BMJ 301:513–515, 1990.

48. Canga C, III, Vakil N: Upper GI malignancy, uncomplicated dyspepsia, and the age threshold for early endoscopy. Am J Gastroenterol 97:600–603, 2002.

49. Fjøsne U, Kleveland PM, Waldum H, et al: The clinical benefit of routine upper gastrointestinal endoscopy. Scand J Gastroenterol 21:433–440, 1986.

50. Hansen JM, Bytzer P, Bondesen S, Schaffalitzky de Muckadell OB: Efficacy and outcome of an open access endoscopy service. Dan Med Bull 38:288–290, 1991.

51. Hungin APS, Idle N, Thomas PR, et al: What happens to patients following open access gastroscopy? An outcome study from general practice. Br J Gen Pract 44:519–521, 1994.

52. Mitchell RM, Collins JS, Watson RG, Tham TC: Differences in the diagnostic yield of upper gastrointestinal endoscopy in dyspeptic patients receiving proton-pump inhibitors and H_2-receptor antagonists. Endoscopy 34:524–526, 2002.

53. Venables TL, Newland RD, Patel AC, et al: Omeprazole 10 milligrams once daily, omeprazole 20 milligrams once daily, or ranitidine 150 milligrams twice daily, evaluated as initial therapy for the relief of symptoms of gastro-oesophageal reflux disease in general practice. Scand J Gastroenterol 32:965–973, 1997.

54. Ofman JJ, Rabeneck L: The effectiveness of endoscopy in the management of dyspepsia: A qualitative systematic review. Am J Med 106:335–346, 1999.

55. Bytzer P: Cost-effectiveness of gastroscopy. Ital J Gastroenterol 31:749–760, 1999.

Role of Gastric Acid in Functional Dyspepsia

*Frank Friedenberg, M.D.,
and Robert S. Fisher, M.D.*

Over the past 25 years, great advances have been made in the diagnosis and treatment of peptic ulcer disease. *Helicobacter pylori* has emerged as a key pathogen in the development of both duodenal and gastric ulcers, and proton pump inhibitors have proven to be highly efficacious for treatment. Despite these advances, little has been accomplished in determining the origin of pain in ulcer disease. Although the role of gastric acid as a precipitant of pain has been investigated, no conclusive evidence has emerged. Confusion exists because of the high prevalence of individuals who are diagnosed with peptic ulcer disease who are pain free. Conversely, many patients with ulcers do not develop pain even with instillation of dilute hydrochloric acid into the stomach.[1] To further confound the situation, many patients develop ulcer-like pain but are found on endoscopic examination to have no macroscopic mucosal disease. These patients are referred to as having functional, or nonulcer dyspepsia. In some individuals with normal findings by endoscopic examination who fulfill the criteria of functional dyspepsia, acid suppression therapy provides prompt relief of symptoms, but in many others there is no improvement. This chapter discusses the role of gastric acid as one of perhaps many stimuli precipitating symptoms in patients with functional dyspepsia. Also, the potential role that *Helicobacter pylori* may play in this complex interaction is discussed.

Mechanism of Acid-Induced Pain

To understand how acid may cause pain in individuals with functional dyspepsia, it is important to recognize acid's role in ulcer disease (Fig. 1). In peptic ulcer disease, it is presumed that *H. pylori* or the use of nonsteroidal antiinflammatory drugs in conjunction with acid leads to ulceration. Gastric acid then activates local nociceptive chemoreceptors, causing pain. As mentioned, in patients without the presence of an ulcer, the origin of pain is unclear. These patients' symptoms are often

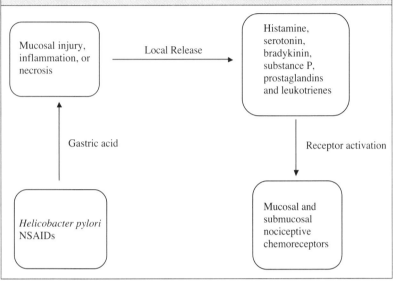

Figure 1. Mechanism of acid-induced pain in patients with peptic ulcer disease. NSAIDs = nonsteroidal anti-inflammatory drugs. (Adapted from Bonica J: The Management of Pain. Philadelphia, Lea & Febiger, 1990; and Higashi H: Pharmacological aspects of visceral sensory receptors. In Cervero F, Morrison JFB (eds): Visceral Sensation. Amsterdam, Elsevier, 1986, p 21.)

identical to the symptoms of patients with ulcer disease, suggesting that a similar mechanism may play a role. Table 1 highlights the prevailing theories that link gastric acid to functional dyspepsia.

Acid Secretory Abnormalities in Functional Dyspepsia

Patients with duodenal ulcer disease have a substantial increase in basal and maximal acid output. Infection with *H. pylori* augments gastrin release, causing an increase in parietal cell mass and acid output. Abnormalities of acid secretion in patients with functional dyspepsia have also been identified.

TABLE 1.   Potential Relationships Between Gastric Acid and Abdominal Symptoms in Patients with Functional Dyspepsia
Increased gastric acid secretion
Increased response to gastrin releasing peptide
Increased visceral sensitivity to luminal acid
Altered release or response to secretin and cholecystokinin
Alterations in phase II and III of migrating motor complex due to acid

Collen and Loebeberg[4] studied 66 consecutive patients with a diagnosis of nonulcer dyspepsia. Performed in 1989, this study included many patients with duodenitis (including erosions) and therefore these patients might not meet the current case definition of functional dyspepsia. Nonulcer dyspepsia patients were compared to healthy control subjects and to patients with duodenal ulcers; however, their *H. pylori* status was not determined. The authors found no difference in basal acid output between patients with dyspepsia (whether or not they had duodenitis) and normal control subjects. As expected, duodenal ulcer patients had a three-fold increase in basal acid output.

A subsequent study further examined whether patients with functional dyspepsia have inherent abnormalities of acid secretion and considered the effect of *H. pylori* status.[5] This study included three groups of *H. pylori*-positive patients (asymptomatic positive control subjects, duodenal ulcer patients, and those with nonulcer dyspepsia) who were compared to healthy, *H. pylori*-negative control subjects. All three *H. pylori*-positive groups were found to have higher basal gastrin concentrations and higher basal acid output than *H. pylori*-negative controls. The basal acid output in duodenal ulcer patients was increased sixfold, whereas the increase in *H. pylori*-positive nonulcer dyspepsia and *H. pylori*-positive normal control subjects was threefold. All *H. pylori*-positive groups had a more pronounced rise in gastrin after an infusion with gastrin-releasing peptide (GRP) than *H. pylori*-negative patients. *H. pylori*-positive, nonulcer dyspepsia patients had a 60% greater GRP-stimulated acid output in comparison to *H. pylori*-positive, asymptomatic control subjects, but this increase was far less than that seen in the ulcer patients. In conclusion, although there is no difference in basal acid output, patients with nonulcer dyspepsia have a heightened level of GRP-stimulated acid output that is between the output of *H. pylori*-positive healthy control subjects and the output of duodenal ulcer patients.

Visceral Perception During Acid Infusion

Although increased amounts of intraluminal acid may not be the cause of pain in some patients with functional dyspepsia, it is possible that there may be an increase in visceral sensitivity to this stimulus. Nearly 20 years ago, Joffe and Primrose[6] explored this possibility by studying patients with duodenal ulcer, duodenitis, and nonulcer dyspepsia. They performed direct infusions of 100 mL of 0.1 N hydrochloric acid, 8.5% sodium bicarbonate, or saline into the duodenal bulb in these three groups of patients. In all patients with nonulcer dyspepsia ($n = 8$), acid infusion did not reproduce their characteristic discomfort. In contrast, patients with either duodenitis or duodenal ulcer typically experienced pain with acid infusion. Misra and Broor[7] performed a similar study in a larger group of patients with functional dyspepsia; 300 mL of either 0.1M hydrochloric acid or saline were infused in a double-blind fashion into the gastric antrum. A positive test result was defined as the reproduction of dyspeptic symptoms with infusion. *H. pylori* status was not determined in either patients with dyspepsia or healthy control subjects. Approximately 20% ($n = 11$) of patients with nonulcer dyspepsia experienced pain with acid infusion, as compared to no occurrences with saline ($P <.05$). Of the 11 patients with positive results, 91% had a positive result when rechallenged with acid. None of the control subjects had symptoms with either saline or acid infusion.

George et al[8] studied the role of acid and duodenogastric reflux of pancreaticobiliary contents as a potential source of pain in patients with nonulcer dyspepsia. Eighteen patients with nonulcer dyspepsia (83% *H. pylori* positive) underwent aspiration of their small bowel juices before and after infusion of cholecyotkinin by a fluoroscopically placed catheter. In a blinded fashion, patients were infused with saline, 0.1N hydrochloric acid, or their own pancreaticobiliary fluid into the stomach. The definition of a positive result was similar to the definition in previous studies. These authors found no relationship between the contents of the infusate and the production of dyspeptic symptoms. They concluded that neither acid nor small bowel refluxate could be responsible for pain in patients with functional dyspepsia.

Samsom et al[9] performed the most recent study exploring the potential link between acid sensitivity and symptoms in patients with functional dyspepsia. The principle objective was to determine whether the clearance of exogenous acid from the duodenal bulb and proximal duodenum differed between patients with functional dyspepsia ($n = 12$) and healthy control subjects ($n = 10$). All patients were *H. pylori* negative and underwent duodenal bulb infusion with either saline or 0.1 N hydrochloric acid in a double-blind study. The procedure was repeated during fasting and after a standardized meal. In patients with functional dyspepsia, acid infusion, not saline, produced an increase in dyspepsia scores.

The balance of data indicates that a significant subset of patients with functional dyspepsia have a hypersensitivity to the infusion of acid. This effect appears to be independent of *H. pylori* status and is typically present during rechallenge. Several hypotheses have been suggested to explain acid hypersensitivity in patients with nonulcer dyspepsia.[10] First, acid hypersensitivity may be the result of peripheral sensitization of primary spinal afferent neurons after local tissue injury by acid. This would lead to the recruitment of "silent" nociceptors and ultimately central sensitization. Alternatively, some patients may develop acid hypersensitivity due to a relative loss of bulbospinal inhibitory modulation. Perhaps mechanoreceptors are involved to a greater degree than chemoreceptors in this population, or perhaps an as yet unknown stimulus in the gastroduodenal mucosal microenvironment plays an important role. The obvious limitation of studies to date is that acid delivered through an infusion catheter acidifies only a very focal area within the gastrointestinal tract; this does not reproduce normal physiologic conditions. Also, infusion of acid into either the stomach or the duodenum can produce symptoms; therefore, the location of acid hypersensitivity remains unclear.

Motility Abnormalities Precipitated by Acid

Based on the cited data, clearly neither an increase in acid secretion nor heightened acid sensitivity is the cause of pain in many patients with functional dyspepsia. An additional hypothesis is that secondary effects of acid, such as its ability to alter upper gastrointestinal tract motility, could cause pain in patients with dyspepsia. To study these relationships, Houghton et al[11] attempted to reproduce older studies that demonstrated delayed gastric emptying after duodenal acidification. They recruited 18 healthy volunteers (*H. pylori* status unknown) and subjected them to duodenal infusions of either saline or 0.1 M hydrochloric acid. Pressures in the gastric antrum, pylorus, and duodenum were measured during alternating infusions. The authors demonstrated that repetitive infusions of acid were associated with a decrease in antral contractility and a change from normal, coordinated contractile activity of the proximal duodenum to random, poorly coordinated contractions. In addition, there was an increase in isolated pyloric pressure waves. All of these motor changes could potentially result in a delay in emptying of acidic gastric contents.

Samsom et al[9] also sought to identify changes in antroduodenal motility related to the infusion of acid. After infusion of acid into the bulb during fasting, the number of pressure waves and pH in the proximal duodenum were found to be significantly lower in patients with functional dyspepsia than in healthy control subjects. These differences were not seen after the ingestion of a standard meal. It was concluded that patients with functional dyspepsia have defective acid clearance of the proximal small bowel and that the prolongation of acidity in that location may contribute to their symptoms.

Theoretically, based on this research, acid suppression therapy could reverse the antroduodenal motor abnormalities identified in patients with functional dyspepsia. One study utilized ranitidine and measured its effect on the interdigestive migrating motor complex (MMC).[12] Sixteen patients with nonulcer dyspepsia (*H. pylori* status unknown), found to have an increased basal acid output, underwent antroduodenal manometry. At least two complete MMCs were recorded in each patient. Under basal conditions, the duration of the complete MMC was significantly longer in patients with nonulcer dyspepsia when compared to a group of healthy control subjects. Patients with nonulcer dyspepsia were then treated with either intravenous ranitidine or intravenous cimetidine followed by ranitidine during phase II (period of irregular motor activity) of the MMC. Acid suppression therapy, after a significant lag period, produced a marked increase in the number and duration of MMC phase III contractions (a period of coordinated aboral contractions termed "activity fronts" by the authors) while shortening phase II. This same group performed a similar study using omeprazole.[13] Nine patients with nonulcer dyspepsia (*H. pylori*–negative) were studied, along with nine healthy control subjects. Omeprazole again shortened the duration of the MMC. In addition, omeprazole-related phase III activity was significantly longer than spontaneous phase III cycle length in patients with dyspepsia.

A more recent study used pantoprazole in a small but carefully selected patient group with functional dyspepsia, all negative for *H. pylori*.[14] The purpose of the study was twofold. First, the authors tested to see whether prior treatment with acid suppression therapy could reverse the decrease in proximal duodenal pressure waves induced by acid infusion in dyspeptic patients. They also studied whether acid suppression could relieve acid hypersensitivity in those patients previously found to be acid hypersensitive (developed typical dyspeptic pain during acid infusion into the antrum). Nineteen patients were randomized to pantoprazole 40 mg per day or placebo for 2 weeks and underwent antroduodenal manometry and acid-saline blinded infusions. Neither pantoprazole nor placebo resulted in a significant change in the number of duodenal pressure waves or antegrade propagated pressure wave sequences, including the preinfusion period and after acid or saline infusion. Pretreatment with pantoprazole did not ameliorate symptoms during acid infusion in patients who were previously identified as "acid-hypersensitive." Interestingly, there was little overlap in patients recruited for the study with an impaired motor response and those with acid hypersensitivity. The authors concluded that different motor and/or sensory impairments coexist in the heterogeneous group of patients labeled as having functional dyspepsia.

Potential Role of Cholecystokinin and Secretin

Gastric acid may cause dyspepsia indirectly through a delay in gastric emptying by virtue of its effect on cholecystokinin and secretin release (Fig. 2). Plasma levels of secretin rise in response to acidification

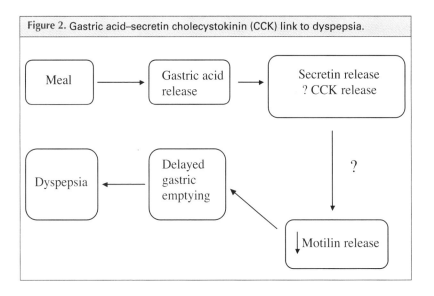

Figure 2. Gastric acid–secretin cholecystokinin (CCK) link to dyspepsia.

of the proximal duodenum. Secretin is responsible for the buffering of duodenal contents through the stimulation of pancreatic bicarbonate secretion. This allows for the optimal duodenal pH for lipolytic and proteolytic activity to occur. A lesser studied action of secretin is its role in increasing the half-time of gastric emptying, consequently allowing for more time to buffer acid. Mitznegg et al[15] were able to demonstrate that serum motilin levels declined in response to injections of secretin and that this fall was linearly related to pancreatic bicarbonate output. Kleibeuker et al[16] subsequently found that secretin may play a role in human gastric motility. In their study, nine healthy male subjects were fed 8% peptone formulas. The gastric pH was maintained at 5.5, 2.5, or 2.0 by intragastric titration. Plasma secretin levels were measured at each pH level by radioimmunoassay. Patients subsequently received an exogenous dose of secretin equivalent to the level produced when the gastric pH was acidified to 2.5. A small but detectable inhibition of gastric emptying was produced. In a follow-up study, these authors randomized healthy male subjects to saline, continuous secretin, or bolus secretin infusion after a standard meal.[17] Both continuous and bolus secretin infusion increased the gastric emptying half-time by 133% and 55%, respectively. It was concluded that secretin, at physiologic plasma concentrations, retards solid food emptying in humans. In an elegant study, Ho et al[18] demonstrated similar physiologic responses in a canine model. Secretin was shown to inhibit gastric emptying at physiologic concentrations along with the inhibition of gastric acid output, possibly through feedback inhibition of gastrin.

Much less information exists concerning the interaction of gastric acid and cholecystokinin. Whereas duodenal acidification is a well recognized stimulus for secretin release, this relationship is less clear for cholecystokinin. In a rat model, Raybould et al[19] were able to show that blockade of the cholecystokinin-A receptor caused a 30% reduction in the inhibition of gastric emptying induced by a duodenal infusion with 0.1 N hydrochloric acid.[19] In rats that had undergone functional ablation of the vagus nerve, there was no effect on the motility response to an acid load through cholecystokinin-A receptor blockade.

In conclusion, although never demonstrated, the indirect effects of gastric acid in patients with functional dyspepsia may be through the release of secretin or cholecystokinin. There may be increased release or sensitivity to these hormones. This may lead to a delay in gastric emptying in response to an acid load in the duodenum resulting in dyspepsia. Perhaps in some patients with functional dyspepsia responsive to antisecretory therapy, therapeutic effect is through an inhibition of the release of secretin or cholecystokinin. Future studies in this area are warranted, especially with the availability of highly accurate assays for these hormones and commercially available antagonists.

Evidence from Studies of Histamine-2 Receptor Blockers and Proton Pump Inhibitors

Effective therapy for functional dyspepsia is very important for the individual patient and has been shown to impact health care utilization, days at work, and overall quality of life.[20] Because acid may play an important role in some patients with functional dyspepsia, acid suppression therapy has been examined. Older studies utilized H_2-receptor antagonists and liquid antacids, whereas more recent information comes from trials utilizing proton pump inhibitors. The efficacy of medical therapy is difficult to show because of the relatively high incidence of a placebo effect (up to 45%) and by the heterogeneous, overlapping, and shifting symptoms of patients with functional dyspepsia. Table 2 reviews high-quality, prospective, randomized, double-blinded, placebo-controlled studies performed with acid suppression therapy for the treatment of functional dyspepsia. Several studies characterized patients as having reflux-like, ulcer-like, or motility-like dyspepsia. The magnitude of benefit from acid suppression over placebo has been marginal in most studies and of little clinical importance. A recent meta-analysis performed by Finney et al[29] examined all studies that utilized

TABLE 2. Selected Randomized, Prospective, Double-Blind, Placebo-Controlled Trials of Acid Suppression Therapy for Functional Dyspepsia

Study	Patients, n	Treatment Duration	Medication(s) studied	Results
Nyren[21] (1986)	159	3 weeks	Cimetidine 400 mg bid, liquid antacids	All reduced pain, no difference between study drugs and placebo
Talley[22] (1986)	62	4 weeks	Cimetidine 200 mg qid, pirenzepine 50 mg bid	Cimetidine marginally superior to placebo; pirenzipine inferior to placebo
Johannessen[23] (1988)	123	12 days	Cimetidine 400 mg tid	Multi-crossover study design; cimetidine superior to placebo
Singal[24] (1989)	56	4 weeks	Cimetidine 400 mg bid	Cimetidine superior to placebo
Farup[25] (1991)	115	6 weeks	Ranitidine 150 mg bid	Multi-crossover design; ranitidine superior to placebo
Lauritsen[26] (1996)	197	2 weeks	Omeprazole 20 mg bid	Omeprazole superior to placebo
Farup[27] (1997)	226	4 weeks	Ranitidine 150 mg bid	Multi-crossover design; ranitidine superior to placebo
Talley[28] (1998)	1262	4 weeks	Omeprazole 20 mg, omeprazole 10 mg once daily	Omeprazole at both doses marginally superior to placebo

cimetidine or ranitidine for the treatment of functional dyspepsia. Three of six studies ultimately included in the analysis demonstrated superiority of medication over placebo. The combined benefit from all six trials was 24 % (95% CI, 17–31), although the absolute benefit was quite small.

Proton pump inhibitors have not performed much better in clinical studies. Talley et al[28] highlight this point in the BOND and OPERA studies in which nearly 1300 patients were randomized to omeprazole 20 mg, omeprazole 10 mg, or placebo and followed for a total of 4 weeks. The authors were able to demonstrate symptom relief in 38% of patients on omeprazole 20 mg, 36% on omeprazole 10 mg, and 28% on placebo. A larger difference in improvement was identified in the groups with ulcer-like and reflux-like dyspepsia, however.

Key Points: Role of Gastric Acid in Functional Dyspepsia

∞ Several lines of evidence support the potential role of acid as an important etiologic factor in functional dyspepsia.

∞ In normal concentrations, acid may cause epigastric or retrosternal pain, possibly due to visceral hypersensitivity mediated by nociceptive afferent neurons.

∞ In some dyspeptic patients, acid has been shown to cause motor changes in the antroduodenal region, which may delay acid clearance from the proximal small intestine.

∞ Changes in the cycle length of the MMC and duration of phase II and phase III activity related to acid infusion are produced in these patients, possibly due to the direct effect of gastric acid or indirectly through the release of secretin or cholecystokinin.

∞ Empiric acid suppression therapy appears warranted but high failure rates can be expected.

Suggested Reading

1. Harrison A, Isenberg JI, Schapira M, et al: Most patients with active symptomatic duodenal ulcers fail to develop ulcer-type pain in response to gastroduodenal acidification. J Clin Gastroenterol 4:105–108, 1982.
2. Bonica J: The Management of Pain. Philadelphia, Lea & Febiger, 1990.
3. Higashi H: Pharmacological aspects of visceral sensory receptors. In Cervero F, Morrison JFB (eds): Visceral Sensation. Amsterdam, Elsevier, 1986, p 21.
4. Collen MJ, Loebenberg MJ. Basal gastric acid secretion in non-ulcer dyspepsia with or without duodenitis. Dig Dis Sci 34:246–250, 1989.
5. El-Omar E, Penman I, Ardill JES, et al: A substantial proportion of non-ulcer dyspepsia patients have the same abnormality of acid secretion as duodenal ulcer patients. Gut 36:534–538, 1995.
6. Joffee SN, Primrose JN. Pain provocation test in peptic duodenitis. Gastrointest Endosc 29:282–284, 1983.
7. Misra SP, Broor L: Is gastric acid responsible for the pain in patients with essential dyspepsia? J Clin Gastroenterol 12:624–627, 1990.
8. George AA, Tsuchiyose M, Dooley CP: Sensitivity of the gastric mucosa to acid and duodenal contents in patients with nonulcer dyspepsia. Gastroenterology 101:3–6, 1991.
9. Samson M, Verhagen MAMT, Henegouwen GPV, et al: Abnormal clearance of exogenous acid and increased acid sensitivity of the proximal duodenum in dyspeptic patients. Gastroenterology 116:515–520, 1999.
10. Mayer EA, Gebhart GF: Basic and clinical aspects of visceral hyperalgesia. Gastroenterology 107:271–293, 1994.
11. Houghton LA, Kerrigan DD, Read NW: Effect of intraduodenal infusion of acid on the antropyloroduodenal motor unit in human volunteers. J Gastrointest Motil 2:202–208, 1990.
12. Bortolotti M, Cucchiara S, Sarti P, et al: Interdigestive gastroduodenal motility in patients with ulcer-like dyspepsia: effect of ranitidine. Hepatogastroenterol 39:31–33, 1992.

13. Bortolotti M, Brunelli F, Sarti P, et al: Effect of omeprazole on interdigestive gastro-duodenal motility of patients with ulcer-like dyspepsia. Hepatogastroenterology 46:588–593, 1999.
14. Schwartz MP, Samson M, Verhagen MAMT, et al: Effect of inhibition of gastric acid secretion on antropyloroduodenal motor activity and duodenal acid hypersensitivity in functional dyspepsia. Aliment Pharmacol Ther 15:1921–1928, 2001.
15. Mitznegg P, Bloom SR, Domschke W, et al: Effect of secretin on plasma motilin in man. Gut 18:468–471, 1977.
16. Kleibeuker JH, Eysselein VE, Maxwell VE, et al: Role of endogenous secretin in acid-induced inhibition of human gastric function. J Clin Invest 73:526–532, 1984.
17. Kleibeuker JH, Beekhuis H, Piers DA, et al: Retardation of gastric emptying of solid foods by secretin. Gastroenterology 94:122–126, 1988.
18. Ho J, Lee KY, Chang TM, et al: Secretin: a physiological regulator of gastric emptying and acid output in dogs. Am J Physiol 267:G702–708, 1994.
19. Raybould HE, Holzer HH: Duodenal acid-induced inhibition of gastric motility and emptying in rats. Am J Physiol 265:G540–546, 1993.
20. Meineche-Schmidt V, Talley NJ, Pap A, et al: Impact of functional dyspepsia on quality of life and health care consumption after cessation of antisecretory treatment. Scand J Gastroenterol 34:566–574, 1999.
21. Nyren O, Adami H, Bates S, et al: Absence of therapeutic benefit from antacids or cimetidine in non-ulcer dyspepsia. N Eng J Med 314:339–343, 1986.
22. Talley NJ, McNeil D, Hayden A, et al: Randomized, double-blind, placebo-controlled crossover trial of cimetidine and pirenzipine in nonulcer dyspepsia. Gastroenterol 91:149–156, 1986.
23. Johannessen T, Fjosne U, Kleveland PM, et al: Cimetidine responders in non-ulcer dyspepsia. Scand J Gastroenterol 23:327–336, 1988.
24. Singal AK, Kumar A, Broor SL: Cimetidine in the treatment of non-ulcer dyspepsia: results of a randomized double-blind, placebo-controlled study. Curr Med Res Opin 11:390–397, 1989.
25. Farup PG, Larsen S, Ulshagen K, et al: Ranitidine for non-ulcer dyspepsia: a clinical study of the symptomatic effect of ranitidine and a classification and characterization of the responders to treatment. Scand J Gastroenterol 26:1209–1216, 1991.
26. Lauritsen K, Aalykke C, Havelund T, et al: Effect of omeprazole in functional dyspepsia: a double-blind randomized, placebo-controlled study. Gastroenterology 110(suppl):A702, 1996.
27. Farup PG, Weitterhus S, Osnes M, et al: Ranitidine effectively relieves symptoms in a subset of patients with functional dyspepsia. Scand J Gastroenterol 32:755–759, 1997.
28. Talley NJ, Meineche-Schmidt V, Pare P, et al: Efficacy of omeprazole in functional dyspepsia: double-blind, randomized, placebo-controlled trials (the BOND and OPERA studies). Aliment Pharmacol Ther 12:1055–1065, 1998.
29. Finney JS, Kinnersley NC, O'Bryan-Tear CG, et al: Meta-analysis of antisecretory and gastrokinetic compounds in functional dyspepsia. J Clin Gastroenterol 26:312–320, 1998.

Role of Motility and Accommodation Abnormalities in Functional (Nonulcer) Dyspepsia

*Hrair P. Simonian, M.D.,
and Henry P. Parkman, M.D.*

The 1999 Rome II criteria for the diagnosis of functional dyspepsia (Table 1) have been useful in standardizing the diagnosis of functional dyspepsia for clinical studies.[1] The Rome group also suggested subcategorizing patients with dyspepsia based on the predominant symptom into ulcer-like, dysmotility-like, and nonspecific dyspepsia (Table 2). Dysmotility-like functional dyspepsia has predominant symptoms of abdominal fullness, early satiety, bloating, and nausea. Specific symptoms that are used for categorizing patients into these subgroups, however, do not always correlate with pathophysiologic abnormalities and response to treatment.

A number of mechanisms have been proposed for the pathogenesis of functional dyspepsia.[2] These include inflammation, motility disturbances, visceral hypersensitivity, and psychological factors (Table 3). The gastric acid/inflammation hypothesis suggests that gastric acid and/or inflammation from acid, bile, or *Helicobacter pylori* infection is responsible for symptoms. This acid/inflammation hypothesis would also include occult gastroesophageal reflux disease and postinfectious dyspepsia.[3] The motor disorder hypothesis suggests that gastric dysmotility, such as delayed gastric emptying, impaired fundic accommodation, antral distension, or gastric dysrhythmias, is important. The visceral hypersensitivity hypothesis suggests exaggerated symptoms in response to physiochemical stimuli such as distension, contraction, acid, and bile. The psychological/psychiatric hypothesis proposes that symptoms are related to depression, anxiety, or a somatization disorder.

TABLE 1.   Rome II Criteria (1999) for Functional Dyspepsia
Persistent or recurrent abdominal pain or discomfort centered in the upper abdomen. Discomfort is defined as an unpleasant sensation and may include fullness, bloating, early satiety, and nausea.
Symptom duration of at least 12 weeks, which need not be consecutive, within the preceding 12 months.
No evidence of organic disease (including at time of upper endoscopic examination) that is likely to explain the symptoms.
No evidence that dyspepsia is exclusively relieved by defecation or associated with the onset of a change in stool frequency or stool form (i.e., not irritable bowel syndrome).

This chapter discusses the role of gastric motility and accommodation abnormalities in the pathogenesis of functional dyspepsia.

Gastrointestinal Dysmotility in Functional Dyspepsia

Motility abnormalities of the stomach have been found in many patients with unexplained dyspepsia. Gastric dysmotility, including delayed gastric emptying, impaired gastric accommodation to a meal, and gastric dysrhythmias, appear to be important pathophysiologic factors in some patients with functional dyspepsia. Each of these abnormalities may be present in 25% to 40% of patients, depending on the particular study. One or more of these factors may be detected in one half to two thirds of patients with functional dyspepsia.[4] However, nearly half of patients do not have these gastric motor abnormalities, suggesting that other factors, such as visceral hypersensitivity or inflammation, are important in the pathogenesis of functional dyspepsia.

TABLE 2. Rome II Subgroups for Functional Dyspepsia*	
Subtype	**Predominant Symptom**
Ulcer-like	Pain in upper abdomen
Dysmotility-like	Discomfort, fullness, early satiety, bloating, nausea
Nonspecific	No predominant symptom
Overlap syndromes (not primarily dyspepsia, if main symptom):	
Gastroesophageal reflux disease	Heartburn, acid regurgitation
Irritable bowel syndrome	Pain relieved with defecation
Biliary tract disease	Right upper quadrant abdominal pain
*Based on predominant or most bothersome symptom	

TABLE 3.	Pathophysiologic Factors Linked to Functional Dyspepsia
Inflammation	
Gastric acid sensitivity	
Helicobacter pylori gastritis	
Enterogastric (bile) reflux	
Motility disturbances	
Delayed gastric emptying/antral hypomotility	
Impaired fundic relaxation/antral distension to meal	
Gastric dysrhythmias	
Visceral hypersensitivity	
Gastric	
Duodenal	
Psychological factors	

Abnormalities in Gastric Emptying

Delayed gastric emptying is present in approximately 35% of patients with functional dyspepsia, with results of studies ranging from 25% to 80%.[4-6] Differentiation between "dysmotility-like" functional dyspepsia and idiopathic gastroparesis may be arbitrary: in cases of functional dyspepsia, the predominant symptom is often abdominal discomfort or pain; whereas in a patient labeled with gastroparesis, the predominant symptom is nausea or vomiting. Specific dyspeptic symptoms and their severity have generally correlated poorly with the degree of gastric stasis.[7] However, in a series of 343 patients with functional dyspepsia, in whom delayed gastric emptying was present in 34%, moderate to severe postprandial fullness and/or vomiting correlated with the presence of delayed gastric emptying.[5]

Recent studies from several groups, including our own, have shown that extending the conventional time of the gastric emptying scintigraphy (GES) test from 2 hours to 4 hours hours detects more patients with an abnormality of gastric emptying.[6] The 4-hour GES test appears to be more reliable in assessing overall gastric emptying. In our study, GES was performed in 66 patients with functional dyspepsia after ingestion of a radiolabelled egg sandwich meal, with imaging at 2, 3, and 4 hours.[6] The percentage of functional dyspeptic patients with delayed gastric emptying found by the conventional 2-hour test was 32%. Extending the GES test to 4 hours and using the results of the 2-, 3-, and 4-hour scans detected delayed gastric emptying in 42 of 66 patients (64%) with functional dyspepsia (Fig. 1). These data suggest that the proportion of patients with functional dyspepsia who have gastroparesis may

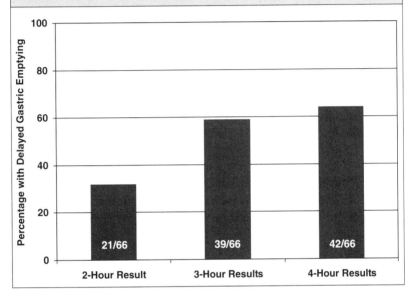

Figure 1. Extending the gastric emptying scintigraphy (GES) test from 2 to 4 hours detects more patients with gastroparesis. These data indicate that the proportion of patients with functional dyspepsia who have gastroparesis may be underestimated when only a 2-hour GES test is used. (Data from Guo J-P, Maurer AH, Urbain J-L, et al: Extending gastric emptying scintigraphy from two to four hours detects more patients with gastroparesis. Digest Dis Sci 46:24–29, 2001.)

be underestimated when only a 2-hour GES test is used. In our study, we found that symptoms of early satiety, nausea, and vomiting, but not abdominal pain, were more severe in functional dyspeptic patients with delayed gastric emptying than in functional dyspeptic patients with normal gastric emptying.

Regional Gastric Dysfunction: Impaired Fundic Accommodation and Antral Distension

Regional gastric function abnormalities may be present in many dyspeptic patients and appear to correlate with dyspeptic symptoms. Normally, the stomach accommodates a meal by relaxation of the gastric fundus and corpus, providing the meal with a reservoir and enabling a volume increase without a rise in intragastric pressure. Reduced postprandial fundic relaxation with impaired accommodation was found in 40% of patients with functional dyspepsia.[8] Impaired proximal gastric accommodation was associated with early satiety and subsequent weight loss and may be related to a vagal defect.[9–13] Impaired fundic ac-

Figure 2. Regional gastric emptying abnormalities in functional dyspepsia. Shown are early images from gastric emptying scintigraphy tests in a normal subject and a patient with functional dyspepsia. In the normal subject, food remains in the proximal half of the stomach immediately after ingestion. It is subsequently redistributed to the distal half over time. In the dyspeptic patient, the activity is quickly distributed to the distal half of the stomach.

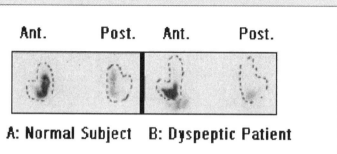

Ant.   Post.   Ant.   Post.

A: Normal Subject   B: Dyspeptic Patient

commodation causes a rapid transit from the proximal stomach into the antrum, leading to early antral distension (Fig. 2). Antral distension, in several studies, has correlated with symptoms.

A subset of dyspeptic patients (17–25%) have a history suggestive of postinfectious dyspepsia.[3] These are patients who have a sudden onset of dyspeptic symptoms, often initially accompanied with symptoms of an acute gastrointestinal infection such as fever, myalgia, or vomiting. Compared to patients with dyspepsia of unspecified onset, these patients are younger and have more symptoms of early satiety, nausea, and vomiting. In a recent study, patients with acute onset "postinfectious" dyspepsia were found to have a high prevalence of impaired accommodation attributable to a dysfunction at the level of gastric nitrergic neurons.[3] The studies showed that in these patients, gastric relaxation measured by a barostat occurred after the administration of amyl nitrate, which acts directly on the muscle, but did not occur after administration of sumatriptan, a 5-HT$_1$ agonist that releases nitric oxide from NO nerves. In contrast, gastric relaxation was obtained after administration of each of these agents in normal subjects and patients with dyspepsia of unspecified onset.

Radionuclide imaging of the gastric wall with single photon emission computed tomography to calculate gastric volumes has been used as a noninvasive measure of gastric accommodation.[14] Single photon emission computed tomography imaging in 32 patients with functional dyspepsia suggested that impaired gastric accommodation (41%) may occur more commonly than delayed emptying (9%) in dyspeptic patients referred to tertiary centers. The majority of the dyspeptic patients were found to have normal gastric emptying and accommodation.[14]

Satiety testing with water or a nutrient drink has also been suggested as a noninvasive technique to evaluate impaired accommodation and sensation. One example is the water load test, in which the subject drinks water until full.[15] Functional dyspeptic patients have reduced consumption. Another is a slow caloric drinking test, in which a nutrient drink is ingested at 15 mL/min.[16] The results of this satiety test are correlated with gastric accommodation to a meal as measured by the barostat. These satiety tests offer the potential to evaluate gastric accommodation in a noninvasive way. A reduced tolerated volume, however, may reflect either impaired accommodation or hypersensitivity of the stomach.[17]

Abnormalities in Antroduodenal Manometry

Antroduodenal manometry provides information about the amplitude, frequency, and coordination of gastric and duodenal motor function in both fasting and postprandial periods (Fig. 3). Antroduodenal manometry has been utilized to study patients with functional dyspepsia. The most common abnormality, present in about half of patients, is postprandial antral hypomotility.[19] Antral hypomotility correlates with delayed gastric emptying.[20]

Several studies have also suggested that small bowel motor dysfunction occurs in a proportion of patients with nonulcer dyspepsia[19]; other investigators have reported small intestinal dysmotility in only a small percentage.[21] Abnormalities of the small intestine may include retrograde, simultaneous, or a reduced frequency of fasting migrating motor complex activity as well as a reduced percentage of migrating motor complexes that start in the antrum. In the fed state, decreased or low-amplitude duodenal contractions may occur. In a study of 41 consecutive patients with severe chronic dyspepsia, a neuropathic disorder (contractions of normal amplitude but abnormal propagation) was present in 39%, myopathy (low-amplitude contractions with normal coordination) in 2%, and normal small bowel motility in 59%.[22]

Decreased antral contractility and phase III migrating motor complexes originating in the small intestine rather than in the stomach can be seen in cases of gastroparesis (see Fig. 3). Occasionally, pylorospasm or irregular bursts of small intestinal contractions, which increase outflow resistance, can be seen. Antroduodenal manometry can help confirm or exclude a gastrointestinal motility disorder if the gastric emptying test result is normal or borderline.[18]

Abnormalities on Gastric Myoelectric Activity in Functional Dyspepsia

Electrogastrography (EGG) is the recording of gastric myoelectrical activity, using cutaneous electrodes on the anterior abdomen overlying

Figure 3. Antroduodenal manometry. **A**, Normal antroduodenal manometry reading in the fasting state. Antral motor activity is recorded in the proximal three leads and duodenal activity is recorded in the distal three leads. A migrating motor complex is seen, starting in the antrum, which propagates into small intestine as recorded in the lower three leads. **B**, Antral hypomotility is seen with essentially no antral motility in the top three antral leads. A spontaneous phase-3 migrating motor complex (MMC) originates in the small intestine (bottom three leads).

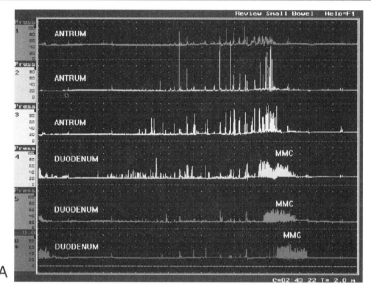

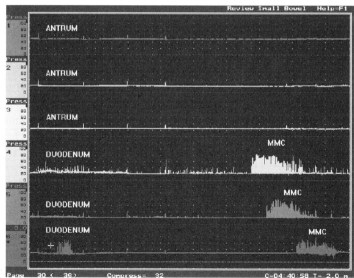

the stomach (Fig. 4). The dominant frequency of the EGG corresponds to the gastric electrical rhythm, or frequency of the gastric slow wave.[23] The normal gastric slow wave frequency is approximately three cycles per minute. Meal ingestion increases the amplitude of the EGG signal due to increases in gastric electrical activity and contractility and/or gas-

Figure 4. Electrogastrography (EGG). **A,** Normal EGG activity with three-cycle/minute activity. **B,** Period of tachygastria. In these figures, multichannel EGG was recorded using Medtronic Polygram ID EGG system with Polygram NET 311224 using 2.5-dB thresholds and 1.8-cpm high-pass filter.

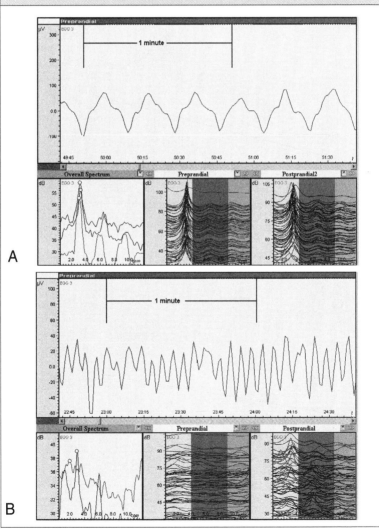

tric distension from the meal. EGG measures the frequency and regularity of gastric myoelectrical activity, detects abnormal rhythms of gastric myoelectrical activity, and assesses the amplitude/power increase after a meal.[18]

Electrogastrography is used to demonstrate gastric myoelectric abnormalities in patients with unexplained nausea and vomiting or functional dyspepsia (see Fig. 4). The EGG is generally used as an adjunct to gastric emptying scintigraphy as part of a comprehensive evaluation of patients with refractory symptoms.[18] Studies have suggested a good correlation between delayed gastric emptying by scintigraphy and an abnormal EGG.[24] The EGG abnormalities seen in delayed gastric emptying are primarily postprandial dysrhythmias and a lack of the normal postprandial increase in the power of the dominant frequency. EGG abnormalites are is present in 75% of patients with gastroparesis, as compared to only 25% of symptomatic patients with normal gastric emptying. Gastric dysrhythmias may be better predictors of symptoms than delayed gastric emptying and may correlate better with symptomatic response to medications.[25] In diabetic patients, hyperglycemia may itself provoke dysrhythmias, primarily tachygastrias.[26]

Gastric myoelectrical abnormalities measured by EGG, such as tachygastria and bradygastria and decreased postprandial to fasting power ratio, are found in about 40% of patients with functional dyspepsia.[24,27–29] This prevalence of EGG abnormalities is similar to that of delayed gastric emptying in functional dyspepsia. However, there is not a one-to-one correlation between an abnormal GES finding and an abnormal EGG: some patients with delayed gastric emptying may have a normal EGG, and some patients with a normal GES finding may have an abnormal EGG. The two tests, EGG and GES, appear to complement each other in attributing symptoms to gastric dysmotility.[30] In our study evaluating the EGGs of patients with dyspeptic symptoms, an abnormal EGG was seen in 22 of 72 (31%) patients: 11 of 22 (50%) patients with delayed gastric emptying and 11 of 50 patients (22%) with normal gastric emptying. Symptoms of upper abdominal discomfort and anorexia were more severe in patients with an abnormal EGG compared to patients with a normal EGG. Symptom scores were significantly higher in patients with both delayed gastric emptying and abnormal EGG compared with patients with normal gastric emptying and EGG, normal gastric emptying and abnormal EGG, and delayed gastric emptying and normal EGG (Fig. 5).

How EGG results affect patient management is controversial. In two small studies, dyspeptic patients with an abnormal EGG had a more favorable response to treatment with prokinetic agent than did patients with a normal EGG.[31,32]

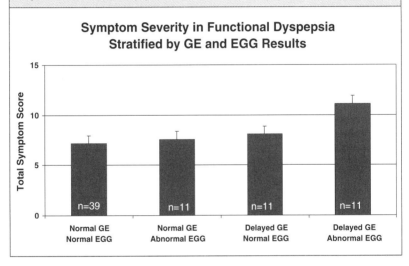

Figure 5. Electrogastrography (EGG) and gastric emptying scintigraphy (GES) are complementary for assessment of dyspepsia. In this study, a 2-hour GES and a 2-hour EGG were performed in 72 patients with dyspeptic symptoms. Delayed gastric emptying was detected in 22 of 72 patients (31%). An abnormal EGG was detected in 22 of 72 patients (31%). In addition, their symptoms of upper abdominal discomfort, early satiety, postprandial abdominal distension, nausea, vomiting, and anorexia were graded by the patient as none (0), mild (1), moderate (2), or severe (3). A total symptom score was calculated as the sum of these six individual symptoms scores. This figure shows their total symptom score with the patients stratified by their GES and EGG results. Symptoms scores were significantly higher in patients with both delayed gastric emptying and abnormal EGG compared with patients with normal gastric emptying and EGG, normal gastric emptying and abnormal EGG, and delayed gastric emptying and normal EGG. (Data from Parkman HP, Miller MA, Trate D, et al: Electrogastrography and gastric emptying scintigraphy are complementary for assessment of dyspepsia. J Clin Gastroenterol 24:214–219., 1997.)

Recently, multichannel EGG recording using electrodes placed at several positions overlying the stomach has been suggested to assess slow-wave propagation and coupling.[33] Patients with functional dyspepsia were found to have inconsistencies in frequency and regularity of gastric slow waves, suggesting impaired slow-wave propagation and coupling.[33]

Thus, there are several pathophysiologic alterations of gastric motility and sensation in functional dyspepsia. Distinct pathophysiologic abnormalities may be present in subgroups of patients, perhaps causing different symptoms, and may predict different responses to treatment. One recent study found that 23% of patients with functional dyspepsia had delayed gastric emptying with associated symptoms of nausea, vomiting, and postprandial fullness, 35% of patients had hypersensitivity to gastric distension associated with symptoms of pain, belching, and weight loss, and 40% had impaired accommodation associated with symptoms of early satiety and weight loss.[4] Twenty-three percent of patients had two or three of these abnormalities, whereas 26% had none, suggesting still another as yet unidentified mechanism of functional dyspepsia. Unfortunately, individual symptoms do not strongly predict underlying pathophysiology.[4] These disorders may be interrelated: reduced fundic accommodation may lead to increased wall tone in response to distension or meal ingestion and may lead to stimulation of visceral afferent nerves and cerebral perception of gastric events/symptoms.[14]

Treatment Focusing on Gastric Motility Abnormalities

There is much literature, although inconsistent, on the treatment of functional dyspepsia. Methodologic shortcomings are present in many studies, including suboptimal study design, unclear inclusion criteria, unvalidated outcome measures, and a short duration of follow-up.[34] In addition, the placebo response in patients with functional dyspepsia can be substantial, approximating 45%.[35] Treatment modalities that have been tested extensively include acid suppressive agents, promotility compounds, and H. pylori eradication. At this time, in part due to the current lack of effective promotility compounds, treatment of functional dyspepsia is aimed at either gastric acid suppression with proton pump inhibitors or visceral hypersensitivity with low-dose antidepressant agents.

Detection of delayed gastric emptying or an abnormal EGG in patients with functional dyspepsia may have prognostic important, since these patients may respond better to prokinetic agents than patients with normal emptying. However, this link of prokinetic agent treatment improving gastric emptying and symptoms has not been well shown. In some studies, both delayed emptying and symptoms may be improved by prokinetic therapy; at other times, emptying or symptoms have improved, but not both.[36]

Promotility Agents

The lack of available promotility compounds at present limits agressive treatment with promotility agents. Promotility agents including metoclopramide, cisapride, and domperidone, have improved dyspeptic symptoms more effectively than placebo in the majority of studies[34,37]; improvement in symptoms with promotility agents has been 40% to 45% greater than placebo.[37] The few studies that compare the effects of acid-suppressing and promotility agents on dyspeptic symptoms have favored the promotility agents.[38]

Several meta-analyses of the prokinetic agent studies in functional dyspepsia have been published.[37,39,40] In a recent meta-analysis of 17 cisapride studies and four domperidone studies, both cisapride and domperidone seemed to be efficacious.[40] For cisapride, there were overall reductions in epigastric pain, early satiety, abdominal distension, and nausea. Another recent meta-analysis found a funnel plot of study results to suggest that publication bias may be skewing the data on the efficacy of prokinetic agents.[41]

Erythromycin and other motilin receptor agonists are potent stimulants of gastric motor function. They have not yet demonstrated efficacy in functional dyspepsia. The motilin receptor agonist, ABT-229, was ineffective in dyspeptic patients with delayed gastric emptying.[42] It is speculated that since motilin receptor agonists increase proximal gastric tone, they may aggravate the impaired fundic accommodation in functional dyspepsia, which could explain the worsening of postprandial symptoms with ABT-229.[42]

Future treatments being evaluated for functional dyspepsia include newer prokinetic agents. These include $5-HT_4$ agonists (tegaserod and cilansetron), dopamine receptor antagonists (levosulpiride), cholecystokinin antagonists (loxiglumide and its dextroisomer, dexloxiglumide), and several motilin agonists. The $5-HT_4$ agonist tegaserod has been found to accelerate gastric emptying as well as to have an effect on visceral afferent sensation.[43] Tegaserod may be helpful in some patients with functional dyspepsia, but studies are available only in abstract form.[44]

Fundic Relaxing Agents

Agents that relax the fundus and improve the accommodation response may be helpful in some patients with functional dyspepsia, perhaps those with early satiety. $5-HT_1$ agonists (sumatriptan, buspirone), α-adrenergic receptor agonists (clonidine), and nitric oxide donors (glyceryl trinitrate) have been tried in several small series.[45]

The $5-HT_1$ agonists, such as sumatriptan, induce relaxation of the gastric fundus through a nitric oxide-mediated pathway. Sumatriptan allows larger volumes to be accommodated before perception or discomfort is reached and improves meal-induced satiety in patients with functional dyspepsia.[46] It is given primarily by injection. Recently, it has become available as an oral agent. Buspirone, an oral $5-HT_1$ agonist, may have effects similar to sumatriptan. It also has anxiolytic properties.

The α-adrenergic agonist, clonidine, reduces proximal gastric tone and pain perception during gastric distension in normal subjects.[47]

Thus, clonidine has the potential to reduce gastric sensation and/or increase gastric compliance without altering other physiologic motor functions. Some studies have suggested that clonidine may delay gastric emptying.[48]

Sildenafil (Viagra) has been shown to increase gastric accommodation.[49] In animal models, it also relaxes the pylorus and improves gastric emptying.[50] In humans, however, it slows gastric emptying.[49]

Recent studies suggest that 5-HT$_3$ receptor agonists relax the gastric fundus without inhibiting antral motility.[51] These may be useful for impaired accommodation.

Gastric Antidysrhythmics

The area of antidysrhythmics has recently been receiving attention because of the increased availability of EGG. Many of the prokinetic agents, such as metoclopramide, cisapride,[52] and domperidone,[25] have been shown to correct gastric dysrhythmias. Prostaglandin inhibitors have been shown to resolve tachygastrias in vitro and in vivo during hyperglycemia.[53] In several patients, indomethacin has improved symptoms and gastric myoelectrical abnormalities.[54] Unfortunately, indomethacin is also ulcerogenic.

Key Points: Role of Motility and Accommodation Abnormalities in Functional (Nonulcer) Dyspepsia

- The initial approach to patients with functional dyspepsia initially involves excluding ulcer disease, followed by empiric treatment trials. Further evaluation, such as gastric emptying and EGG, can be performed to identify delayed gastric emptying and gastric dysrhythmias.
- These tests can demonstrate abnormalities in approximately 30% to 45% of patients with functional dyspepsia.
- Detection of delayed gastric emptying or an abnormal EGG in patients with functional dyspepsia may provide prognostic information, since these patients may respond better to prokinetic agents than patients with normal emptying, although this remains controversial.
- At this time, there is a paucity of available effective promotility agents to aggressively treat gastric dysmotility in patients with functional dyspepsia.

Key Points (*Continued*)

∞ Newer agents that target specific pathophysiologic abnormalities, such as impaired gastric accommodation, gastric dysrhythmias, and visceral hypersensitivity, are involved in clinical research studies.

∞ New techniques using satiety testing to assess impaired accommodation/hypersensitivity and gastric mucosal labeling with scintigraphy to assess changes in gastric volume after a meal offer diagnostic potential to evaluate gastric accommodation and/or hypersensitivity in practical, noninvasive ways.

Suggested Reading

1. Talley NJ, Stanghellini V, Heading RC, et al: Functional gastrointestinal disorders. Gut 45(Suppl II):1137–1142, 1999.

2. Fisher RS, Parkman HP: Management of nonulcer dyspepsia. N Engl J Med 339:1376–1381, 1998.

3. Tack J, Demedts I, Dehondt G, et al: Clinical and pathophysiological characteristics of acute-onset functional dyspepsia. Gastroenterology 122:1738–1747, 2002.

4. Tack J, Bisschops R, Degreef T, et al: Can symptoms predict underlying pathophysiological mechanisms in functional dyspepsia? Gastroenterology 120:A80, 2001.

5. Stanghellini V, Tosetti C, Paternico A, et al: Risk indicators of delayed gastric emptying of solids in patients with functional dyspepsia. Gastroenterology 110:1036–1042, 1996.

6. Guo J-P, Maurer AH, Fisher RS, Parkman HP: Extending gastric emptying scintigraphy from two to four hours detects more patients with gastroparesis. Dig Dis Sci 46:24–29, 2001.

7. Talley NJ, Verlinden M, Jones M: Can symptoms discriminate among those with delayed or normal gastric emptying in dysmotility-like dyspepsia? Am J Gastroenterol 96:1422–1428, 2001.

8. Tack J, Piessevaux H, Coulie B, et al: Role of impaired gastric accommodation to a meal in functional dyspepsia. Gastroenterology 115:1346–1352, 1998.

9. Troncon LEA, Bennett RM, Ahluwalia NK, Thompson DC: Abnormal distribution of food during gastric emptying in functional dyspepsia patients. Gut 35:327–332, 1994.

10. Gilja OH, Hausken T, Wilhelmsen I, Berstad A: Impaired accommodation of proximal stomach to a meal in functional dyspepsia. Dig Dis Sci 41:689–696, 1996.

11. Salet CAM, Samsom M, Roelofs IMM, et al: Responses to gastric distention in functional dyspepsia. Gut 42:823–829, 1998.

12. Tack J, Piessevaux H, Coulie B, et al: Role of impaired gastric accommodation to a meal in functional dyspepsia. Gastroenterology 115:1346–1352, 1998.

13. Scott AM, Kellow JE, Shuter B, et al: Intragastric distribution and gastric emptying of solids and liquids in functional dyspepsia. Dig Dis Sci 38:2247–2254, 1993.

14. Kim D-Y, Delgado-Aros S, Camilleri M, et al: Noninvasive measurement of gastric in patients with idiopathic nonulcer dyspepsia. Am J Gastroenterol 96:3099–3105, 2001.

15. Koch KL, Hong S-P, Xu L: Reproducibility of gastric myoelectrical activity and the

water load test in patients with dysmotility-like dyspepsia symptoms and in control subjects. J Clin Gastroenterol 31:125–129, 2000.

16. Tack JF, Caenepeel P, Vos R, Janssens J: A satiety test to assess gastric accommodation in functional dyspepsia. Gastroenterology 118:A389, 2000.

17. Kim D-Y, Myung S-J, Camilleri M: Novel testing of human gastric motor and sensory functions: Rationale, methods, and potential applications in clinical practice. Am J Gastroenterol 95:3365–3373, 2000.

18. Camilleri M, Hasler W, Parkman HP, et al: Measurement of gastroduodenal motility in the GI laboratory. Gastroenterology 115:747–762, 1998.

19. Malagelada J-R, Stanghellini V: Manometric evaluation of functional upper gut symptoms. Gastroenterology 88:1223–1231, 1985.

20. Camilleri M, Brown ML, Malagelada J-R: Relationship between impaired gastric emptying and abnormal gastrointestinal motility. Gastroenterology 91:94–99, 1986.

21. Stanghellini V, Ghidini C, Ricci Maccarini M, et al: Fasting and postprandial gastrointestinal motility in ulcer and nonulcer dyspepsia. Gut 33:184–190, 1992.

22. Bjornsson ES, Abrahamsson H: Contractile patterns in patients with severe chronic dyspepsia. Am J Gastroenterol 94:54–64, 1999.

23. Chen JZ, McCallum RW: Clinical applications of electrogastrography. Am J Gastroenterol 88:1324–1336, 1993.

24. Lin X, Levanon D, Chen JDZ: Impaired postprandial gastric slow waves in patients with functional dyspepsia. Dig Dis Sci 43:1678–1684, 1998.

25. Koch KL, Stern RM, Stewart WR, et al: Gastric emptying and gastric myoelectrical activity in patients with diabetic gastroparesis: effect of long-term domperidone treatment. Am J Gastroenterol 84:1069–1075, 1989.

26. Jebbink RJA, Samsom M, Bruus PPM, et al: Hyperglycemia induces abnormalities of gastric myoelectrical activity in patients with type 1 diabetes mellitus. Gastroenterology 107:1390–1397, 1994.

27. Ghoos YF, Maes BD, Geypens BJ, et al: Measurement of gastric emptying rate of solids by means of a carbon-labeled octanoic acid breath test. Gastroenterology 104:1640–1647, 1993.

28. Koch KL, Hong S-P, Xu L: Reproducibility of gastric myoelectrical activity and the water load test in patients with dysmotility-like dyspepsia symptoms and in control subjects. J Clin Gastroenterol 31:125–129, 2000.

29. Lin Z, Eaker EY, Sarosiek I, et al: Gastric myoelectrical activity and gastric emptying in patients with functional dyspepsia. Am J Gastroenterol 94:2384–2389, 1999.

30. Parkman HP, Miller MA, Trate D, et al: Electrogastrography and gastric emptying scintigraphy are complementary for assessment of dyspepsia. J Clin Gastroenterology 24:214–219, 1997.

31. Chen JDZ, Ke MY, Lin XM, et al: Cisapride provides symptomatic relief in functional dyspepsia associated with gastric myoelectrical abnormality. Aliment Pharmacol Ther 14:1041–1047, 2000.

32. Besherdas K, Leahy A, Mason I, et al: The effect of cisapride on dyspepsia symptoms and the electrogastrogram in patients with non-ulcer dyspepsia. Aliment Pharm Ther 12:755–759, 1998.

33. Lin X, Chen JZ: Abnormal gastric slow waves in patients with functional dyspepsia assessed with multichannel electrogastrography. Am J Physiol 280:G1370-G1375, 2001.

34. Veldhuyzen van Zanten SJO, Cleary C, Talley NJ, et al: Drug treatment of functional dyspepsia: a systematic analysis of trial methodology with recommendations for design of future trials. Am J Gastroenterol 91:660–673, 1996.

35. Mearin F, Balboa A, Zarate N, et al: Placebo in functional dyspepsia: symptomatic,

gastrointestinal motor, and gastric sensorial responses. Am J Gastroenterol 94:116–125, 1999.

36. Jian R, Ducrot F, Ruskone A, et al: Symptomatic, radionuclide and therapeutic assessment of chronic idiopathic dyspepsia. Dig Dis 34:657–664, 1989.

37. Dobrilla G, Comberlato M, Steele A, et al: Drug treatment of functional dyspepsia: a meta-analysis of randomized controlled clinical trials. J Clin Gastroenterol 11:169–177, 1989.

38. Halter F, Miazza B, Brignoli R: Cisapride or cimetidine in the treatment of functional dyspepsia. Scand J Gastroenterol 29:618–623, 1994.

39. Finney JS, Kinnersley N, Hughes M, et al: Meta-analysis of antisecretory and gastrokinetic compounds in functional dyspepsia. J Clin Gastroenterol 26:312–320, 1998.

40. Veldhuyzen van Zanen SJOV, Jones MJ, Verlinden M, et al: Efficacy of cisapride and domperidone in functional dyspepsia: a meta-analysis. Am J Gastroenterol 96:689–696, 2001.

41. Soo S, Deeks JJ, Delaney BC, et al: A systematic review of pharmacological therapies in non-ulcer dyspepsia. Gastroenterology 118:A440, 2000.

42. Talley NJ, Verlinden M, Snape W, et al: Failure of a motilin receptor agonist (ABT-229) to relieve the symptoms of functional dyspepsia in patients with and without delayed gastric emptying. Aliment Pharmacol Ther 14:1653–1661, 2000.

43. Degen L, Matzinger D, Merz M, et al: Tegaserod, a 5-HT4 receptor partial agonist, accelerates gastric emptying and gastrointestinal transit in healthy male subjects. Aliment Pharmacol Ther 15:1745–1751, 2001.

44. Tack J, Delia T, Ligozio G, et al: A phase II placebo controlled randomized trial with tegaserod in functional dyspepsia patients with normal gastric emptying. Gastroenterology 122:A20, 2002.

45. Thumshirn M, Cho M-G, Zinsmeister AR, et al: Modulation of gastric sensory and motor functions by nitrergic and alpha-2 adrenergic agents. Gastroenterology 116:573–585, 1999.

46. Tack J, Coulie B, Andrioli A, et al: Influence of sumatriptan on gastric fundus tone and of the perception of gastric distension in man. Gut 46:468–473, 2000.

47. Thumshirn M, Cho M-G, Zinsmeister AR, et al: Modulation of gastric sensory and motor functions by nitrergic and alpha-2 adrenergic agents. Gastroenterology 116:573–585, 1999.

48. Gullikson GW, Virina MA, Loeffler R, et al: Alpha-2-adrenergic model of gastroparesis. Am J Physiol 261:G426-G432, 1991.

49. Sarnelli G, Vos R, Sifrim D, et al: Influence of sildenafil on fasting and postprandial gastric tone in man [abstract]. Gastroenterology 120:A285-A286, 2001.

50. Watkins CC, Sawa A, Jaffrey S, et al: Insulin restores neuronal nitric oxide synthase expression and function that is lost in diabetic gastropathy. J Clin Invest 106:373–384, 2000.

51. Coleman NS, Marciani L, Blackshaw PE, et al: MKC-733, a selective 5-HT3 receptor agonist, stimulates small bowel transit and relaxes the gastric fundus in man. Gastroenterology 120:A71, 2001.

52. Rothstein RD, Alavi A, Reynolds JC: Electrogastrography in patients with gastroparesis and effect of long-term cisapride. Dig Dis Sci 38:1518–1524, 1993.

53. Hasler WL, Soudah HC, Dulai G, et al: Mediation of hyperglycemia-evoked gastric slow-wave dysrhythmias by endogenous prostaglandins. Gastroenterology 108:727–736, 1995.

54. Pimentel M, Sam C, Lin HC: Indomethacin improves symptoms and electrogastrographic findings in patients with gastric dysrhythmias. Neurogastroenterol Motil 13:422, 2001.

Role of
Helicobacter pylori
in Dyspepsia

chapter
20

Wai-Man Wong, M.D.,
and Benjamin Chun-Yu Wong, M.D.

Nonulcer dyspepsia (NUD), or functional dyspepsia, is a common problem encountered in gastroenterology. According to Rome II criteria, it is defined as persistent or recurrent pain or discomfort centered in the upper abdomen for at least 12 weeks in the preceding 12 months[1] and in the absence of clinical, biochemical, endoscopic, or ultrasonographic evidence of organic disease that would explain the symptoms. Dyspepsia affects 25% of the U.S. population annually and accounts for up to 5% of all visits to primary care physicians.[2,3] The prevalence of dyspepsia in the community has been found to be 21% in the United Kingdom, where 2% of the population consults their primary care physician with a new or first episode of dyspepsia each year, accounting for 40% of all gastroenterologic consultations. Community surveys have suggested that only 35% of sufferers consult their doctor, although this proportion rises with age.[4] In the Asia-Pacific region, dyspepsia is as common as in the rest of the world, with prevalence rates varying from 10% to 20%.[5–8] The pathophysiology of dyspepsia is not fully understood. However, several factors have been identified as relevant, including the roles of gastric acid secretion, gastroduodenal dysmotility, visceral hypersensitivity, the effects of stress and psychological factors, and *Helicobacter pylori* infection. This chapter focuses on the role of *H. pylori* infection in dyspepsia.

Pathogenesis

The role of *H. pylori* infection on the pathogenesis of NUD is still unclear. *H. pylori* infection invariably causes chronic gastritis, which is characterized by a neutrophilic infiltration of the gastric mucosa and the production of inflammatory mediators, which may

- affect gastric acid secretion
- lead to gastric dysmotility
- possibly affect visceral perception

The consensus from the literature, however, is that *H. pylori* infection is not associated with impaired gastric emptying.[9,10] Furthermore, gastric accommodation to meal ingestion was reduced in patients with dyspepsia, irrespective of their *H. pylori* status.[11] The impaired accommodation was associated with an increased perception of distension stimuli in both *H. pylori*–positive and *H. pylori*–negative patients.

Dyspepsia Symptoms

There is no specific set of dyspeptic complaints indicative of *H. pylori* gastritis.[12] Given the fact that 50% to 60% of patients with functional dyspepsia are *H. pylori*–positive, and that this is also the case in 25% to 28% of asymptomatic individuals,[13,14] it is reasonable to assume that a certain subset of patients with dyspepsia will have symptoms due to *H. pylori* infection. However, a detailed and validated questionnaire failed to identify upper gastrointestinal symptoms suggestive of *H. pylori* infection, although patients with *H. pylori* infection had a higher overall symptom score.[15]

Epidemiologic Studies

A meta-analysis documented a higher prevalence of *H. pylori* in patients with NUD compared with control subjects, with an odds ratio of 2.3.[16] Danesh et al.[17] identified 30 observational studies comprising 3392 cases of NUD; although small studies often reported associations between *H. pylori* and NUD, potential confounders were not adequately considered and the results were not usually confirmed in larger, better controlled studies.

Randomized Controlled Trials

Although some epidemiologic studies have suggested a higher prevalence of *H. pylori* infection in patients with dyspepsia, these studies could not prove a causal relationship between *H. pylori* infection and dyspepsia. Double-blinded, randomized controlled studies are required to solve the issue.

Four well-designed, randomized, double-controlled clinical trials have been performed so far. Three reported failure of symptomatic improvement after *H. pylori* eradication,[18,20,21] but one showed improvement in dyspepsia symptoms (Fig. 1).[19] The negative studies were multicenter studies with a high selection bias; the study with the positive result was a single-center study. How can the discrepancies between

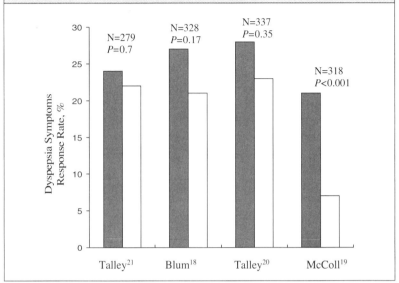

Figure 1. Complete dyspepsia symptoms response rate of the four randomized controlled trials of *H. pylori* eradication (*shaded bars*) versus placebo (*white bars*) for the treatment of nonulcer dyspepsia.

these high-quality trials be explained? McColl[22] suggested that the symptomatic benefit of eradicating *H. pylori* in patients with NUD is probably related to the background prevalence of *H. pylori*-related ulcer disease in the population being studied. In areas with a high prevalence of *H. pylori*–related ulcer disease, the symptomatic benefit reported in patients with NUD may be explained by the inclusion of patients with either unrecognized peptic ulcer disease or ulcer diathesis in which *H. pylori* eradication does prevent the development of peptic ulcer diseases. Because of geographic and national differences in the causes of both ulcer disease and NUD, treatment that is beneficial in one country may be ineffective in another.[22]

A U.S. systematic review suggested that *H. pylori* eradication had no effect on the symptoms of NUD,[23] whereas a Cochrane Collaboration systematic review found a small but statistically significant effect of *H. pylori* eradication on NUD.[24] The main discrepancy between the two systematic reviews appears to be the time-frame of the search. The U.S. systematic review assessed trials until December 1999 and identified seven trials involving 1544 patients, whereas the Cochrane Collaboration systematic review evaluated studies through May 2000 and identified a further 1000 patients that allow the small benefit due to *H. pylori*

Figure 2. Algorithm for the management of patients with nonulcer dyspepsia. (*Age cut-off varies with age-specific incidence of gastric cancer in each country [35 to 55 years]. †In a country with a high incidence of gastric cancer, *H. pylori* testing followed by endoscopy in positive patients may be appropriate.)

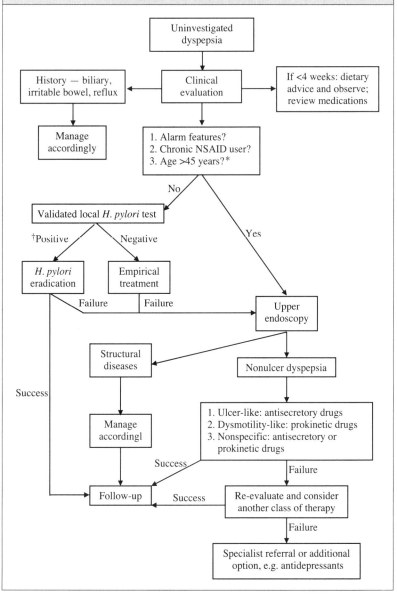

eradication to be detected. These data have led the Maastricht II consensus meeting to suggest that *H. pylori* eradication is advisable in patients with NUD.[25]

Helicobacter pylori Test-and-Treat Strategy

Data are now available from direct comparative studies of early endoscopy and an *H. pylori* test-and-treat strategy for patients with low risk of underlying diseases.[26–29] Three trials measured dyspepsia symptom resolution and found the *H. pylori* test-and-treat strategy to be at least as effective as prompt endoscopy. Quality of life assessment was similar between the two treatment strategies. A decision analysis model showed that the *H. pylori* test-and-treat strategy is more cost-effective than prompt endoscopy, however, costing US$134 per patient per year, as compared with US$240 per patient per year for endoscopy.[30] However, relative cost-effectiveness is likely to be dependent on the local cost of the two interventions and the prevalence of *H. pylori* infection in the local population. It should be noted that as the prevalence of *H. pylori* infection falls, the benefit of a test-and-treat strategy may also decline, and the recommendation of this approach to treatment may require future modification. There are also concerns that a test-and-treat strategy may miss cases of gastric cancer. Thus, in areas with a high incidence of gastric cancer and where endoscopy is affordable and available, *H. pylori* testing followed by endoscopy in positive patients (test-and-referral strategy) may be appropriate.[6] A suggested algorithm for the primary management of uninvestigated dyspepsia is given in Figure 2.

Key Points: Role of *Helicobacter pylori* in Dyspepsia

☞ Controversy continues about the role of *H. pylori* infection in nonulcer dyspepsia.

☞ Even in well-conducted randomized controlled trials, the results are still conflicting and may be related to the prevalence of *H. pylori*–related peptic ulcer diseases. There is evidence to suggest that the *H. pylori* test-and-treat strategy is at least as effective as prompt endoscopy for patients with no alarm symptoms.

Acknowledgment

This article is supported by the Simon KY Lee Gastroenterology Research Fund.

Suggested Reading

1. Talley NJ, Stanghellini V, Heading RC, et al: Functional gastroduodenal disorders. Gut 45(Suppl 2):37–42, 1999.
2. Talley NJ, Zinsmeister AR, Schleck CD, Melton LJ 3rd: Dyspepsia and dyspepsia subgroups: a population-based study. Gastroenterology 102:1259–1268, 1992.
3. Fisher RS, Parkman HP: Management of nonulcer dyspepsia. N Engl J Med 339:1376–1381, 1998.
4. Jones RH, Lydeard SE, Hobbs FD, et al: Dyspepsia in England and Scotland. Gut 31:401–405. 1990.
5. Lam SK, Talley NJ: Report of the 1997 Asia Pacific Consensus Conference on the management of *Helicobacter pylori* infection. J Gastroenterol Hepatol 13:1–12, 1998.
6. Talley NJ, Lam SK, Goh KL, et al: Management guidelines for uninvestigated and functional dyspepsia in the Asia-Pacific region: First Asian Pacific Working Party on Functional Dyspepsia. J Gastroenterol Hepatol 13:335–353, 1998.
7. Hu WHC, Wong WM, Lam CLK, et al: Anxiety but not depression determines health seeking behaviour in Chinese patients with dyspepsia and irritable bowel syndrome: a population based study. Aliment Pharmacol Ther 16:2081–2088, 2002.
8. Ho KY, Kang JY, Seow A: Prevalence of gastrointestinal symptoms in a multiracial Asian population, with particular reference to reflux-type symptoms. Am J Gastroenterol 93:1816–1822, 1998.
9. Troncon LE, Bennett RJ, Ahluwalia NK, Thompson DG: Abnormal intragastric distribution of food during gastric emptying in functional dyspepsia patients. Gut 35:327–332, 1994.
10. Stanghellini V, Tosetti C, Barbara G, et al: Risk indicators of delayed gastric emptying of solids in patients with functional dyspepsia. Gastroenterology 110:1036–1042, 1996.
11. Thumshirn M, Camilleri M, Saslow SB, et al: Gastric accommodation in non-ulcer dyspepsia and the roles of *Helicobacter pylori* infection and vagal function. Gut 44:55–64, 1999.
12. Loffeld RJ, Potters HV, Arends JW, et al: Campylobacter associated gastritis in patients with non-ulcer dyspepsia. J Clin Pathol 41:85–48, 1988.
13. Loffeld RJ, Stobberingh E, van Spreeuwel JP, et al: The prevalence of anti-*Helicobacter (Campylobacter) pylori* antibodies in patients and healthy blood donors. J Med Microbiol 32:105–109, 1990.
14. Barthel JS, Westblom TU, Havey AD, et al: Gastritis and *Campylobacter pylori* in healthy, asymptomatic volunteers. Arch Intern Med 148:1149–1151, 1988.
15. Werdmuller BF, van der Putten TB, Balk TG, et al: Clinical presentation of *Helicobacter pylori*-positive and -negative functional dyspepsia. J Gastroenterol Hepatol 15:498–502, 2000.
16. Armstrong D: *Helicobacter pylori* infection and dyspepsia. Scand J Gastroenterol Suppl 215:38–47, 1996.
17. Danesh J, Lawrence M, Murphy M, et al: Systematic review of the epidemiological evidence on *Helicobacter pylori* infection and nonulcer or uninvestigated dyspepsia. Arch Intern Med 160:1192–1198, 2000.
18. Blum AL, Talley NJ, O'Morain C, et al: Lack of effect of treating *Helicobacter pylori* infection in patients with nonulcer dyspepsia. Omeprazole plus Clarithromycin and Amoxicillin Effect One Year after Treatment (OCAY) Study Group. N Engl J Med 339:1875–1881, 1998.
19. McColl KEL, Murray L, El-Omar E, et al: Symptomatic benefit from eradicating *He-*

licobacter pylori infection in patients with nonulcer dyspepsia. N Engl J Med 339:1869–1874, 1998.

20. Talley NJ, Vakil N, Ballard ED 2nd, Fennerty MB: Absence of benefit of eradicating *Helicobacter pylori* in patients with nonulcer dyspepsia. N Engl J Med 341:1106–1111, 1999.

21. Talley NJ, Janssens J, Lauritsen K, et al: Eradication of *Helicobacter pylori* in functional dyspepsia: randomised double blind placebo controlled trial with 12 months' follow up. The Optimal Regimen Cures Helicobacter Induced Dyspepsia (ORCHID) Study Group. BMJ 318:833–837, 1999.

22. McColl KE: Absence of benefit of eradicating *Helicobacter pylori* in patients with nonulcer dyspepsia. N Engl J Med 342:589, 2000.

23. Laine L, Schoenfeld P, Fennerty MB: Therapy for *Helicobacter pylori* in patients with nonulcer dyspepsia: a meta-analysis of randomized, controlled trials. Ann Intern Med 134:361–369, 2001.

24. Moayyedi P, Soo S, Deeks J, et al: Systematic review and economic evaluation of *Helicobacter pylori* eradication treatment for non-ulcer dyspepsia. Dyspepsia Review Group. BMJ 321:659–664, 2000.

25. Malfertheiner P, Megraud F, O'Morain C, et al: Current concepts in the management of *Helicobacter pylori* infection: the Maastricht 2–2000 Consensus Report. Aliment Pharmacol Ther 16:167–180, 2002.

26. Heaney A, Collins JSA, Watson RGP, et al: A prospective randomised trial of a "test and treat" policy versus endoscopy based management in young *Helicobacter pylori* positive patients with ulcer-like dyspepsia, referred to a hospital clinic. Gut 45:186–190, 1999.

27. Jones RH, Tait CL, Sladen G, et al: A *Helicobacter* test and treat strategy: costs and outcomes in a randomised controlled trial in primary care. Gut 42(Suppl 1):A81, 1998.

28. Lassen AT, Pedersen FM, Bytzer P, et al: *Helicobacter pylori* test-and-eradicate versus prompt endoscopy for management of dyspeptic patients. Lancet 356:455–460, 2000.

29. Duggan A, Elliott C, Logan RPH, et al: Does near patient *H. pylori* testing in primary care reduce referral for endoscopy? Results from a randomised trial. Gut 42(Suppl 1):A82, 1998.

30. Moayyedi P: *Helicobacter pylori* test and treat strategy for young dyspeptic patients: new data. Gut 50(Suppl 4):47–50, 2002.

Role of Visceral Hypersensitivity in Dyspepsia

Uri Ladabaum, MD, M.S.

Dyspepsia is defined as pain or discomfort centered in the upper abdomen that may be associated with fullness, early satiety, bloating, belching, nausea, or vomiting.[1] Several important clinical entities must be distinguished from dyspepsia, including biliary, pancreatic, or mesenteric vascular pathologic conditions as well as nongastrointestinal disease such as myocardial ischemia (Fig. 1). Patients with dyspepsia should be distinguished from those with predominant retrosternal burning (heartburn), who are very likely to suffer from gastroesophageal reflux disease and can be treated with antisecretory medication. When referring to patients with dyspepsia, some clinicians use the term *gastritis,* which is a term that should be restricted to histologically demonstrated inflammation of the stomach. The relationship between gastritis and dyspepsia remains controversial.

When patients with dyspepsia first present for evaluation, they have *uninvestigated dyspepsia.* The causes of dyspepsia include peptic ulcer disease, gastroesophageal reflux disease, malignancy, and medications. In as many as 60% of patients with dyspepsia, however, no explanation for dyspepsia is identified during conventional clinical testing (see Fig. 1).[2] These patients are diagnosed with *functional dyspepsia,* which is defined as persistent or recurrent dyspepsia without evidence of organic disease (including at upper endoscopic examination) that is likely to explain the symptoms.[1] Functional gastrointestinal disorders, including functional dyspepsia, irritable bowel syndrome (IBS), and functional (noncardiac) chest pain are among the most common gastrointestinal conditions seen in clinical practice.

In recent years, investigators have attempted to identify physiologic abnormalities in patients with functional dyspepsia. Among these abnormalities, *visceral hypersensitivity,* which refers to increased sensation in response to a visceral stimulus, has received much attention.[3] It has been hypothesized that sensory dysfunction may lead to the experience of clinical symptoms in response to physiologic stimuli that normally

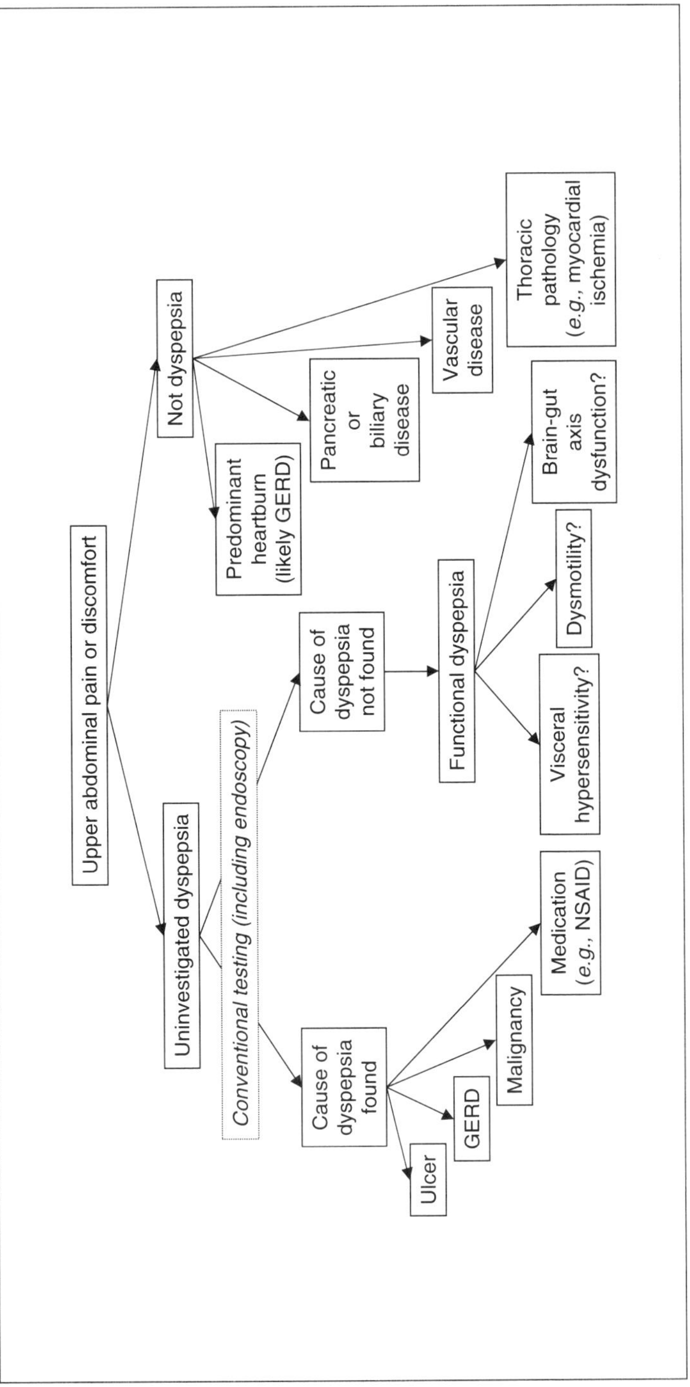

Figure 1. Differential diagnosis of upper abdominal pain or discomfort. Visceral hypersensitivity is present in some patients with functional dyspepsia. (GERD = gastroesophageal reflux disease, NSAID = nonsteroidal anti-inflammatory drug)

would be unperceived or not perceived as noxious. Although many patients with functional gastrointestinal disorders display visceral hypersensitivity, it remains to be determined what role, if any, visceral hypersensitivity plays in the pathophysiology underlying the experience of symptoms in these disorders.

Is Functional Dyspepsia a Single Disorder?

Symptom-Based Classification

Attempts to classify patients into distinct subgroups of "functional dyspepsia" based on symptoms (ulcer-like, dysmotility-like, reflux-like) have been of little utility due to the significant overlap between subgroups and the failure of these subgroups to guide clinical management. More recently, researchers have aimed to define specific physiologic abnormalities in patients with functional dyspepsia that some day could be the targets of therapeutic interventions.

Physiologic Abnormalities in Functional Dyspepsia

As a group, patients with functional gastrointestinal disorders display differences in gastrointestinal motility, visceral sensation, and brain-gut axis function as compared to healthy subjects. In subgroups of patients with functional dyspepsia, investigators have described various abnormalities, including delayed gastric emptying,[4,5] decreased antral motility,[6] impaired gastric fundic accommodation to a meal,[7,8] abnormal intragastric meal distribution,[9] abnormal visceral reflexes,[10] hypersensitivity to gastric and intestinal distension,[4,11–13] hypersensitivity to exogenous gastric and duodenal acid perfusion,[14,15] and hypersensitivity to concomitant duodenal lipid perfusion and gastric distension.[16] It is conceivable that sensory, motor, and reflex regulatory abnormalities could coexist and contribute to clinical symptoms.[17] A provocative set of recent studies suggests that intestinal gas handling may be abnormal in patients with IBS, reflecting subtle abnormalities in motility, and possibly relating to the clinical problems of abdominal distension and bloating, which can be prominent symptoms in patients classified as having functional dyspepsia.[18–20]

A specific abnormality, such as visceral hypersensitivity, is not always demonstrable in a specific patient who carries the diagnosis of functional dyspepsia. Therefore, *functional dyspepsia* should be considered an umbrella term that encompasses what is probably a heterogeneous group of physiologic abnormalities (see Fig. 1). For instance, recent investigations have found that 40% of functional dyspeptic patients displayed impaired accommodation to a meal, which was associated with early satiety,[7] and that 34% displayed hypersensitivity to gastric distension, which was associated with postprandial pain, belching, and weight loss.[21]

How Is Visceral Hypersensitivity Demonstrated Experimentally?

Visceral hypersensitivity and visceral hyperalgesia, which denotes specifically increased pain sensation in response to a visceral stimulus, have been recognized in a significant fraction of patients with functional gastrointestinal disorders, including gastric hypersensitivity in cases of functional dyspepsia,[11–13] rectal hypersensitivity in cases of IBS,[22–23] and esophageal hypersensitivity in cases of functional chest pain.[24,25] Most of the research on visceral sensation has used visceral distension (that is, mechanical stimulation) as the stimulus, usually by means of a balloon mounted on a tube that is placed in the viscus of interest and is attached to a distending device, such as a barostat, which controls distensions at specified pressures. Some studies have used electrical stimulation and some have investigated chemical stimulation, such as with nutrients or acid.

Visceral hypersensitivity in groups of patients with functional gastrointestinal disorders has most often been identified as a decrease in the mean pressure thresholds for sensations, or as an increase in the mean levels of sensation (e.g., visual analogue scale ratings) at various distending pressures as compared with control subjects (Fig. 2). Notably, although visceral balloon distension is not a physiologic stimulus, it tends to induce sensations that are reminiscent of patients' clinical symptoms.[10]

How Sensitive Is Visceral Hypersensitivity for Functional Dyspepsia?

It has been proposed that altered rectal perception, including hypersensitivity or abnormal sensation referral patterns or quality, is a biological marker of IBS.[23] However, not all individuals with IBS have exhibited abnormal rectal sensitivity across studies.[3] As a group, patients with functional dyspepsia display visceral hypersensitivity compared to control subjects, but there is significant overlap between the perceptual responses of individuals in the two groups. For instance, one study demonstrating group differences in pain thresholds between functional dyspeptic patients and control subjects (5.5 ± 4.0 mm Hg vs. 10.2 ± 2.2 mm Hg above the minimal pressure required to begin distending the stomach, $P < 0.004$) reported that the perception scores of more than 50% of functional dyspeptic patients were in the control range at most

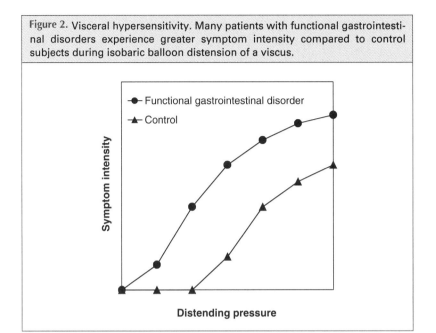

Figure 2. Visceral hypersensitivity. Many patients with functional gastrointestinal disorders experience greater symptom intensity compared to control subjects during isobaric balloon distension of a viscus.

distension levels.[26] Thus, the fraction of patients with a particular functional gastrointestinal disorder who are classified as "hypersensitive" depends on how "normal" is defined.

Experimentally, "normal" has often been determined as the lower end of the distribution of responses recorded for healthy volunteers. Based on a large study of 160 functional dyspeptic patients and 80 healthy volunteers, the increase in intragastric pressure over minimal distending pressure has been proposed as the most appropriate measure of gastric hypersensitivity, because a lower end of normal could be defined and because the measure was not dependent on age and body mass index.[21] In this study, with the normal range of sensitivity thresholds defined as the mean ± 2 standard deviations in the healthy volunteers, hypersensitivity to gastric distension was found in 34% of functional dyspeptic patients. This subgroup did not differ from the other functional dyspeptic patients in terms of demographic or clinical characteristics.

Because visceral hypersensitivity can be demonstrated in functional dyspeptic patients as a group compared to healthy volunteers, but only a fraction of functional dyspeptic patients are labeled as "hypersensitive" once a lower end of normal is defined, visceral hypersensitivity cannot be considered to be a very sensitive marker at the level of an individual for "functional dyspepsia" as this term is currently (broadly) defined. On the other hand, when considering the subgroup of functional dyspeptic patients who have decreased tolerance to gastric distension as compared with control subjects, then visceral hypersensitivity is, by definition, an extremely sensitive marker.

How Specific Is Visceral Hypersensitivity for Functional Dyspepsia?

The following questions all address different aspects of the specificity of visceral hypersensitivity in functional dyspepsia.

Can visceral hypersensitivity differentiate functional disease not only from normal, but also from "organic disease"? Visceral perception appears to be different in patients with functional dyspepsia and in patients with severe organic dyspepsia associated with tissue injury. However, some overlap exists even among patients in these groups, with 87% of functional dyspeptic patients displaying reduced perception thresholds or altered sensory referral patterns compared with 20% of organic dyspeptic patients ($P = 0.014$).[27]

Is hypersensitivity specific for visceral perception or do patients with functional gastrointestinal disorders have generalized hypersensitivity? Most studies have found patients with functional gastrointestinal disorders to have normal, and in some cases decreased, somatic sensitivity.[10,11,28] A recent study that revisited this question, however, found that 33 patients with functional gastrointestinal disorders had decreased pain thresholds for immersion of the nondominant hand into water at 4°C compared with healthy volunteers (pain at 41 $\pm$ 3 seconds vs. 76 $\pm$ 6 sec, and hand withdrawal at 62 $\pm$ 6 seconds vs. 102 $\pm$ 4 sec, $P <$ 0.05).[29] On balance, it has generally been considered that hypersensitivity in patients with functional gastrointestinal disorders is specific for the viscera.

Is visceral hypersensitivity restricted to a specific type of stimulus, such as mechanical distension? It has been reported that patients with IBS display hypersensitivity to mechanical stimulation of the small intestine but normal perception of transmucosal electrical stimulation.[28] Electrical stimulation may "bypass" an end-organ site of hypersensitivity (e.g., involving mechanoreceptors) by nonspecifically stimulating afferent nerves.

In various studies of functional dyspeptic patients, hypersensitivity to chemical stimulation has been demonstrated. Eleven of 50 patients (22%) with functional dyspepsia developed pain with infusion of 0.1 M hydrochloric acid into the antrum, compared with none with saline infusion ($P < 0.05$) and none of 25 healthy volunteers with acid infusion.[14] Notably, in 10 of these 11 patients, pain was again elicited on acid rechallenge and was relieved with bicarbonate infusion. In a similar study, 0.1 N hydrochloric acid but not saline infused into the antrum reproduced patients' clinical pain in 42% of 12 patients with ulcer-like functional dyspepsia ($P < 0.05$) and in none of seven control subjects.[30] Acid instillation into the duodenum has been shown to elicit nausea in functional dyspeptic patients, who also demonstrated reduced duodenal acid clearance, but not in healthy control subjects.[15] The potential clinical relevance of these findings is highlighted by studies in which complete symptom relief was achieved in 38% of functional dyspeptic patients treated with the proton pump inhibitor omeprazole 20 mg every day, 36% of functional dyspeptic patients treated with omeprazole 10 mg every day, and 28% of functional dyspeptic patients on placebo ($P = 0.002$ and $P = 0.02$ for the two doses of omeprazole compared to placebo, respectively).[31]

Nutrients in the intestine may also sensitize the stomach to distension in healthy volunteers as well as patients with functional dyspepsia (see later).

Is visceral hypersensitivity restricted to persons who seek medical care for their symptoms? Many people who have symptoms fulfilling the diagnostic criteria for functional gastrointestinal disorders do not seek medical attention. Such individuals with dyspepsia can be referred to as nonconsulter dyspeptics. It has been reported that nonconsulter dyspeptic individuals display visceral hypersensitivity as compared with control subjects,[32] just as has been demonstrated for consulters with dyspepsia. This suggests that visceral hypersensitivity is not specific to those who seek medical care, which is consistent with research suggesting that psychosocial factors are important determinants of healthcare seeking for gastrointestinal symptoms.

Is visceral hypersensitivity "site-specific" in the gastrointestinal tract in a given disorder? The current definitions of the functional gastrointestinal disorders describe different syndromes primarily to promote uniformity in research. Patients with functional dyspepsia, for instance, must not have pain or discomfort that is exclusively relieved with defecation or that is associated with altered defecation (which are features of IBS).[1] However, it is well recognized that functional gastrointestinal symptoms can fluctuate over time and that patients who at one point fit the criteria for one disorder, such as functional dyspepsia, may at another point fit the criteria for another, such as IBS.[33] In this light, it is of interest that patients with functional gastrointestinal disorders may display visceral hypersensitivity in regions of the gastrointestinal tract distant to those where their symptoms are presumed to originate.[34] It is therefore conceivable that patients diagnosed with various of the currently defined functional gastrointestinal disorders could be exhibiting different manifestations of a generalized disorder of visceral sensation.

Where Does the Abnormality Responsible for Visceral Hypersensitivity Reside?

Visceral hypersensitivity could result from end-organ abnormalities such as mechanoreceptor hypersensitivity,[35] afferent pathway abnormalities such as sensitization of neurons in the dorsal horn of the spinal cord, or abnormalities in processing of visceral afferent stimuli at the level of the central nervous system.[36] Hyporeactive visceral reflexes could be considered evidence of peripheral abnormalities.[4,10] It has been suggested that the increased area of viscerosomatic referral in patients with functional dyspepsia could result from abnormalities in dorsal horn neurons.[37] Differences in central nervous system responses (regional brain blood flow) during visceral stimulation have been reported in patients with IBS as compared with control subjects.[36,38,39] An important finding in IBS patients seems to be abnormal activation of the anterior cingulate cortex, a brain region whose functions are believed to include mediating the emotional response to pain. The brain activation pattern during gastric distension in healthy volunteers bears important similarities to activation patterns with stimulation of other viscera.[40] The results of studies comparing the brain activation patterns during visceral stimulation in functional dyspeptics and healthy volunteers are awaited.

Just as functional dyspepsia is probably a collection of heterogeneous disorders, it is conceivable that the subgroup of patients with visceral hypersensitivity could itself include patients with abnormalities of visceral sensory processing at different levels in the brain-gut axis.

What Could Cause Visceral Hypersensitivity?

The factors determining the onset of functional gastrointestinal symptoms remain poorly understood. Acute infectious insults, inflammation, and stress may play a role.[41–43] In a subgroup of patients, there appears to be a postinfectious syndrome.[44,45] These patients often report that they were well until a clearly identifiable, acute gastrointestinal illness.

Presumed Postinfectious Dyspepsia

In a recent study using a screening questionnaire answered by 400 consecutive dyspeptic patients, 66 patients (17%) were classified as having presumed postinfectious dyspepsia based on acute onset and associated symptoms such as fever, myalgias, diarrhea, or vomiting.[46] In these patients, impaired gastric accommodation to a meal was more common than in those without presumed postinfectious dyspepsia (67% vs. 30%, $P < 0.05$), but sensitivity to gastric distension was not different between these groups.

Helicobacter pylori

With the recognition of the role of *Helicobacter pylori* in the pathogenesis of peptic ulcer disease, there was great enthusiasm over the prospect of curing dyspepsia by treating *H. pylori* infection. It has become clear that *H. pylori* infection cannot explain symptoms in the majority of patients with functional dyspepsia, many of whom do not even harbor *H. pylori*. However, *H. pylori* eradication may be beneficial in a small fraction of functional dyspeptic patients,[47] although this remains controversial.[48] Whether *H. pylori* infection could be related to gastric hypersensitivity remains unclear.[8,49] A provocative recent study using a murine model demonstrated *H. pylori*–induced changes in neural function, some of which persisted after *H. pylori* eradication.[50] It remains to be determined whether *H. pylori* infection in humans could cause neural or other changes that may not resolve with eradication therapy or that may resolve only over a longer time period than has generally been studied.

Are Patients with Functional Dyspepsia Hypersensitive to Specific Foods?

In many patients with functional dyspepsia, symptoms are meal-related. Patients often search in vain for specific food triggers for their symptoms. Strict exclusionary diets are rarely beneficial and may in fact be detrimental if nutrition is compromised. However, there is experimental evidence that some food components may exacerbate dyspeptic symptoms. Duodenal lipid perfusion has been shown to sensitize the stomach to distension in healthy subjects[51,52] and in patients with functional dyspepsia.[16] It is conceivable that this effect could contribute to clinical symptoms.

Patients may complain of dyspepsia with coffee ingestion. Intragastric administration of coffee has been reported to increase gastric relaxation compared to water in healthy volunteers, but it did not affect gastric compliance or sensitivity to distension.[53] Of note, it is possible for coffee to exacerbate gastroesophageal reflux disease, which some patients can experience as dyspepsia.

Does Visceral Sensitivity Play a Role in Drug-Induced Dyspepsia?

Aspirin and nonsteroidal anti-inflammatory drugs are widely used medications that commonly cause dyspepsia in the absence of frank peptic ulceration. The mechanisms underlying the development of drug-induced dyspepsia are not well understood. Even when there is mucosal injury, there is no clear relationship with the development of pain or discomfort, as exemplified by patients whose initial presentation of peptic ulceration is gastrointestinal bleeding in the absence of preceding pain or discomfort.

A recent small study investigating the effects of aspirin on gastric mechanosensitivity found that sensory thresholds to gastric distension increased in functional dyspeptic patients as well as healthy control subjects who did not develop dyspepsia on aspirin, but not in those who did develop dyspepsia.[54] Gastric mechanosensitivity and clinical symptoms were not explained by the degree of mucosal damage or gastric emptying. The authors suggest that normal antinociceptive pathways may have failed to become activated in those subjects who developed dyspepsia.

Should Visceral Sensitivity Be Tested in Patients with Functional Dyspepsia in the Clinical Setting?

Visceral distension testing has not been adopted as a diagnostic tool for specific functional gastrointestinal disorders because of many reasons, including uncertainty regarding its sensitivity and specificity, the unclear relationship between visceral hypersensitivity and clinical symptoms, the lack of specific therapies aimed at visceral hypersensitivity, and the invasive nature of the procedure. Whether visceral sensory testing will be applied in the clinical setting in the future will depend on the availability of therapies aimed at different physiologic disturbances in subgroups of patients with functional dyspepsia, the ability of testing to guide clinical management, and the relative merits of treatment directed by specific testing versus empiric medication trials based on clinical presentation.

Noninvasive tests of gastric function that could identify patients with functional dyspepsia and guide management would be of great interest.[3]

Does the Concept of Visceral Hypersensitivity Have Implications for Clinical Practice?

Even in the subgroup of patients that could be defined as viscerally hypersensitive based on comparisons to healthy volunteers and patients with organic disease, a fundamental question remains: Does visceral hypersensitivity explain clinical symptoms? That is, even if visceral hypersensitivity could be considered a disease marker, it may not necessarily be the cause of symptoms. At present, few therapies are available for the gastrointestinal disorders, and it has not been demonstrated that medications that yield clinical benefit also decrease visceral sensitivity. In addition, there appear to be only weak correlations between clinical symptoms and rectal sensory thresholds in IBS.[55]

Pharmacologic Treatment of Symptoms and Modulation of Physiology

The serotonin 5-HT$_3$ receptor antagonist alosetron has a modest benefit over placebo in achieving adequate relief in diarrhea-predominant IBS.[56,57] In patients with IBS, alosetron increased the perception and pain thresholds to volume distension, in association with an increase in colonic compliance.[58] However, there was no change in the sensory thresholds with respect to distending pressure. On the other hand, a recent study raised the possibility that alosetron's clinical benefit could be due in part to modulation of central nervous system networks involved in emotional expression.[59] In functional dyspepsia, alosetron showed a modest benefit compared to placebo in achieving adequate relief of symptoms, but the difference was statistically significant only in a specific subanalysis, and only for the 1 mg twice daily dosage (51% vs. 40% for placebo, $P = 0.05$). Notably, gastric sensitivity does not seem to be affected by 5-HT$_3$ receptor antagonists.[52,60]

The serotonin 5-HT$_1$ receptor agonist sumatriptan has been shown to increase the gastric volume, but not the gastric pressure, at the thresholds for perception and discomfort in healthy humans.[61] This effect appears to be due to induction of fundic relaxation. Furthermore, sumatriptan has been shown to restore gastric accommodation in functional dyspeptic patients with impaired accommodation.[7] The α_2-adrenergic agonist clonidine has been found to increase gastric compliance but also reduce gastric sensation in response to distension in healthy humans, but its role in the treatment of functional dyspepsia remains undefined.[62] An intriguing study has found that red pepper powder may decrease functional dyspeptic symptoms more than placebo, perhaps through desensitization of gastric nociceptive C-fibers by the capsaicin contained in the red pepper, but this mechanistic hypothesis was not tested directly in this study.[63] These interventions have not reached widespread clinical application. Further studies are needed assessing clinical end-points.

Antidepressants

Antidepressants are among the most commonly used medications to treat the functional gastrointestinal disorders. These agents often achieve symptomatic benefit in patients without concomitant psychiatric disease and at doses lower than needed to treat depression.[64,65] A recent meta-analysis concluded that the summary odds ratio for improvement in functional gastrointestinal disorder symptoms with the use of antidepressants compared to placebo was 4.2 (95% CI; 2.3–7.9), with the average standardized mean improvement in pain equaling 0.9 SD units (95% CI; 0.6–1.2 SD units); that is, pain ratings decreased from the mean rating by nearly 1 SD on average.[66]

Most available studies of antidepressants and functional gastrointestinal disorders have used a tricyclic antidepressant. Notably, it appears that tricyclic antidepressants do not affect visceral sensitivity.[67] A small crossover study of amitriptyline in functional dyspepsia found that seven out of seven patients studied reported significantly less severe gastrointestinal symptoms with amitriptyline than with placebo, but this clinical effect was not accompanied by changes in gastric sensitivity to distension.[68] Although they are widely used in clinical practice to treat functional gastrointestinal disorders because of their favorable side effect profile, the selective serotonin reuptake inhibitors have only recently been the subject of systematic study in the field of visceral sensation. In a recent blinded, placebo-controlled crossover study, the selective serotonin reuptake inhibitor sertraline had no effect on gastric compliance, sensitivity, or somatic pain tolerance in healthy volunteers.[69] Thus, it appears that any benefit of antidepressants in the functional gastrointestinal disorders may not depend on modulation of visceral sensitivity, at least not those aspects of visceral sensation that are generally assessed experimentally with barostat-controlled distension of a viscus. It is conceivable that the central nervous system effects of these medications could affect the evaluation of visceral afferent stimulation, rather than the perceived intensity of a stimulus.

In clinical practice, treatments for functional dyspepsia (limited as they may be) are currently chosen based on their impact on symptoms and not because of a presumed or proven effect on visceral sensation. It cannot be ruled out, however, that some of the clinical benefit of therapy could relate to changes in processing of visceral afferent information.

Key Points: Role of Visceral Hypersensitivity in Dyspepsia

- ☞ In a large fraction of patients with dyspepsia, no identifiable cause for their symptoms is found during routine clinical evaluation. These patients are diagnosed with functional dyspepsia.
- ☞ Numerous physiologic abnormalities, including visceral hypersensitivity, have been described in subgroups of patients with functional dyspepsia.

Key Points (*Continued*)

∞ Although visceral hypersensitivity has consistently been identified as a feature of the functional gastrointestinal disorders, it remains to be determined what role, if any, visceral hypersensitivity plays in the genesis of symptoms in patients with these disorders.

∞ Whether visceral sensory testing and specific visceral antinociceptive therapies will be applied in the clinical setting in the future will depend on the availability of such therapies, the ability of testing to guide clinical management for subgroups of patients with different physiologic disturbances, and the relative merits of treatment guided by testing compared to empirical treatment.

Suggested Reading

1. Talley NJ, Stanghellini V, Heading RC, et al: Functional gastroduodenal disorders. In Drossman DA (ed): The Functional Gastrointestinal Disorders; 2nd ed. McLean VA, Degnon Associates, 2000, pp 299–350.

2. American Gastroenterological Association: Medical position statement: evaluation of dyspepsia. Gastroenterology 114:579–581, 1998.

3. Camilleri M, Coulie B, Tack JF: Visceral hypersensitivity: facts, speculations, and challenges. Gut 48:125–131, 2001.

4. Geydanus MP, Vassallo M, Camilleri M, et al: Neurohormonal factors in functional dyspepsia: insights on pathophysiological mechanisms. Gastroenterology 100: 1311–1318, 1991.

5. Tucci A, Corinaldesi R, Stanghellini V, et al: Helicobacter pylori infection and gastric function in patients with chronic idiopathic dyspepsia. Gastroenterology 103: 768–774, 1992.

6. Stanghellini V, Ghidini C, Maccarini MR, et al: Fasting and postprandial gastrointestinal motility in ulcer and non-ulcer dyspepsia. Gut 33:184–190, 1992.

7. Tack J, Piessevaux H, Coulie B, et al: Role of impaired gastric accommodation to a meal in functional dyspepsia. Gastroenterology 115:1346–1352, 1998.

8. Thumshirn M, Camilleri M, Saslow SB, et al: Gastric accommodation in non-ulcer dyspepsia and the roles of Helicobacter pylori infection and vagal function. Gut 44:55–64, 1999.

9. Troncon LE, Bennett RJ, Ahluwalia NK, Thompson DG: Abnormal intragastric distribution of food during gastric emptying in functional dyspepsia patients. Gut 35:327–332, 1994.

10. Coffin B, Azpiroz F, Guarner F, Malagelada JR: Selective gastric hypersensitivity and reflex hyporeactivity in functional dyspepsia. Gastroenterology 107:1345–1351, 1994.

11. Mearin F, Cucala M, Azpiroz F, Malagelada JR: The origin of symptoms on the brain-gut axis in functional dyspepsia. Gastroenterology 101:999–1006, 1991.

12. Lemann M, Dederding JP, Flourie B, et al: Abnormal perception of visceral pain in response to gastric distension in chronic idiopathic dyspepsia: the irritable stomach syndrome. Dig Dis Sci 36:1249–1254, 1991.

13. Bradette M, Pare P, Douville P, Morin A: Visceral perception in health and functional

dyspepsia: crossover study of gastric distension with placebo and domperidone. Dig Dis Sci 36:52–58, 1991.

14. Misra SP, Broor SL: Is gastric acid responsible for the pain in patients with essential dyspepsia? J Clin Gastroenterol 12:624–627, 1990.

15. Samsom M, Verhagen MA, vanBerge Henegouwen GP, Smout AJ: Abnormal clearance of exogenous acid and increased acid sensitivity of the proximal duodenum in dyspeptic patients. Gastroenterology 116:515–520, 1999.

16. Barbera R, Feinle C, Read NW: Nutrient-specific modulation of gastric mechanosensitivity in patients with functional dyspepsia. Dig Dis Sci 40:1636–1641, 1995.

17. Azpiroz F: Hypersensitivity in functional gastrointestinal disorders. Gut 51(Suppl 1): i25–28, 2002.

18. Serra J, Azpiroz F, Malagelada JR: Mechanisms of intestinal gas retention in humans: impaired propulsion versus obstructed evacuation. Am J Physiol 281:G138–143, 2001.

19. Serra J, Azpiroz F, Malagelada JR: Impaired transit and tolerance of intestinal gas in the irritable bowel syndrome. Gut 48:14–19, 2001.

20. Serra J, Salvioli B, Azpiroz F, Malagelada JR: Lipid-induced intestinal gas retention in irritable bowel syndrome. Gastroenterology 123:700–706, 2002.

21. Tack J, Caenepeel P, Fischler B, et al: Symptoms associated with hypersensitivity to gastric distention in functional dyspepsia. Gastroenterology 121:526–535, 2001.

22. Whitehead WE, Holtkotter B, Enck P, et al: Tolerance for rectosigmoid distention in irritable bowel syndrome. Gastroenterology 98:1187–1192, 1990.

23. Mertz H, Naliboff B, Munakata J, et al: Altered rectal perception is a biological marker of patients with irritable bowel syndrome. Gastroenterology 109:40–52, 1995.

24. Richter JE, Barish CF, Castell DO: Abnormal sensory perception in patients with esophageal chest pain. Gastroenterology 91:845–852, 1986.

25. Vantrappen G, Janssens J, Ghillebert G: The irritable oesophagus: a frequent cause of angina-like pain. Lancet 1:1232–1234, 1987.

26. Klatt S, Pieramico O, Guethner C, et al: Gastric hypersensitivity in nonulcer dyspepsia: an inconsistent finding. Dig Dis Sci 42:720–723, 1997.

27. Mertz H, Fullerton S, Naliboff B, Mayer EA: Symptoms and visceral perception in severe functional and organic dyspepsia. Gut 42:814–822, 1998.

28. Accarino AM, Azpiroz F, Malagelada JR: Selective dysfunction of mechanosensitive intestinal afferents in irritable bowel syndrome. Gastroenterology 108:636–643, 1995.

29. Bouin M, Meunier P, Riberdy-Poitras M, Poitras P: Pain hypersensitivity in patients with functional gastrointestinal disorders: a gastrointestinal-specific defect or a general systemic condition? Dig Dis Sci 46:2542–2548, 2001.

30. Son HJ, Rhee PL, Kim JJ, et al: Hypersensitivity to acid in ulcer-like functional dyspepsia. Korean J Intern Med 12:188–192, 1997.

31. Talley NJ, Meineche-Schmidt V, Pare P, et al: Efficacy of omeprazole in functional dyspepsia: double-blind, randomized, placebo-controlled trials (the Bond and Opera studies). Aliment Pharmacol Ther 12:1055–1065, 1998.

32. Holtmann G, Gschossmann J, Neufang-Huber J, et al: Differences in gastric mechanosensory function after repeated ramp distensions in non-consulters with dyspepsia and healthy controls. Gut 47:332–336, 2000.

33. Agreus L, Svardsudd K, Nyren O, Tibblin G: Irritable bowel syndrome and dyspepsia in the general population: overlap and lack of stability over time. Gastroenterology 109:671–680, 1995.

34. Trimble KC, Farouk R, Pryde A, et al: Heightened visceral sensation in functional

gastrointestinal disease is not site-specific: evidence for a generalized disorder of gut sensitivity. Dig Dis Sci 40:1607–1613, 1995.

35. Gebhart GF: Peripheral contributions to visceral hyperalgesia. Can J Gastroenterol 13(Suppl A):37A–41A, 1999.

36. Mertz H: Role of the brain and sensory pathways in gastrointestinal sensory disorders in humans. Gut 51(Suppl 1):i29–33, 2002.

37. Thumshirn M: Pathophysiology of functional dyspepsia. Gut 51(Suppl 1):i63–66, 2002.

38. Silverman DH, Munakata JA, Ennes H, et al: Regional cerebral activity in normal and pathological perception of visceral pain. Gastroenterology 112:64–72, 1997.

39. Mertz H, Morgan V, Tanner G, et al: Regional cerebral activation in irritable bowel syndrome and control subjects with painful and nonpainful rectal distention. Gastroenterology 118:842–848, 2000.

40. Ladabaum U, Minoshima S, Hasler WL, et al: Gastric distention correlates with activation of multiple cortical and subcortical regions. Gastroenterology 120:369–376, 2001.

41. Collins SM, Piche T, Rampal P: The putative role of inflammation in the irritable bowel syndrome. Gut 49:743–745, 2001.

42. Collins SM: A case for an immunological basis for irritable bowel syndrome. Gastroenterology 122:2078–2080, 2002.

43. Mayer EA, Collins SM: Evolving pathophysiologic models of functional gastrointestinal disorders. Gastroenterology 122:2032–2048, 2002.

44. Gwee KA, Graham JC, McKendrick MW, et al: Psychometric scores and persistence of irritable bowel after infectious diarrhoea. Lancet 347:150–153, 1996.

45. Neal KR, Hebden J, Spiller R: Prevalence of gastrointestinal symptoms six months after bacterial gastroenteritis and risk factors for development of the irritable bowel syndrome: postal survey of patients. BMJ 314:779–782, 1997.

46. Tack J, Demedts I, Dehondt G, et al: Clinical and pathophysiological characteristics of acute-onset functional dyspepsia. Gastroenterology 122:1738–1747, 2002.

47. Moayyedi P, Soo S, Deeks J, et al: Systematic review and economic evaluation of *Helicobacter pylori* eradication treatment for non-ulcer dyspepsia. Dyspepsia Review Group. BMJ 321:659–664, 2000.

48. Laine L, Schoenfeld P, Fennerty MB: Therapy for *Helicobacter pylori* in patients with nonulcer dyspepsia: a meta-analysis of randomized, controlled trials. Ann Intern Med 134:361–369, 2001.

49. Mearin F, de Ribot X, Balboa A, et al: Does *Helicobacter pylori* infection increase gastric sensitivity in functional dyspepsia? Gut 37:47–51, 1995.

50. Bercik P, De Giorgio R, Blennerhassett P, et al: Immune-mediated neural dysfunction in a murine model of chronic *Helicobacter pylori* infection. Gastroenterology 123:1205–1215, 2002.

51. Feinle C, D'Amato M, Read NW: Cholecystokinin-A receptors modulate gastric sensory and motor responses to gastric distension and duodenal lipid. Gastroenterology 110:1379–1385, 1996.

52. Ladabaum U, Brown MB, Pan W, et al: Effects of nutrients and serotonin 5-HT3 antagonism on symptoms evoked by distal gastric distension in humans. Am J Physiol 280:G201–208, 2001.

53. Boekema PJ, Samsom M, Roelofs JM, Smout AJ: Effect of coffee on motor and sensory function of proximal stomach. Dig Dis Sci 46:945–951, 2001.

54. Holtmann G, Gschossmann J, Buenger L, et al: Do changes in visceral sensory function determine the development of dyspepsia during treatment with aspirin? Gastroenterology 123:1451–1458, 2002.

55. Whitehead WE, Diamant N, Meyer K, et al: Pain thresholds measured by the barostat predict the severity of clinical pain in patients with irritable bowel syndrome [abstract]. Gastroenterology 114:A858, 1998.

56. Camilleri M, Northcutt AR, Kong S, et al: Efficacy and safety of alosetron in women with irritable bowel syndrome: a randomised, placebo-controlled trial. Lancet 355:1035–1040, 2000.

57. Camilleri M, Chey WY, Mayer EA, et al: A randomized controlled clinical trial of the serotonin type 3 receptor antagonist alosetron in women with diarrhea-predominant irritable bowel syndrome. Arch Intern Med 161:1733–1740, 2001.

58. Delvaux M, Louvel D, Mamet JP, et al: Effect of alosetron on responses to colonic distension in patients with irritable bowel syndrome. Aliment Pharmacol Ther 12:849–855, 1998.

59. Berman SM, Chang L, Suyenobu B, et al: Condition-specific deactivation of brain regions by 5-HT3 receptor antagonist alosetron. Gastroenterology 123:969–977, 2002.

60. Klatt S, Beock W, Rentschler J, et al: Effects of tropisetron, a 5-HT3 receptor antagonist, on proximal gastric motor and sensory function in nonulcer dyspepsia. Digestion 60:147–152, 1999.

61. Tack J, Coulie B, Wilmer A, et al: Influence of sumatriptan on gastric fundus tone and on the perception of gastric distension in man. Gut 46:468–473, 2000.

62. Thumshirn M, Camilleri M, Choi MG, Zinsmeister AR: Modulation of gastric sensory and motor functions by nitrergic and alpha2-adrenergic agents in humans. Gastroenterology 116:573–585, 1999.

63. Bortolotti M, Coccia G, Grossi G, Miglioli M: The treatment of functional dyspepsia with red pepper. Aliment Pharmacol Ther 16:1075–1082, 2002.

64. Clouse RE, Lustman PJ, Geisman RA, Alpers DH: Antidepressant therapy in 138 patients with irritable bowel syndrome: a five-year clinical experience. Aliment Pharmacol Ther 8:409–416, 1994.

65. Clouse RE: Antidepressants for functional gastrointestinal syndromes. Dig Dis Sci 39:2352–2363, 1994.

66. Jackson JL, O'Malley PG, Tomkins G, et al: Treatment of functional gastrointestinal disorders with antidepressant medications: a meta-analysis. Am J Med 108:65–72, 2000.

67. Gorelick AB, Koshy SS, Hooper FG, et al: Differential effects of amitriptyline on perception of somatic and visceral stimulation in healthy humans. Am J Physiol 275:G460–466, 1998.

68. Mertz H, Fass R, Kodner A, et al: Effect of amitriptyline on symptoms, sleep, and visceral perception in patients with functional dyspepsia. Am J Gastroenterol 93:160–165, 1998.

69. Ladabaum U, Glidden D: Effect of the selective serotonin reuptake inhibitor sertraline on gastric sensitivity and compliance in healthy humans. Neurogastroenterol Motil 14:395–402, 2002.

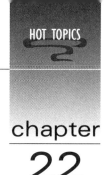

Current Treatment for Dyspepsia

Brooks D. Cash, M.D., and William D. Chey, M.D.

chapter 22

The distinction between uninvestigated dyspepsia and functional dyspepsia is very important. Uninvestigated dyspepsia refers to the condition of all symptomatic patients in whom an evaluation has not yet been performed and a specific cause of symptoms has not been identified. On the other hand, a diagnosis of functional dyspepsia is rendered only after an evaluation has excluded potential structural or biochemical causes of dyspeptic symptoms. Understanding the difference between uninvestigated dyspepsia and functional dyspepsia is important on a number of different levels, particularly as it pertains to selection of, and expected outcomes associated with, specific therapies.

Patients with dyspepsia need to be distinguished from those with predominant retrosternal burning or "heartburn." Patients suffering from heartburn are very likely to suffer from gastroesophageal reflux disease and thus are likely to benefit from antisecretory medication. In clinical practice, however, it is important to point out that some patients considered to have dyspepsia in reality suffer with an atypical presentation of gastroesophageal reflux disease. The inclusion of patients with pathologic gastroesophageal reflux in clinical trials is likely to have contributed to the finding of a modest benefit of proton pump inhibitor (PPI) therapy in functional dyspepsia.[1,2] Other causes of abdominal pain, including biliary pain, pancreatic pain, mesenteric ischemia, and atypical angina pectoris, are often associated with characteristics that can help to differentiate them from dyspepsia (Table 1).

Treatment of Uninvestigated Dyspepsia

Dietary Recommendations

There is often a relationship between dyspeptic symptoms and eating a meal. As such, many patients ask about the potential benefits of dietary restrictions for dyspeptic symptoms. A number of conditions, including

TABLE 1.   Characteristics of Identifiable Causes of Upper Abdominal Pain

Cause	Characteristics
Gastroesophageal reflux disease	Heartburn, regurgitation, typically substernal, worse after large meals, temporary relief with antacids
Peptic ulcer disease	Epigastric abdominal pain, typically better with meals, history of NSAID use, *Helicobacter pylori* infection, temporary relief with antacids
Mesenteric ischemia	Replicable, severe abdominal pain, worse after meals (intestinal angina), associated with weight loss, diarrhea; history of vascular disease
Biliary pain	Pain in right upper quadrant, epigastrium, back, or shoulder, may or may not be related to meals, crescendo-decrescendo pattern, may last hours
Pancreatic pain	Boring pain, epigastrium radiating to back, steatorrhea when pancreatic dysfunction is severe
Atypical angina pectoris	Exertional, often radiating to shoulder, improves with rest
Abdominal wall pain	Reproducible with physical examination, trigger points, associated with movement or bending
Gastroparesis	Early satiety, bloating, fullness, emesis, weight loss, coexisting diabetes mellitus

NSAID = nonsteroidal anti-inflammatory drug

carbohydrate malabsorption, celiac sprue, gastroparesis, and gastroesophageal reflux disease, can cause meal-related dyspeptic symptoms. In patients with such disorders, specific dietary interventions can be very useful. In the absence of such disorders, however, there is no convincing evidence that highly restrictive diets will lead to symptom resolution in patients with dyspeptic symptoms. If there is a clear relationship between meals and symptom onset, it can be helpful for the patient to keep a diet diary for 2 to 3 weeks. During such an exercise, patients keep a record of dietary constituents and any postprandial symptoms in the hopes of identifying specific foods that exacerbate their symptoms.

Management Strategies

The available initial management strategies for individuals with uninvestigated dyspeptic symptoms include the "test-and-treat" strategy for *Helicobacter pylori* infection, empiric therapy with an antisecretory medication, or prompt visualization of the upper gastrointestinal tract (Fig. 1). Each strategy offers advantages as well as disadvantages (Tables 2 and 3).

Test-and-Treat Strategy for Helicobacter pylori Infection

The best choice of noninvasive diagnostic test for the test-and-treat strategy has been the subject of some debate. Most older guidelines ad-

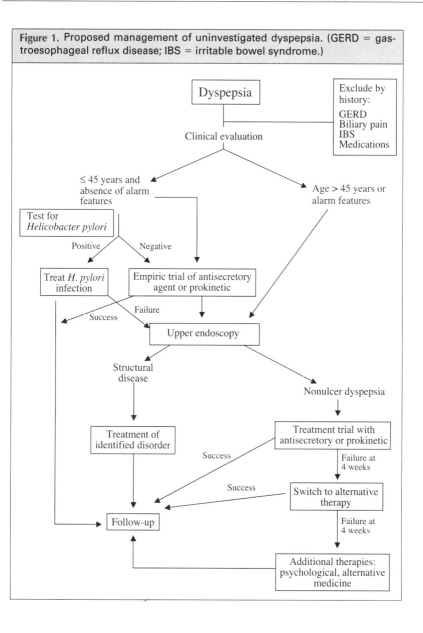

Figure 1. Proposed management of uninvestigated dyspepsia. (GERD = gastroesophageal reflux disease; IBS = irritable bowel syndrome.)

vocate the use of antibody testing. Advantages of antibody testing include wide availability and relatively low cost. A recent meta-analysis of 21 studies that evaluated a variety of different serum-based enzyme-linked immunosorbant assays for *H. pylori* found the overall sensitivity and specificity to be 85% and 79%, respectively.[3] A recent multicenter

TABLE 2. Pros and Cons of Empiric Antisecretory Therapy
Advantages
• Inexpensive for those with few recurrences
• H_2RAs and PPIs safe even when used long-term
Disadvantages
• Can mask serious disease
• May only postpone investigation
• Can lead to inappropriate chronic medication use by denying curative therapy in those with *Helicobacter pylori* infection
Utility
• Young dyspeptic patients with no warning signs
• Populations with a low *H. pylori*/ulcer prevalence
H_2RAs = histamine-2 receptor antagonists, PPIs = proton pump inhibitors

study from the United States reported that the available finger stick, whole blood, qualitative antibody tests may be even less sensitive than the enzyme-linked immunosorbent assays.[4] Based on these performance characteristics, the positive predictive value [PPV = true-positives ÷ true-positives + false positives] of antibody testing should be profoundly influenced by the background prevalence of *H. pylori* infection in a given population (Fig. 2).[3] For example, in a population with a *H. pylori* prevalence of 50%, antibody testing would be expected to yield a PPV of greater than 80%, whereas in a population with a *H. pylori* prevalence of 15%, the PPV of antibody testing is likely to be less than 50%. Given the falling prevalence of *H. pylori* infection in most developed nations, this point takes on particular relevance. The noninvasive alternatives to antibody tests are the "active tests," which identify only patients with active *H. pylori* infection. These tests include the urea breath test, the urea blood test, and the fecal antigen test. Each of these tests has been reported to yield sensitivity and specificity of greater than 90%.[5] Because of their

TABLE 3. Pros and Cons of Immediate Endoscopy
Advantages
• Provides reassurance to patient and doctor
• Allows targeted therapy and the potential for fewer prescriptions
Disadvantages
• Expensive
• Invasive with small risk of complications
• Lack of infrastructure to provide endoscopy to all patients with dyspepsia
Utility
• Patients with symptom onset after age 45 or 50 years or with alarm features
• Nonresponders to initial test-and-treat and/or empiric therapy

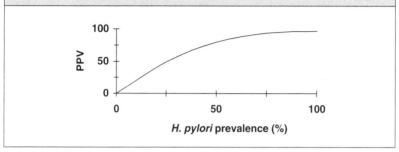

Figure 2. Effect of *Helicobacter pylori* prevalence on the positive predictive value (PPV) of antibody testing (where sensitivity = 85% and specificity = 79%). (Adapted from Loy CT, Irwig LM, Kateralis PH, et al. Do commercial serological kits for *Helicobacter pylori* infection differ in accuracy? A meta-analysis. Am J Gastroenterol 91:1138–1144, 1996.)

high sensitivity and specificity, the active tests remain accurate even in populations with a low prevalence of *H. pylori* infection. The major disadvantages of the active tests are their limited availability and their cost, which is considerably greater than the cost of the antibody tests.[6] Related to these points, antibody tests are likely to be most useful in populations with a higher *H. pylori* prevalence, whereas active tests are likely to be of greater value in populations with a lower *H. pylori* prevalence. If antibody testing is to be used in a low-prevalence population, some practitioners have suggested that a positive result be confirmed with an active test before antibiotic therapy is offered.

If the clinician embarks on the test-and-treat strategy, he or she should be prepared to offer treatment if *H. pylori* infection is identified. If a patient is penicillin allergic, the use of a PPI, tetracycline, metronidazole, and bismuth is a reasonable option. If the patient is not allergic to penicillin, the combination of a PPI, clarithromycin, and amoxicillin is appropriate (Table 4). Treatment should be offered for 7 to 14 days. With either of these therapies, cure of *H. pylori* infection can be expected in 80% to 85% of cases.[7,8]

Empiric Antisecretory Therapy

Empiric therapy with an antisecretory or prokinetic agent has long been employed as an initial management option in patients with uninvestigated dyspepsia. At present in the United States, the only available prokinetic agent is metoclopramide, which is associated with significant side effects in a substantial minority of patients. Most patients with uninvestigated dyspepsia are empirically treated with agents that suppress gastric acid secretion. In a systematic review reported in the Cochrane data base, PPIs were found to be more effective than histmaine-2 re-

TABLE 4.	Initial Treatment Regimens for *Helicobacter pylori* Infection

Not penicillin allergic: Clarithromycin-based triple therapy (7–14 days)
Proton pump inhibitor bid or qd (for Nexium)

plus

Clarithromycin 500 mg bid

plus

Either amoxicillin 1000 mg bid or metronidazole 500 mg bid

Penicillin allergic: Bismuth-based quadruple therapy (7–14 days)
Bismuth subsalicylate 2 tabs or 2 tablespoons qid

plus

Tetracycline 500 mg qid

plus

Metronidazole 250 mg qid

plus

Proton pump inhibitor given bid or qd

ceptor antagonists (H$_2$RAs) or antacids in relieving dyspeptic symptoms.[9] In one of the few large, randomized, double-blind trials to have compared the effectiveness of an H$_2$RA with that of a PPI in patients with uninvestigated dyspepsia, Jones and Baxter[10] found that treatment with a PPI (lansoprazole 30 mg/d) was more likely to result in symptom resolution than treatment with an H$_2$RA (ranitidine 150 mg bid). In the *H. pylori* era, however, empiric antisecretory therapy has been criticized because patients with *H. pylori*–associated peptic ulcer disease are denied the benefits of reduced recurrence of the disease after successful cure of the infection.[11]

Treatment of Functional Dyspepsia

General Considerations

One of the critically important features of successfully managing functional dyspepsia is an interactive, constructive patient-physician relationship. The physician should acknowledge that the symptoms that the patient is experiencing are real and understandably bothersome. The patient's fears and concerns regarding his or her health status should also receive attention. This should be followed by education and reassurance that nonulcer dyspepsia is both common and not life threatening. Setting reasonable treatment goals and empowering the patient to take responsibility for his or her own health care are also important features of supportive care. This can be done through use of a symptom diary that allows the patient to examine and understand possible triggers or behaviors that exacerbate symptoms.

Medical Therapy

Antisecretory Therapy

As previously discussed, antisecretory agents (H$_2$RAs or PPIs) and *H. pylori* eradication therapy have a central role in the initial treatment approach to patients with uninvestigated dyspepsia. In patients with nonulcer dyspepsia, in whom acid hypersensitivity may play a role, PPIs are the antisecretory agents of choice, since they have been shown, in many studies, to provide a more robust and prolonged acid suppression than H$_2$RAs.[12] Whereas H$_2$RAs remain the primary antisecretory therapies of choice for many primary care physicians, a Cochrane review of randomized controlled trials demonstrated the superiority of PPI therapy to H$_2$RA therapy with symptom relief in the 40% to 70% range.[13] Antisecretory therapy may not be equally effective in all patients with dyspeptic symptoms, however. In a recent trial evaluating the effectiveness of omeprazole in functional dyspepsia,[14] only patients with "ulcer-like" or "reflux-like" dyspepsia derived benefit (on omeprazole 20 mg and 10 mg every day, complete relief in 40% and 35% for ulcer-like dyspepsia compared to 27% with placebo, and 54% and 45% for "reflux-like" dyspepsia compared to 23% with placebo; all $P < 0.05$ compared to placebo except 10 mg dose in ulcer-like dyspepsia, $P = 0.08$). Patients with dysmotility-like dyspepsia (nausea, bloating, early satiety) experienced no benefit on omeprazole compared to placebo. Among the five available PPIs, none has proven to be more effective than the others for relief of dyspeptic symptoms. Because PPIs only bind active proton pumps, they should be taken 30 to 60 minutes before a meal to maximize their effect on acid suppression. Although most studies report that PPIs are more effective than placebo for the treatment of patients with functional dyspepsia, it is important to understand that the majority of patients will not experience symptom resolution. This is undoubtedly related to the diverse pathogenesis of symptoms reported by patients carrying the diagnosis of functional dyspepsia.

Promotility Agents

Promotility agents are thought to improve symptoms in patients with functional dyspepsia through their effects on gastric motility and accommodation. Delayed gastric emptying has long been thought to contribute to symptoms in a subset of patients with functional dyspepsia. There is some evidence to suggest that patients with predominant symptoms of dysmotility (fullness, early satiety, bloating, nausea) are more likely to have abnormalities in gastric emptying.[15] There is also emerging evidence to suggest that impaired reflex relaxation of the proximal stomach in response to eating a meal (accommodation reflex) is common in patients with functional dyspepsia.[16] Unfortunately, the relationship between these abnormalities in gastric motor and reflex function and symptoms in patients with functional dyspepsia remains poorly defined. In other words, correction of abnormalities in gastric motor or reflex function does not consistently lead to symptom improvement [17]

Promotility agents available in the United States include metoclopramide and erythromycin. Metoclopramide is a peripherally acting dopamine antagonist with antiemetic properties and effects on gastric emptying. Erythromycin is a motilin receptor agonist with gastric prokinetic properties. Neither of these agents has been proven to be effective for functional dyspepsia. In addition, both are limited by potentially serious adverse effects and, in the case of erythromycin, the rapid development of tachyphylaxis. Metoclopramide crosses the blood-brain barrier and is associated with significant central nervous system side effects, including drowsiness, agitation, depression, dystonic reactions, and, rarely, tardive dyskinesia.

Two additional promotility agents that have shown promise for nonulcer dyspepsia are cisapride and domperidone. Cisapride stimulates gastrointestinal motility through its action as a partial 5-HT_4 agonist. Domperidone, like metoclopramide, is a peripherally acting dopamine antagonist, and it accelerates gastric emptying and stimulates antropyloric motility. Domperidone has antiemetic properties but, unlike metoclopramide, does not cross the blood-brain barrier. As such, domperidone is not associated with the central nervous system side effects that commonly occur with metoclopramide. In addition to their effects on gastric motility, it is also possible that these agents may have effects on gastric sensation or accommodation, or both. Both of these agents appear to benefit a subset of patients with functional dyspepsia. A recent meta-analysis of placebo-controlled trials by van Zanten et al.[18] found both agents to be effective for global improvement in dyspeptic symptoms as well as individual symptoms such as bloating or early satiety. An important caveat to this conclusion is that the outcomes from many of the trials included in this meta-analysis were derived from the investigator's rather than the patient's assessment of symptoms. In trials of therapy for functional gastrointestinal disorders, the Rome II consensus committee recommended that patient-reported outcomes, in particular patient global assessment of well being, serve as the primary outcome measure.[19]

Unfortunately, for different reasons, neither of these agents is available in the United States. Cisapride was voluntarily withdrawn from the market due to concerns about effects on cardiac conduction and rare but sometimes fatal cardiac arrhythmias. Domperidone has not been approved by the Food and Drug Administration (FDA) for use in the United States. Domperidone is available in most other countries, however, including Canada and Mexico. Domperidone is used at doses of 10 to 20 mg given orally 30 minutes before a meal. Other motilin agonists, 5-HT$_4$ agonists, and dopamine receptor antagonists (levosulpiride) are in various stages of development. Tegaserod, a recently approved partial 5-HT$_4$ agonist for irritable bowel syndrome–constipation predominant, is currently undergoing evaluation for a potential therapeutic role in nonulcer dyspepsia [20] In addition, recent studies suggest that drugs that modify gastric accommodation may also hold promise in functional dyspepsia.[21,22]

Antinociceptive Agents

Antidepressant therapies have been used in treating functional gastrointestinal disorders for several years, with varying degrees of success. In low doses, tricyclic antidepressants (TCAs) appear to have effects on visceral pain perception and, in this way, may serve as a "visceral analgesic" for patients with functional gastrointestinal disorders such as functional dyspepsia. Numerous small studies have evaluated the potential benefits of TCAs for noncardiac chest pain, functional dyspepsia, and the irritable bowel syndrome. A recent meta-analysis of antidepressant therapy for functional gastrointestinal disorders by Jackson et al[23] demonstrated a treatment benefit from TCAs (odds ratio, 4.2; 95% CI, 2.3–7.9). Based on the therapeutic gain reported in this trial, the number of patients that would need to be treated to achieve one positive outcome was 3.2 (95% CI, 2.1–6.5 patients). However, these data must be viewed with caution, since the trials analyzed included patients with a variety of functional gastrointestinal disorders and most of the studies utilized significantly flawed methodology. Few studies have specifically evaluated the use of antidepressants for functional dyspepsia. In a small randomized trial of seven patients with functional dyspepsia, amitriptyline (50 mg at bedtime) was found to be more effective than placebo in improving symptoms.[24] This benefit did not correlate with changes in perception of gastric balloon distention, suggesting that the analgesic effect was likely mediated centrally, perhaps through effects on the cortical processing of painful visceral sensations.[25]

The TCAs are typically reserved for patients with moderate to severe symptoms who have failed antisecretory therapy. When TCAs are used for the functional gastrointestinal disorders, lower doses are typically necessary than when treating depression (Table 5). For functional gastrointestinal disorders, target doses for the TCAs range from 10 to 100 mg per day. Of course, higher doses are necessary in the presence of comorbid psychological conditions such as depression. These drugs are usually given in the evening to minimize problems related to their sedative effects. Patients should also be warned about the possibility of dry mouth and eyes as well as weight gain. Secondary amines such as nor-

TABLE 5. Antidepressant Therapy for Functional Gastrointestinal Disorders

Antidepressant	Dose, mg	Range, mg/d	Anti-cholinergic	Drowsi-ness	Agitation	Hypo-tension	Weight gain
Amitriptyline	10–100	50–300	++++	++++	0	++++	++++
Desipramine	10–100	50–300	+	+	+	++	+
Doxepin	10–200	50–300	+++	++++	0	++	+++
Imipramine	10–100	50–300	+++	+++	+	++++	+++
Nortriptyline	10–100	50–300	+	+	0	++	+
Fluoxetine	5–20	20–80	0	0	++	0	0
Paroxetine	10–20	20–50	0	0	++	0	0
Sertraline	25–50	50–200	0	0	++	0	00
Trazodone	25–50	50–400	0	++++	0	+	+

Adapted from Budavari AJ, Olden KW: The use of antidepressants in irritable bowel syndrome. Pract Gastroenterol 26:13–24, 2002.

triptyline and desipramine may be better tolerated than the older tertiary amines (amitriptyline, imipramine).

There are currently no published randomized controlled trials that have evaluated the effectiveness of the selective serotonin reuptake inhibitors in patients with functional dyspepsia. The selective serotonin reuptake inhibitors are as or more effective in treating anxiety and depression and better tolerated than the TCAs. For this reason, it makes sense to consider these agents in patients with significant comorbid psychological disease. Other classes of drugs that hold promise related to their antinociceptive effects in functional dyspepsia include the peripheral opioid agonists[26] and the 5-HT$_3$ receptor antagonists.[27]

Psychological Therapies

The relationship between comorbid psychological conditions and the functional gastrointestinal disorders is well established.[28] Patients with functional dyspepsia are more likely to report increased life stress and score higher for traits such as anxiety, tension, and neuroticism than the general population.[29] A history of verbal, physical, or sexual abuse is also more common in patients with frequent dyspepsia than in a control population.[30] While patients often do not demonstrate these traits through impaired social functioning, psychological factors can result in increased health care seeking[31] and may contribute to alterations in visceral perception via the central and enteric nervous systems.

Psychotherapy has been examined in patients with functional gastrointestinal disorders. Most of these studies have evaluated the effects of psychotherapy on IBS symptoms. Different psychotherapeutic modalities used to treat functional gastrointestinal disorders include insight-oriented psychotherapy, relaxation and stress management training, cognitive based behavioral therapy, biofeedback, and hypnotherapy.[32,33] The best studied of these techniques is cognitive-behavioral therapy. This form of psychotherapy is designed to teach patients how to identify maladaptive behaviors and manage their responses to emotional and life stresses. Haug et al.[34] randomized 100 patients to cognitive psychotherapy or no therapy and found that the psychotherapy patients experienced significant improvement in symptoms such as bloating, epigastric pain, and nausea. Mine at al.[35] randomized 198 patients with nonulcer dyspepsia to a combination of medical, psychiatric, and psychotherapeutic treatments versus medical therapy alone and found that the multimodality therapy afforded significantly improved outcomes compared with medical therapy alone. Hamilton et al.[36] sought to determine whether brief psychodynamic-interpersonal psychotherapy was superior to reassurance alone. At the end of the therapy period, patients in the psychotherapy group had significant symptom reduction compared to the group treated with reassurance alone. A post-hoc analysis at 1 year, removing patients with severe heartburn symptoms, indicated a potential benefit for the psychotherapy group. Another recent study found that hypnotherapy yielded a greater improvement in symptoms, reduced antidepressant medication, and reduced consultation rates as compared with supportive therapy or medical therapy.[32]

Although the data regarding the effectiveness of psychological therapies for dyspepsia are still too sparse to draw absolute conclusions, it does appear that addressing life stresses and improving coping mechanisms can be a useful adjunct to traditional therapies once organic gastrointestinal disease has been excluded. Several factors make the use of psychological therapy challenging in clinical practice. In addition to overcoming the stigma of referring patients for psychological therapy and the failure of many insurance plans to cover this form of outpatient treatment, it can be difficult to find mental health professional with the training and/or willingness to take on patients with functional gastrointestinal disorders.

Alternative Therapies

Given the limited efficacy of conventional medical therapy for functional dyspepsia, patients frequently seek out "alternative" therapies. The use of these therapies has dramatically increased in the last decade. In 1997, it was estimated that 42% of U.S. citizens were using alternative therapies, and out-of-pocket expenses totaled more than US $12 billion.[37] Common alternative therapies include acupuncture, massage therapy, herbal remedies, probiotics, therapeutic touch, aromatherapy, and color therapy. There have been very few methodologically acceptable trials that have evaluated alternative therapies in functional dyspepsia. A recent systematic review found only three trials of herbal therapies for patients with functional dyspepsia.[38] One trial reported significant benefit in overall well-being with peppermint oil extract.[39] Two others evaluated traditional Chinese herbal therapies and reported treatment benefits.[40,41] Importantly, all of the trials were limited by small sample size, short duration, and a failure to use validated symptom assessment tools. Thus, at the current time, there is not enough evidence to recommend the routine use of alternative therapies for functional dyspepsia. Further well-designed clinical trials are eagerly awaited.

Key Points: Current Treatment for Dyspepsia

- ⤷ The optimal treatment of dyspepsia has yet to be determined. Dietary and lifestyle recommendations as well as a careful review of medication use can be helpful.
- ⤷ Young patients with dyspeptic symptoms who do not exhibit alarm features can be managed by either the test-and-treat strategy for *H. pylori* infection or empiric antisecretory therapy.
- ⤷ Patients presenting with new symptoms after the age of 45 years or those with alarm features should be referred for early evaluation with upper endoscopy.
- ⤷ A structural evaluation that reveals no cause for a patient's symptoms confirms the diagnosis of functional dyspepsia.
- ⤷ Most patients with functional dyspepsia are managed initially with antisecretory agents. In patients with dysmotility-related symptoms, the use of a promotility agent may be preferred.
- ⤷ Patients with moderate to severe symptoms, particularly if associated with comorbid psychological distress, often benefit from therapy with antidepressants. Another consideration in patients with co-morbid psychological disease are the psychological therapies.
- ⤷ Multimodality treatment may be more effective for patients with severe symptoms, as is often encountered in the tertiary care setting.
- ⤷ Despite the popularity of alternative therapies among lay persons, there is currently a paucity of data to support their routine use.

Disclaimer

The opinions and assertions contained herein are the sole views of the authors and should not be construed as official or as representing the view of the U.S. Navy, Department of Defense, or Department of Veteran Affairs.

Suggested Reading

1. Farup PG, Hovde O, Torp R, et al: Patients with functional dyspepsia responding to omeprazole have a characteristic gastro-oesophageal relfux pattern. Scand J Gastroenterol 34:575–579, 1999.

2. Farup PG, Wetterhus S, Osnes M, et al: Ranitidine effectively relieves symptoms in a subset of patients with functional dyspepsia. Scand J Gastroenterol 32:755–759, 1997.

3. Loy CT, Irwig LM, Kateralis PH, et al: Do commercial serological kits for *Helicobacter pylori* infection differ in accuracy? A meta-analysis. Am J Gastroenterol 91:1138–1144, 1996.

4. Chey WD, Linscheer W, Zawadski A, et al: A comparison of three fingerstick whole blood antibody tests for *Helicobacter pylori:* a United States, multicenter trial. Am J Gastroenterol 94:1512–1516, 1999.

5. Lake JM, Chey WD: Testing for *Helicobacter pylori* in the clinical setting. Frontiers Biosci 6:e129–136, 2001.

6. Chey WD, Fendrick AM: Noninvasive *Helicobacter pylori* testing for the "test-and-treat" strategy. Arch Intern Med 161:2129–2132, 2001.

7. Katelaris PH, Forbes GM, Talley NJ, et al: A randomized comparison of quadruple and triple therapies for Helicobacter pylori eradication: the QUADRATE study. Gastroenterology 123:1763–1769, 2002.

8. Peterson WL, Fendrick AM, Cave DR, et al: *Helicobacter pylori*-related disease: guidelines for testing and treatment. Arch Intern Med 160:1285–1291, 2000.

9. Delaney BC, Innes MA, Deeks J, et al: Initial management strategies for dyspepsia. Cochrane Database Sys Rev 2CD001961, 2000.

10. Jones RH, Baxter G: Lansoprazole 30 mg daily versus ranitidine 150 b.d. in the treatment of acid-related dyspepsia in general practice. Aliment Pharmacol Ther 11:541–546, 1997.

11. Talley NJ, Azon A, Bytzer P, et al: Management of uninvestigated and functional dyspepsia: a working party report for the World Congress of Gastroenterology 1998. Aliment Pharm Ther 13:1135–1148, 1999.

12. Hunt RH: Importance of pH control in the management of GERD. Arch Intern Med 159:649–657, 1999.

13. Delaney BC, Innes MA, Deeks J, et al: Initial management strategies for dyspepsia (Cochrane Review). Cochrane Database Sys Rev 3CD001961, 2002.

14. Talley NJ, Meineche-Schmidt V, Pare P, et al: Efficacy of omeprazole in functional dyspepsia: double-blind, randomized, placebo-controlled trials (the Bond and Opera studies). Aliment Pharmacol Ther 12:1055–1065, 1998.

15. Stanghellini V, Tosetti C, Paternico A, et al: Predominant symptoms identify different subgroups in functional dyspepsia. Am J Gastroenterol 94:2080–2085, 1999.

16. Tack J, Piessevaux H, Coulie B, et al: Role of impaired gastric accommodation to a meal in functional dyspepsia. Gastroenterology 115:1346–1352, 1998.

17. Fisher RS, Parkman HP: Management of nonulcer dydpepsia. N Engl J Med 339:1376–1381, 1998.

18. van Santen SJOV, Jones MJ, Verlindin M, et al: Efficacy of cisapride and domperidone in functional (nonulcer) dyspepsia: a meta-analysis. Am J Gastroenterol 96:689–696, 2001.

19. van Santen S, Talley NJ, Bytzer P, et al: Design of treatment trials for functional gastrointestinal disorders. Gut 45(Suppl II):II69–II77, 1999.

20. Tack J, Delia T, Ligozio G, et al: A phase II placebo controlled randomized trial with tegaserod in functional dyspepsia patients with normal gastric emptying. Gastroenterology 122:AB154, 2002.

21. Tack J, Coulie B, Wilmer A, et al: Influence of sumatriptan on gastric fundus tone and on the perception of gastric distention in man. Gut 46:468–473, 2000.

22. Thumshirn M, Camilleri M, Choi MG, et al: Modulation of gastric sensory and motor functions by nitrergic and α2-adrenergic agents in humans. Gastroenterology 116:573–585, 1999.

23. Jackson J, O'Malley P, Tomkins G, et al: Treatment for functional pastrointestinal disorders and antidepressant medications: a meta-analysis. Am J Med 169:65–72, 2000.

24. Mertz H, Fass R, Kodner A, et al: Effect of amitriptyline on symptoms, sleep, and visceral perception in patients with functional dyspepsia. Am J Gastroenterol 93:160–165, 1998.

25. Fioramonti J, Bueno L: Centrally acting agents and visceral sensitivity. Gut 51(suppl 1):i91–95, 2002.

26. Fraitag B, Homerin M, Hecketsweiler P: Double-blind dose-response multicenter comparison of fedotozine and placebo in treatment of nonulcer dyspepsia. Dig Dis Sci 39:1072–1077, 1994.

27. Mayer EA: Alosetron. Clin Perspect Gastroenterol Sept/Oct:299–303, 1999.

28. Drossman DA (ed): Rome II: The Functional Gastrointestinal Disorders. McLean, VA; Degnon Associates, 2000; pp 157–246, 299–350.

29. Alpers DH: Why should psychotherapy be a useful approach to management of patients with nonulcer dyspepsia? Gastroenterology 119:869–871, 2000.

30. Talley NJ, Fett SL, Zinsmeister AR, et al: Gastrointestinal tract symptoms and self-reported abuse: a population-based study. Gastroenterology 107:1040–1049, 1994.

31. Koloski NA, Talley NJ, Boyce PM: Predictors of health care seeking for irritable bowel syndrome and nonulcer dyspepsia: a critical review of the literature on symptom and psychosocial factors. Am J Gastroenterol 96:1340–1349, 2001.

32. Calvert EL, Houghton LA, Cooper P, et al: Long-term improvement in functional dyspepsia using hypnotherapy. Gastroenterology 123:1778–1785, 2002.

33. Talley NK, Owen BK, Boyce P, et al: Psychological treatments for irritable vowel syndrome: a critique of controlled clinical trials. Am J Gastroenterol 91:277–286, 1996.

34. Haug TT, Wilhelmsen I, Svebak S, et al: Psychotherapy in functional dyspepsia. J Psychosom Res 38:735–744, 1994.

35. Mine K, Kanazawa F, Hosoi M, et al: Treating nonulcer dyspepsia considering both functional disorders of the gastrointestinal tract and psychiatric conditions. Dig Dis Sci 43:1241–1247, 1998.

36. Hamilton J, Guthrie E, Creed F, et al: A randomized controlled trial of psychotherapy in patients with chronic functional dyspepsia. Gastroenterology 119:661–669, 2000.

37. Eisenberg DM, Davis RB, Ettner SL, et al: Trends in alternative medicine use in the United States, 1990–1997. JAMA 280:1569–1575, 1998.

38. Cash B, Schoenfeld P: Alternative medical therapies for dyspepsia: a systematic review of randomized controlled trials. In Johnson DA, Katz PO, Castell DO (eds): Philadelphia, American College of Physicians, 2001, pp 159–175.

39. May B, Kuntz HD, Kieser M, et al: Efficacy of a fixed peppermint oil/caraway oil combination in non-ulcer dyspepsia. Arzneimittelforschung 46:1149–1153, 1996.

40. Tatsuta M, Iishi H: Effect of treatment with Liu-Jun-Zi-Tang (TJ-43) on gastric emptying and gastrointestinal symptoms in dyspeptic patients. Aliment Pharm Ther 7:459–462, 1993.

41. Thamlikitkul V, Dechatiwongse T, Chantrakul C, et al: Randomised double blind study of *Curcuma domestica* for dyspepsia. J Med Assoc Thai 72:614–620, 1989.

Future Treatment of Functional Dyspepsia

chapter

23

Jan Tack, M.D., Ph.D.,
and Kwang-Jae Lee, M.D., Ph.D.

Several possible pathophysiologic mechanisms have been postulated in functional dyspepsia, but until now the real pathophysiology of functional dyspepsia has not been elucidated.

The gastric emptying profile has been studied frequently in patients with functional dyspepsia, and delayed gastric emptying of solids is present in 25% to 40% of patients.[1–3] Large-scale studies have shown that delayed gastric emptying is associated with postprandial fullness, nausea, and vomiting.[3]

Scintigraphic and ultrasonographic studies have demonstrated an abnormal intragastric distribution of food in patients with functional dyspepsia, with preferential accumulation in the distal stomach.[4–6] This finding suggests defective postprandial accommodation of the proximal stomach. Using a gastric barostat in 40 consecutive dyspeptic patients, we showed that impaired gastric accommodation was present in 40% of these patients and that this impairment was associated with early satiety and weight loss.[7] A study using single photon emission computed tomography confirmed the association with weight loss,[8] whereas others could not detect a clear relationship between postprandial symptoms and proximal stomach function.[9] Phasic fundic contractions induce transient increases in gastric wall tension and can be perceived in functional dyspepsia.[10] In a recent study, we found unsuppressed postprandial phasic contractility in the proximal stomach in a small subset of patients (15%). This alteration was associated with *Helicobacter pylori* infection and relevant or severe bloating, but also with the absence of nausea.[11]

Using a gastric barostat, several investigators have demonstrated that, as a group, patients with functional dyspepsia have lower sensory thresholds during balloon distension in the proximal stomach and the duodenum than healthy volunteers.[12-15] In a large study, we observed gastric hypersensitivity in 36% of dyspeptic patients, and this was associated with symptoms of postprandial pain, belching, and weight loss.[16]

383

A recent systematic review of the epidemiologic evidence on a relationship between *H. pylori* infection and functional dyspepsia found no evidence for a strong association. According to the authors, however, there was not enough evidence to rule out a modest association.[17] Mechanistic studies comparing *H. pylori*-positive and -negative patients have failed to demonstrate consistent alterations in motor or sensory function associated with the infection.

Infusion of lipids, but not glucose, in the duodenum sensitizes the stomach to distension in patients with functional dyspepsia, in contrast to control subjects.[18,19] This effect is mediated via lipid digestion and release of cholecystokinin.[20,21] Also, 5-HT$_3$ receptors seem to be involved in this gastric response to duodenal lipids.[22]

Duodenal infusion of hydrochloric acid was found to induce nausea in a subset of functional dyspepsia patients but not in healthy control subjects, suggesting duodenal hypersensitivity to acid. Furthermore, the duodenal motor response to acid was decreased in functional dyspepsia patients, resulting in reduced clearance of exogenous duodenal acid.[23–25] Recently, we confirmed that spontaneous duodenal acid exposure to endogenous acid was increased in functional dyspepsia patients who displayed delayed clearance of exogenous duodenal acid, but the relationship with symptoms is unclear.[26]

There is evidence of an association between psychopathology and functional dyspepsia,[27] but the relevance to symptom pattern is unknown. In a recent factor analysis of dyspepsia symptoms, we demonstrated that nausea, vomiting, early satiety, and weight loss were associated with female sex and sickness behavior and that epigastric pain was associated with several psychosocial dimensions, including medically unexplained symptoms and conditions, as well as with health-related quality of life.[28] It remains to be proven, however, whether the associated psychopathologic abnormalities have a pathogenetic role or whether they are influencing symptom perception or health care seeking behavior in dyspeptic patients.

New Therapeutic Developments in Functional Dyspepsia

Because of the relationship with symptom pattern, it seems logical in the future to target potential therapeutic approaches in patients with functional dyspepsia toward the underlying pathophysiologic abnormality. To be able to achieve this in clinical practice, however, easy, noninvasive methods are needed. The gastric emptying breath test and satiety drinking tests may be valid options.[7,29] Using a rapid drinking test, no correlation between the drinking capacity and pathophysiologic alterations could be observed.[30] With a slow caloric drinking test (15 mL/min; 1.5

kcal/mL), we were able to show a significant relationship between the amount of ingested calories at maximum satiety and the presence of early satiety and the accommodation of the proximal stomach.[31]

An alternative conceivable approach, bypassing underlying pathophysiologic mechanisms, is the use of agents that decrease visceral sensitivity enough to inhibit the occurrence of symptoms of discomfort or pain induced by impaired sensorimotor function.

Acid suppression

Acid suppressive therapy seems valid for patients with gastroesophageal reflux disease who present with symptoms of dyspepsia. On the other hand, recent studies have suggested the role of increased duodenal acid exposure or hypersensitivity to duodenal acid in the pathogenesis of functional dyspepsia.[23–26] In patients with duodenal acid hypersensitivity, a tendency toward a decrease of duodenal acid hypersensitivity was observed after 2 weeks of proton pump inhibitor treatment. However, the potential benefits of acid suppressive treatment for functional dyspepsia patients with increased duodenal acid exposure remain to be defined.

Prokinetics

Recently, tegaserod, a partial 5-HT_4 agonist, was found to accelerate gastric emptying, indicating its possibility as a prokinetic agent.[32] In addition, we showed a trend that tegaserod improved upper gastrointestinal symptoms in female functional dyspepsia patients with normal gastric emptying, suggesting that it may affect pathophysiologic mechanisms other than delayed gastric emptying.[33] Motilin-receptor agonists can also act as prokinetics, but a recent study showed that the motilin agonist ABT-229 was of no value for relief of symptoms in patients with functional dyspepsia and diabetes mellitus with and without delayed gastric emptying.[34,35] Several factors connected with the drug and with the design of the studies might have contributed to the negative outcome.[36] The fact that erythromycin and related compounds reduce the meal-induced relaxation of the proximal stomach[37] and enhance the sensitivity to gastric distension[38] may have influenced the lack of a positive symptomatic effect.

Agents Acting on Visceral Sensitivity

Antidepressants are commonly used in treating functional gastrointestinal disorders and are believed to exert an analgesic rather than an antidepressant effect. However, studies of the effects of antidepressants on visceral sensitivity are rare and the existing data are controversial.[39,40] Agents that modify serotonergic function have therapeutic potential for the treatment of visceral hypersensitivity, either through a direct effect on perception or through modulation of visceral tone or motility. Selective serotonin reuptake inhibitors do not appear to affect sensitivity to gastric distension.[41]

Fedotozine, a peripherally acting κ opioid receptor agonist, influences visceral sensitivity[41,43] and has been shown to increase discomfort thresholds to gastric distension in healthy volunteers.[44] However, development of this drug has not been continued. The concept of using κ opioid agonists is still valid, and other compounds are under evaluation. Asimadoline, another peripherally acting κ opioid receptor agonist, was shown to inhibit meal-induced satiety in humans.[45] It is unclear whether this relates to the visceral analgesic properties of the drug, or whether it is altering gastric accommodation to a meal.

Fundus-Relaxing Drugs

In patients with impaired gastric accommodation, restoring gastric accommodation is likely to improve symptoms of early satiety. Prolonged use of nitrates to treat impaired accommodation is usually associated with undesirable vascular side effects due to the lack of specificity. 5-HT receptors on intrinsic nitrergic neurons are involved in the control of the gastric accommodation. Similar to the central nervous system, serotonin reuptake in the enteric nervous system is also inhibited by selective serotonin reuptake inhibitors.[46] We observed that pretreatment with paroxetine, a selective serotonin reuptake inhibitor, strongly enhanced the meal-induced relaxation of the proximal stomach in humans.[41] Clinical studies addressing its potential benefit in patients with impaired gastric accommodation seem warranted.

Tegaserod, a partial 5-HT$_4$ agonist has been shown to relax the stomach[47] and to accelerate gastric emptying,[32] and promising results from a phase II trial in functional dyspepsia patients with normal gastric emptying rates was recently reported.[33]

We have shown that administration of sumatriptan, a 5-HT$_1$ receptor agonist, relaxes the proximal stomach in healthy subjects[48] and, in short-term studies, restores meal-induced relaxation in patients with impaired gastric accommodation and increases the amount of calories ingested at maximum satiety in patients with early satiety.[7] Owing to its pharmacologic properties, its cost, and its mode of administration, sumatriptan is not suitable for chronic treatment of functional dyspepsia. Buspirone is a nonselective 5-HT$_1$ receptor agonist, used in the treatment of panic attacks. In a placebo-controlled study in patients with functional dyspepsia, we confirmed that buspirone was superior to placebo in alleviating dyspeptic symptoms, and that this was associated with an enhancement of the accommodation to a meal.[49]

Administration of nitric oxide donors also relaxes the proximal stomach,[50] but long-term use is usually limited by vascular side effects. Sildenafil blocks phosphodiesterase type 5, which degrades nitric oxide stimulated $3'5'$-cyclic monophophate thereby relaxing smooth muscle in various organs. It enhances accommodation of the proximal stomach,[51] and trials of this drug in cases of functional dyspepsia are warranted. Clonidine, which is an α_2-receptor agonist, relaxes the stomach and reduces gastric sensation.[50] This drug might also prove to be an interesting treatment option in the future.

Z-338

Z-338 is a blocker of muscarinic autoreceptors. In a pilot study, this drug was shown to provide symptomatic benefit and to improve impaired accommodation in functional dyspepsia.[52] Phase 2 studies are currently in progress.

Other Agents

Studies in animals suggest that 5-HT_3 receptors are putative excitatory mediators in visceral sensory pathways, and thus 5-HT_3 antagonists may reduce the level of perception to visceral distension.[53] However, the selective 5-HT_3 antagonists alosetron and ondansetron do not appear to have any significant effects on sensitivity to gastric distension in humans.[54] A recent study demonstrated a reduction in dyspeptic symptoms in functional dyspepsia patients treated with alosetron.[55] The mechanism underlying this beneficial effect remains to be elucidated, but additional studies with alosetron are unlikely because this drug has been withdrawn due to side effects[56] and later used in a restricted program only. In humans, ondansetron reduces the sensation of nausea provoked by the combined stimuli of intraduodenal lipid infusion and gastric distension.[22] As this drug does not alter gastric tone or sensitivity, it is likely to act at duodenal vagal afferent nerves.[22,55]

Inhibitors of lipid digestion decrease the sensation induced by intraduodenal lipid infusion.[21] Future studies will investigate the therapeutic potential of these drugs. Cholecystokinin receptor antagonists also reduce duodenal lipid sensitivity and might prove to be useful in treating functional dyspepsia in the near future.[20]

A recent study showed that the chronic administration of capsaicin, or red pepper was more effective than placebo in decreasing the intensity of dyspeptic symptoms in patients with functional dyspepsia.[57] This result might be explained by the finding that capsaicin initially produces sensitization, but repeated stimulation of the capsaicin receptor on capsaicin-sensitive primary afferent nerves leads to desensitization.[58] Thus, the visceral analgesic effect of capsaicin warrants investigation in humans.

Key Points: Future Treatment of Functional Dyspepsia

☞ Several possible pathophysiologic mechanisms have been postulated in functional dyspepsia, including delayed gastric emptying, abnormal intragastric distribution of food, lower sensory thresholds, *H. pylori* infection, lipid digestion, pH profile, and psychopathologic factors.

☞ In the future, therapeutic approaches should be targeted at the underlying pathophysiologic abnormality.

☞ Acid suppressive agents, prokinetics, agents acting on visceral sensitivity, fundus-relaxing drugs, and blockers of muscarinic autoreceptors all are being investigated as potentially useful therapies.

☞ Other new therapies may include 5-HT$_3$ antagonists, cholecystokinin receptor antagonists, and capsaisin.

Suggested Reading

1. Maes BD, Ghoos YF, Hiele MI, Rutgeerts PJ: Gastric emptying rate of solids in patients with nonulcer dyspepsia. Dig Dis Sci 42:1158–1162, 1997.
2. Quartero AO, de Wit NJ, Lodder AC, et al: Disturbed solid-phase gastric emptying in functional dyspepsia: a meta-analysis. Dig Dis Sci 43:2028–2033, 1998.
3. Stanghellini V, Tosetti C, Paternico A, et al: Risk indicators of delayed gastric emptying of solids in patients with functional dyspepsia. Gastroenterology 110:1036–1042, 1996.
4. Gilja OH, Hausken T, Wilhelmsen I, Berstad A: Impaired accommodation of proximal stomach to a meal in functional dyspepsia. Dig Dis Sci 41:689–696, 1996.
5. Scott AM, Kellow JE, Shuter B, et al: Intragastric distribution and gastric emptying of solids and liquids in functional dyspepsia. Dig Dis Sci 38:2247–2254, 1993.
6. Troncon LEA, Bennett RJM, Ahluwalia NK, Thompson DG: Abnormal distribution of food during gastric emptying in functional dyspepsia patients. Gut 35:327–332, 1994.
7. Tack J, Piessevaux H, Coulie B, et al: Role of impaired gastric accommodation to a meal in functional dyspepsia. Gastroenterology 115:1346–1352, 1998.
8. Kim DY, Delgado-Aros S, Camilleri M, et al: Noninvasive measurement of gastric accommodation in patients with idiopathic nonulcer dyspepsia. Am J Gastroenterol 96:3099–3105, 2001.
9. Boeckxstaens GE, Hirsch DP, Kuiken SD, et al: The proximal stomach and postprandial symptoms in functional dyspeptics. Am J Gastroenterol 97:40–48, 2002.
10. Tack J, Vos R, Caenepeel P, et al: Fundic tension receptors mediate perception in functional dyspepsia patients with hypersensitivity to gastric distensions. Gastroenterology 120:A-1244, 2001.
11. Simren M, Vos R, Janssens J, Tack J: Unsuppressed postprandial phasic contractility in the proximal stomach in functional dyspepsia: relevance to symptoms? Am J Gastroenterol. In press, 2003.
12. Bradette M, Pare P, Douville P, Morin A: Visceral perception in health and functional dyspepsia: crossover study of gastric distension with placebo and domperidone. Dig Dis Sci 36:52–58, 1991.

13. Coffin B, Azpiroz F, Guarner F, Malagelada JR: Selective gastric hypersensitivity and reflex hyporeactivity in functional dyspepsia. Gastroenterology 107:1345–1351, 1994.

14. Holtmann G, Goebell H, Talley J: Impaired small intestinal peristaltic reflexes and sensory thresholds are independent functional disturbances in patients with chronic unexplained dyspepsia. Am J Gastroenterol 91:485–491, 1996.

15. Lemann M, Dederding JP, Flourie B, et al: Abnormal perception of visceral pain in response to gastric distension in chronic idiopathic dyspepsia: the irritable stomach syndrome. Dig Dis Sci 36:1249–1254, 1991.

16. Tack J, Caenepeel P, Fischler B, et al: Symptoms associated with hypersensitivity to gastric distention in functional dyspepsia. Gastroenterology 121:526–535, 2001.

17. Danesh J, Lawrence M, Murphy M, et al: Systematic review of the epidemiological evidence on *Helicobacter pylori* infection and nonulcer or uninvestigated dyspepsia. Arch Intern Med 160:1192–1198, 2000.

18. Barbera R, Feinle C, Read NW: Nutrient-specific modulation of gastric mechanosensitivity in patients with functional dyspepsia. Dig Dis Sci 40:1636–1641, 1995.

19. Barbera R, Feinle C, Read NW: Abnormal sensitivity to duodenal lipid infusion in patients with functional dyspepsia. Eur J Gastroenterol Hepatol 7:1051–1057, 1995.

20. Feinle C, Meier O, Otto B, et al: Role of duodenal lipid and cholecystokinin A receptors in the pathophysiology of functional dyspepsia. Gut 48:347–355, 2001.

21. Feinle C, Rades T, Otto B, Fried M: Fat digestion modulates gastrointestinal sensations induced by gastric disention and duodenal lipid in humans. Gastroenterology 120:1100–1107, 2001.

22. Feinle C, Read NW: Ondansetron reduces nausea induced by gastroduodenal stimulation without changing gastric motility. Am J Physiol 271:G591–597, 1996.

23. Samsom M, Verhagen MA, van Berge Henegouwen GP, Smout AJPM: Abnormal clearance of exogenous acid and increased acid sensitivity of the proximal duodenum in dyspeptic patients. Gastroenterology 116:515–520, 1999.

24. Schwarz MP, Samsom M, Smout AJPM: Chemospecific alterations in duodenal perception and motor response in functional dyspepsia. Am J Gastroenterol 96:2596–2602, 2001.

25. Schwarz MP, Samsom M, van Berge Henegouwen GP, Smout AJPM: Effect of inhibition of gastric acid secretion on antropyloroduodenal motor activity and duodenal acid hypersensitivity in functional dyspepsia. Aliment Pharmacol Ther 15:1921–1928, 2001.

26. Reference deleted.

27. Wilhelmsen I, Haug TT, Ursin H, Berstad A: Discriminant analysis of factors distinguishing patients with functional dyspepsia from patients with duodenal ulcer. Significance of somatization. Dig Dis Sci 40:1105–1111, 1995.

28. Fischler B, Tack J, De Gucht V, et al: Heterogeneity of symptom pattern, psychosocial factors and pathophysiological mechanisms in severe functional dyspepsia. Gastroenterology 124:903–910, 2003.

29. Maes BD, Ghoos YF, Geypens BJ, et al: Combined carbon-13-glycin/carbon-14-octanoic acid breath test to monitor gastric emptying rates of liquids and solids. J Nucl Med 35:824–831, 1994.

30. Boeckxstaens GE, Hirsch DP, Van Den Elzen BD, et al: Impaired drinking capacity in patients with functional dyspepsia: relationship with proximal stomach function. Gastroenterology 121:1054–1063, 2001.

31. Tack J, Caenepeel P, Piessevaux H, et al: Assessment of meal-induced gastric accommodation by a satiety drinking test in health and in functional dyspepsia. Gut In press, 2003.

32. Degen L, Matzinger D, Merz M, et al: Tegaserod, a 5-HT$_4$ receptor partial agonist, accelerates gastric emptying and gastrointestinal transit in healthy male subjects. Aliment Pharmacol Ther 15:1745–1751, 2001.

33. Tack J, Delia T, Ligozio G, et al: A phase II placebo controlled randomized trial with tegaserod in functional dyspepsia patients with normal gastric emptying. Gastroenterology 122:A154, 2002.

34. Talley NJ, Verlinden M, Snape W, et al: Failure of a motilin receptor agonist (ABT-229) to relieve the symptoms of functional dyspepsia in patients with and without delayed gastric emptying: a randomized double-blind placebo-controlled trial. Aliment Pharmacol Ther 14:1653–1661, 2000.

35. Talley NJ, Verlinden M, Geenen DJ, et al: Effects of a motilin receptor agonist (ABT-229) on upper gastrointestinal symptoms in type 1 diabetes mellitus: a randomised, double blind, placebo controlled trial. Gut 49:395–401, 2001.

36. Tack J, Peeters T: What comes after macrolides and mother motilin stimulants? Gut 49:317–318, 2001.

37. Bruley des Varannes S, Parys V, Ropert A, et al: Erythromycin enhances fasting and postprandial proximal gastric tone in humans. Gastroenterology 109:32–39, 1995,

38. Piessevaux H, Tack J, Wilner A, et al: Perception of changes in wall tension of the proximal stomach in humans. Gut 49:203–208, 2001.

39. Gorelick AB, Koshy SS, Hooper FG, et al: Differential effects of amitriptyline on perception of somatic and visceral stimulation in healthy humans. Am J Physiol 275:G460–466, 1998.

40. Peghini PL, Katz PO, Castell DO: Imipramine decreases oesophageal pain perception in human male volunteers. Gut 42:807–813, 1998.

41. Tack J, Broekaert D, Coulie B, et al: Influence of the selective serotonin re-uptake inhibitor, paroxetine, on gastric sensorimotor function in humans. Aliment Pharmacol Ther 17:603–608, 2003.

42. Diop L, Riviere PJ, Pascaud X, Junien JL: Peripheral kappa-opioid receptors mediate the antinociceptive effect of fedotozine on the duodenal pain reflex in rat. Eur J Pharmacol 27:65–71, 1994.

43. Langlois A, Diop L, Friese N, et al: Fedotozine blocks hypersensitive visceral pain in conscious rats: action at peripheral kappa-opioid receptors. Eur J Pharmacol 324:211–217, 1997.

44. Coffin B, Bouhassira D, Chollet R, et al: Effect of the kappa agonist fedotozine on perception of gastric distension in healthy humans. Aliment Pharmacol Ther 10:919–925, 1996.

45. Delgado-Aros S, Chial HJ, Camilleri M, et al: Effects of a kappa-opioid agonist, asimadoline, on satiation and GI motor and sensory functions in humans. Am J Physiol Gastrointest Liver Physiol 284:G558–66, 2003.

46. Gershon MD, Jonakait GM: Uptake and release of 5-hydroxytryptamine by enteric 5-hydroxytryptaminergic neurons: effects of fluoxetine (Lilley 110140) and chlorimipramine. Br J Pharmacol 66:7–9, 1979.

47. Tack J, Vos R, Janssens J, et al: Influence of tegaserod on proximal gastric tone and on the perception of gastric distention. Submitted for publication.

48. Tack J, Coulie B, Wilmer A, et al: Effect of sumatriptan on gastric fundus tone and on the perception of gastric distension in man. Gut 46:468–473, 2000.

49. Tack J, Piessevaux H, Caenepeel P, et al: A placebo-controlled trial of buspirone, a fundus-relaxing drug, in functional dyspepsia. Submitted for publication.

50. Thumshirn M, Camilleri M, Choi MG, Zinsmeister AR: Modulation of gastric sensory and motor functions by nitrergic and alpha2-adrenergic agents in humans. Gastroenterology 116:573–585, 1999.

51. Sarnelli G, Sifrim D, Janssens J, Tack J: Influence of sildenafil on gastric sensorimotor function in man. Gut In press, 2003.

52. Tack J, Masclee A, Heading R, et al: A phase IIa randomised multicentre double-blind placebo controlled parallel group pilot study with Z-338 in functional dyspepsia patients. Abstract book UEGW 2002.

53. Moss HE, Sanger GJ: The effects of granisetron, ICS 205–930 and ondansetron on the visceral pain reflex induced by duodenal distension. Br J Pharmacol 100:497–501, 1990.

54. Zerbib F, Bruley des Varannes S, Oriola RC, et al: Alosetron does not affect the visceral perception of gastric distension in healthy subjects. Aliment Pharmacol Ther 8:403–407, 1994.

55. Talley NJ, Van Zanten SV, Saez LR, et al: A dose-ranging, placebo-controlled, randomized trial of alosetron in patients with functional dyspepsia. Aliment Pharmacol Ther 15:525–537, 2001.

56. Thompson CA: Alosetron withdrawn from market. Am J Health Syst Pharm 58:13, 2001.

57. Bortolotti M, Coccia G, Grossi G, Miglioli M: The treatment of functional dyspepsia with red pepper. Aliment Pharmacol Ther 16:1075–1082, 2002.

58. Maggi CA: Therapeutic potential of capsaicin-like molecules: studies in animals and humans. Life Sci 51:1777–1781, 1992.

Index

Page numbers in **boldface** type indicate complete chapters.